The Essential Guide to the Nutrition Care Process

Bassim Hamadeh, CEO and Publisher
Jennifer Codner, Senior Field Acquisitions Editor
Michelle Piehl, Senior Project Editor
Christian Berk, Associate Production Editor
Jess Estrella, Senior Graphic Designer
Stephanie Kohl, Licensing Associate
Don Kesner, Interior Designer
Natalie Piccotti, Senior Marketing Manager
Kassie Graves, Vice President of Editorial
Jamie Giganti, Director of Academic Publishing

Cover image Copyright © 2015 Depositphotos/happyroman.
Copyright © 2015 Depositphotos/sn3g.
Copyright © 2016 Depositphotos/PandaVector.
Copyright © 2016 Depositphotos/StudioIcon.
Copyright © 2018 Depositphotos/ylivdesign.
Copyright © 2015 Depositphotos/somen.
Copyright © 2017 Depositphotos/kentoh.

Printed in the United States of America.

ISBN: 978-1-5165-3452-4 (pbk) / 978-1-5165-3453-1 (br)

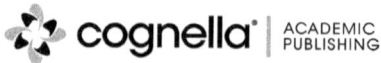

The Essential Guide to the Nutrition Care Process

Tonia Reinhard, MS, RD, FAND and

Mary Width, MS, RD

Wayne State University
Department of Nutrition and Food Science
Coordinated Program in Dietetics
Detroit, Michigan

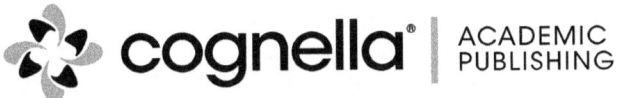

cognella® | ACADEMIC PUBLISHING

CONTENTS

Chapter 1 The Profession and the Process: An Overview.......................................1

Chapter 2 Nutrition Assessment: Data Gathering from the Medical
Record and Determining Nutrient Needs..**47**

Chapter 3 Nutrition Assessment: Data Gathering from the Patient
Using Communication and Interviewing Skills.................................. **109**

Chapter 4 Nutrition Assessment: Nutrition-Focused
Physical Examination.. **141**

Chapter 5 Nutrition Diagnosis: Making Sense of Assessment Data............... **163**

Chapter 6 Nutrition Intervention: Planning Diets and Coordinating Care......... **187**

Chapter 7 Nutrition Intervention: Nutrition Education and
Cultural Competency.. **221**

Chapter 8 Monitoring and Evaluation: Assessing the Nutrition
Interventions and Documenting in the Medical Record...................... **265**

Chapter 9 Case Studies: Practicing the Nutrition Care Process...................... **287**

Appendix A: Answers to "Case Studies: Practicing the Nutrition
Care Process"... **337**

Appendix B: Answers to "Check for Understanding" and
"Put It into Practice"... **367**

Appendix C: Evidence-Based Dietetic Practice: Understanding
Scientific Research... **371**

Appendix D: Vitamin and Mineral Facts...................................... **379**

Appendix E: Laboratory Assessment... **401**

Appendix F: Common Medical Abbreviations.................................. **421**

Appendix G: Nutritionally Relevant Medications............................. **433**

Appendix H: Body Mass Index Table... **463**

CHAPTER 1

The Profession and the Process

AN OVERVIEW

By the end of the chapter, the reader will be able to

- Describe key components of the dietetic profession and the mission of the Academy of Nutrition and Dietetics in relation to their own academic and career path as a nutrition professional
- Plan the steps in their own progress toward achieving the credential of the Registered Dietitian/Nutritionist
- Access the online professional tools of the Academy of Nutrition and Dietetics: Standards of Practice (SOP), Standards of Professional Performance (SOPP), Code of Ethics, and the Evidence Analysis Library
- Describe the nutrition care process: its purpose, application, and all components
- Determine their optimal learning style as applied to the development of a learning assessment portfolio

D ietitians have been applying the principles of nutrition and other sciences to improve the health of people for generations. They just weren't always called dietitians, or when they were, it wasn't always spelled that way. One thing is unambiguous: the knowledge and skills they bring to the health care of individuals and populations is indispensable. In 2003, the introduction of the Nutrition Care Process Model (NCP) with its standardized nutrition terminology revolutionized how dietitians in every practice setting approached their goal of improving human health and systematically communicated their activities. This great advance has added quality to the services they provide and makes it imperative for dietitians and future dietitians to have a thorough knowledge of and skill in the NCP.

THE DIETETIC PROFESSION AND THE REGISTERED DIETITIAN NUTRITIONIST

History of the Profession of Dietetics

The recognition of the importance of nutrition to human health has grown exponentially over the past decades as a result of the burgeoning body of research evidence in this crucial area of study. As nutrition professionals, Registered Dietitians/Nutritionists (RDs/RDNs) have been at the forefront since the inception of the American Dietetic Association in 1917, the professional association of dietetic practitioners (1). What began with only 39 charter members, the Academy of Nutrition and Dietetics, renamed in 2012, now boasts over 100,000 members.

It is the science of nutrition that has inspired many people to undertake study in the profession of dietetics, often not realizing the distinctions, but knowing that they also had a passion for applying this science to helping people. The study of nutrition encompasses food science, nutrient metabolism, and the interaction of foods and nutrients as they relate to health and disease. In contrast, the Academy defines dietetics as "the integration, application and communication of practice principles derived from food, nutrition, social, business and basic sciences, to achieve and maintain optimal nutrition status of individuals and groups" (2). The significant differences between the two definitions include 1) the terms, integration, application and communication; and 2) the inclusion of bringing about optimal nutrition status in people. These distinctions make it necessary for dietetic professionals to gain knowledge and skills in areas outside of nutrition science, such as interpersonal communication, education, and patient and client care.

The dietetic profession has its roots in hospitals, specifically military hospitals beginning in 1917, with the American Red Cross having established qualifications for dietitians in 1916 and later enrolling them in military service (Box 1.1) (3). Over 300 dietitians served during World War I. Prior to that time, dietetic professionals worked in other areas, although without clear qualifications, titles, and role delineations. The profession now encompasses a wide range of venues beyond the traditional practice area categories of clinical, community, and management. And while hospitals were the main employers of dietitians in the profession's early days, the Academy has reported that 32% work in hospitals (inpatient), 17% in ambulatory care (outpatient), 11% in management, 10% in community and public health, 8% in long-term care, 8% in business, and 7% in education and research (Box 1.2) (4). Within these categories, dietitians also practice in several areas of specialization, such as cardiology, diabetes, oncology, renal, nutrition support, and pediatrics.

BOX 1.1

Key Milestones in Dietetics

1839: Dietetics defined by Dunglison Medical Lexicon as "a branch of medicine comprising rules to be followed for preventing, relieving, or curing diseases, by diet."

1916–1917: American Red Cross establishes qualifications for dietitians; enrolls 356 dietitians in military service.

1917: First conference for dietitians in Cleveland, Ohio.

1917: American Dietetic Association established; Lulu G. Graves, Head Dietitian, Lakeside Hospital, Cleveland, Ohio, elected first president 1917–1920.

1920: Federal government issues regulations for dietitians.

1925: First issue of the *Journal of the American Dietetic Association* mailed to members.

1930: The Association adopts official spelling for "dietitian."

1946: *The Handbook of Diet Therapy* published, the precursor to the current *Nutrition Care Manual.*

1974: The first international reciprocity agreement established with the Dietitians of Canada.

1969–1970: National professional registration established with an RD examination.

1986: Standards of Practice published in the journal.

2003: Nutrition Care Process Model developed.

2012: Organization name changed to Academy of Nutrition and Dietetics.

Academy of Nutrition and Dietetics, History of the Academy. http://www.eatrightpro.org/History%20Timeline
Baylor University, History of Military Dietitians. http://www.baylor.edu/graduate/nutrition/index.php?id=68073

BOX 1.2

Where Dietitians Work

Hospitals (inpatient): 32%

Ambulatory care (outpatient): 17%

Management: 11%

Community and public health: 10%

Long-term care: 8%

Business: 8%

Education and research: 7%

Rogers, D. (2015). Compensation and benefits survey. *J Acad Nutr Diet* 2016; *116*(3): 370–388.

Designations and Credentials of Dietetic Professionals

Registered Dietitian (RD) Registered Dietitian Nutritionist (RDN)
The American Dietetic Association established the professional registration system in 1969 for credentialing of dietitians as Registered

Dietitian (RD). The Commission on Dietetic Registration (CDR) is the credentialing agency that regulates the process of both conferring the credential and its maintenance, an autonomous agency separate from the Academy. In 2013, RDs had the option to use an equivalent term, Registered Dietitian Nutritionist (RDN). Based on statistics provided from one state at the time of publication, 84% of dietitians continue to use the "RD" designation. In 2012, CDR announced that the minimum educational degree required to meet eligibility requirements for the RD credentialing exam will be changed from a bachelor's to a graduate degree beginning January 1, 2024, although the requirement is waived for RDs who hold the RD credential prior to that date (5).

The current components of registration include completion of an ACEND-accredited dietetics program and baccalaureate degree, completion of an ACEND-accredited supervised practice program, and successfully passing the national Registration Examination for Dietitians.

Nutrition and Dietetics education programs are accredited by the Accreditation Council for Education in Nutrition and Dietetics (ACEND). As part of dietetics program accreditation and continuing accreditation, programs must ensure and document that their graduates meet ACEND's required Knowledge and Competencies for Nutrition and Dietetics. Didactic Programs in Dietetics and Coordinated Programs are required to provide the didactic coursework to prepare students with the knowledge requirements. Coordinated Programs and Dietetic Internships are required to provide the supervised practice experiences needed to prepare students with the required competencies,). Box 1.3 shows the required knowledge (KRDN) and competencies (CRDN) required for coordinated programs, and for other program standards go to the ACEND website (www.catright pro.org/ACEND) (6). The knowledge and competency statements represent education standards and describe the specific knowledge and skills required for entry-level dietitians. The national Registration Examination content is based on this foundation. An important source for both the examination content and the education standards is the Dietetics Practice Audit (DPA). The DPA is a survey conducted by CDR every five years to assess the current state of dietetic practice.

This enables CDR and ACEND to identify the knowledge and skills needed by entry-level practitioners in order to develop a valid registration examination and education standards that prepare new dietitians for career opportunities that are constantly expanding and evolving (7).

BOX 1.3

ACEND 2017 Knowledge (KRDN) and Competency Statements (CRDN) for Nutrition and Dietetics, Coordinated Programs

Domain 1. Scientific and Evidence Base of Practice: Integration of Scientific Information and Research into Practice.

KRDN 1.1 *Demonstrate how to locate, interpret, evaluate and use professional literature to make ethical, evidence-based practice decisions.*

KRDN 1.2 *Use current information technologies to locate and apply evidence-based guidelines and protocols.*

KRDN 1.3 *Apply critical thinking skills.*

CRDN 1.1 Select indicators of program quality and/or customer service and measure achievement of objectives.

CRDN 1.2 Apply evidence-based guidelines, systematic reviews and scientific literature.

CRDN 1.3 Justify programs, products, services and care using appropriate evidence or data.

CRDN 1.4 Evaluate emerging research for application in nutrition and dietetics practice.

CRDN 1.5 Conduct projects using appropriate research methods, ethical procedures and data analysis.

CRDN 1.6 Incorporate critical-thinking skills in overall practice.

Domain 2. Professional Practice Expectations: Beliefs, Values, Attitudes and Behaviors for the Professional Dietitian Nutritionist Level of Practice.

KRDN 2.1 *Demonstrate effective and professional oral and written communication and documentation.*

KRDN 2.2 *Describe the governance of nutrition and dietetics practice, such as the Scope of Nutrition and Dietetics Practice and the Code of Ethics for the Profession of Nutrition and Dietetics; and describe interprofessional relationships in various practice settings.*

KRDN 2.3 *Assess the impact of a public policy position on nutrition and dietetics practice.*

KRDN 2.4 Discuss *the impact of health care policy and different health care delivery systems on food and nutrition services.*

KRDN 2.5 *Identify and describe the work of interprofessional teams and the roles of others with whom the registered dietitian nutritionist collaborates in the delivery of food and nutrition services.*

KRDN 2.6 *Demonstrate an understanding of cultural competence/ sensitivity.*

KRDN 2.7 *Demonstrate identification with the nutrition and dietetics profession through activities such as participation in professional organizations and defending a position on issues impacting the nutrition and dietetics profession.*

KRDN 2.8 *Demonstrate an understanding of the importance and expectations of a professional in mentoring and precepting others.*

CRDN 2.1 Practice in compliance with current federal regulations and state statutes and rules, as applicable and in accordance with accreditation standards and the Scope of Nutrition and Dietetics Practice and Code of Ethics for the Profession of Nutrition and Dietetics.

CRDN 2.2 Demonstrate professional writing skills in preparing professional communications.

CRDN 2.3 Demonstrate active participation, teamwork and contributions in group settings.

CRDN 2.4 Function as a member of interprofessional teams.

CRDN 2.5 Assign duties to NDTRs and/or support personnel as appropriate.

CRDN 2.6 Refer clients and patients to other professionals and services when needs are beyond individual scope of practice.

CRDN 2.7 Apply leadership skills to achieve desired outcomes.

CRDN 2.8 Demonstrate negotiation skills.

CRDN 2.9 Participate in professional and community organizations.

CRDN 2.10 Demonstrate professional attributes in all areas of practice.

CRDN 2.11 Show cultural competence/sensitivity in interactions with clients, colleagues and staff.

CRDN 2.12 Perform self-assessment and develop goals for self-improvement throughout the program.

CRDN 2.13 Prepare a plan for professional development according to Commission on Dietetic Registration guidelines.

CRDN 2.14 Demonstrate advocacy on local, state or national legislative and regulatory issues or policies impacting the nutrition and dietetics profession.

CRDN 2.15 Practice and/or role play mentoring and precepting others.

Domain 3. Clinical and Customer Services: Development and Delivery of Information, Products and Services to Individuals, Groups and Populations.

KRDN 3.1 *Use the Nutrition Care Process to make decisions, identify nutrition-related problems and determine and evaluate nutrition interventions.*

KRDN 3.2 *Develop an educational session or program/educational strategy for a target population.*

KRDN 3.3 *Demonstrate counseling and education methods to facilitate behavior change and enhance wellness for diverse individuals and groups.*

KRDN 3.4 *Explain the processes involved in delivering quality food and nutrition services.*

KRDN 3.5 *Describe basic concepts of nutritional genomics.*

CRDN 3.1 Perform the Nutrition Care Process and use standardized nutrition language for individuals, groups and populations of differing ages and health status, in a variety of settings.

CRDN 3.2 Conduct nutrition focused physical exams.

CRDN 3.3 Demonstrate effective communications skills for clinical and customer services in a variety of formats and settings.

CRDN 3.4 Design, implement and evaluate presentations to a target audience.

CRDN 3.5 Develop nutrition education materials that are culturally and age appropriate and designed for the literacy level of the audience.

CRDN 3.6 Use effective education and counseling skills to facilitate behavior change.

CRDN 3.7 Develop and deliver products, programs or services that promote consumer health, wellness and lifestyle management.

CRDN 3.8 Deliver respectful, science-based answers to client questions concerning emerging trends.

CRDN 3.9 Coordinate procurement, production, distribution and service of goods and services, demonstrating and promoting responsible use of resources.

CRDN 3.10 Develop and evaluate recipes, formulas and menus for acceptability and affordability that accommodate the cultural diversity and health needs of various populations, groups and individuals.

Domain 4. Practice Management and Use of Resources: Strategic Application of Principles of Management and Systems in the Provision of Services to Individuals and Organizations.

KRDN 4.1 *Apply management theories to the development of programs or services.*

KRDN 4.2 *Evaluate a budget and interpret financial data.*

KRDN 4.3 *Describe the regulation system related to billing and coding, what services are reimbursable by third party payers and how reimbursement may be obtained.*

KRDN 4.4 *Apply the principles of human resource management to different situations.*

KRDN 4.5 *Describe safety principles related to food, personnel and consumers.*

KRDN 4.6 *Analyze data for assessment and evaluate data to be used in decision-making for continuous quality improvement.*

CRDN 4.1 Participate in management of human resources.

CRDN 4.2 Perform management functions related to safety, security and sanitation that affect employees, customers, patients, facilities and food.

CRDN 4.3 Conduct clinical and customer service quality management activities.

CRDN 4.4 Apply current nutrition informatics to develop, store, retrieve and disseminate information and data.

CRDN 4.5 Analyze quality, financial and productivity data for use in planning.

CRDN 4.6 Propose and use procedures as appropriate to the practice setting to promote sustainability, reduce waste and protect the environment.

CRDN 4.7 Conduct feasibility studies for products, programs or services with consideration of costs and benefits.

CRDN 4.8 Develop a plan to provide or develop a product, program or service that includes a budget, staffing needs, equipment and supplies.

CRDN 4.9 Explain the process for coding and billing for nutrition and dietetics services to obtain reimbursement from public or private payers, fee-for-service and value-based payment systems.

CRDN 4.10 Analyze risk in nutrition and dietetics practice.

From Academy of Nutrition and Dietetics, 2017. Standards and Templates. http://www.eatrightpro.org/resources/acend/accreditation-standards-fees-and-policies/2017-standards

The Commission on Dietetic Registration Examination for Dietitians

After program graduates have fulfilled their didactic and supervised practice requirements for registration eligibility, they begin the examination application process. Program directors initiate a file online in CDR's Registration Eligibility Processing System (REPS). Exam candidates review, correct, and/or input their personal demographic and contact information. The program director then adds degree information, uploads transcripts and Verification Statements (VS), which are signed by the program director(s), and the signed acknowledgment of the RDE or RDNE Misuse Form. Graduates from a didactic program in dietetics (DPD) receive the VS from their DPD program director and another VS from their dietetic internship program director, both of which are required to be submitted with their examination eligibility online application.

The program director submits the file electronically to CDR, which in turn verifies the candidate's eligibility to test. Candidates will receive an Authorization to Test e-mail from Pearson VUE containing personal CDR Candidate Identification and dates of initial authorization. It also includes instructions on creating an examination application account with Pearson VUE and a link to the *Candidate Handbook*. The examination is offered at Pearson VUE test centers throughout the nation throughout the year (8).

Content of the examination is based on results of the most current dietetics practice audit (DPA) and covers the four domains of principles of dietetics, nutrition care for individuals and groups, management of food and nutrition programs and services, and foodservice systems (Box 1.4). The Registered Dietitian Examination Test Specifications are updated every five years, based on the results of the DPA and are published on the CDR website (9). The examination format is that of computer-adaptive testing. In this type of testing, the examinee must answer each question before being allowed to go to the next and cannot go back to previous questions that they have already answered.

Another feature of this format is that the content of the questions adapts to the examinee, with a minimum of 125 questions (of which only 100 are scored) and a maximum of 145 (of which 120 are scored). The examinee is presented with a tutorial prior to beginning the test for a total testing time of three hours, including the tutorial. The majority of eligible candidates take an examination review course either online or in person to prepare for the examination, and CDR also offers preparation materials, as does the Academy at their online store.

BOX 1.4

Registered Dietitian Examination—Test Specifications

I.   Principles of Dietetics: 25%

    A.   Food Science and Nutrient Composition of Foods

    B.   Nutrition and Supporting Sciences

    C.   Education, Communication and Technology

D.   D. Research Applications

II.   Nutrition Care for Individuals and Groups: 40%

A.   Screening and Assessment

B.   Diagnosis

C.   Planning and Intervention

D.   Monitoring and Evaluation

III.   Management of Food and Nutrition Programs and Services: 21%

A.   Functions of Management

B.   Human Resources

C.   Financial Management

D.   Marketing and Public Relations

E.   Quality Management and Improvement

IV.   Foodservice Systems: 14%

A.   Menu Development

B.   Procurement, Production, Distribution, and Service

C.   Sanitation and Safety

D.   Equipment and Facility Planning

Data from Commission on Dietetic Registration. Registered Dietitian Examination—Test Specifications. https://www.cdrnet.org/vault/2459/web/files/RDTestSpecs2017.pdf

Some states have separate certification or licensure for dietitians and nutritionists, a process in which the state evaluates and provides a credential of either "licensed" or "certified," based on specific requirements to enable an individual to practice within its jurisdiction. Of the 38 states that license dietitians, 42% include nutritionists, and of the seven states that confer certification, two states include nutritionists (10). Of the states with statutory certification, the specific requirements vary by state as to education, supervised practice, and examination.

Nutrition and Dietetics Technician, Registered (NDTR)

The only other dietetics credential established by CDR is the Nutrition and Dietetics Technician, Registered (NDTR), or the equivalent term of Dietetic Technician, Registered (DTR). The training and education of NDTRs is at the technical level, and their scope of practice permits them to provide numerous nutrition services (11). They can work independently to provide general nutrition education to the healthy public. However, NDTRs must be supervised by RDs when providing direct patient care in hospitals, clinics, long-term care facilities, hospices, home health care, and research facilities.

The NDTR credential is conferred after successful completion of the Registration Examination for Dietetic Technicians preceded by one of three routes, two of which consist of a baccalaureate degree. The NDTR who has completed a baccalaureate degree may also use the designation of BS-DTR or BSNDTR. The three routes for the NDTR credential are:

1. Associate's degree from a US regionally accredited college, university, or foreign equivalent and 450 hours of supervised practice in an ACEND-accredited technician program.

2. Baccalaureate degree from a US regionally accredited college, university, or foreign equivalent; meet academic requirements for an ACEND-accredited Didactic Program in Dietetics; 450 hours of supervised practice in an ACEND-accredited technician program.

3. Baccalaureate degree from a US regionally accredited college or university or foreign equivalent; completion of an ACEND-accredited Didactic Program in Dietetics.

Academy Membership and Maintaining Registration Status

Academy membership and registration status are separate for both RDs and NDTRs, with Academy membership dues paid to the Academy, while registration fees to maintain the credentials are paid to CDR. The benefits of membership are numerous and include automatic membership with state affiliates, reduced conference registration costs (national and state), both mailed copy and online access of the *Journal of the Academy of Nutrition and Dietetics*, reduced cost for Academy publications, and access to several important Academy professional tools, some of which are free to members, and others are available at reduced cost (each described in the next section) (12).

In order to maintain the credentials, both RDs and NDTRs complete the Professional Development Portfolio (PDP) recertification requirement, which involves developing and revising the PDP, and accruing approved continuing professional education (CPE). The requirement for RDs is 75 CPEs and 50 for NDTRs every five years. The PDP is an excellent tool for assessment of one's learning needs, and dietetic students can begin this process early in their academic careers to help guide their path toward specific learning opportunities and prepare for completing the PDP. In addition, a learning portfolio can be taken on job interviews to show prospective employers examples of one's work on assignments and special projects (Put it into Practice 1.1).

Professional Standards and Tools

Standards of Practice (SOP) and Standards of Professional Performance (SOPP)

The highly diverse and continually expanding venues for dietetic practice was the impetus in 2004 for the Academy to establish a task force to develop the Scope of Practice (SOP) Framework. The SOP represents an overview of the profession and outlines the range of roles, activities, and regulations for RDs. For any individual with established credentials, SOP is generally defined by the credentialing agency, such as CDR for RDs, or a state board, in the case of state licensure laws (13, 11). The Standards of Professional Practice (SOPP) in Nutrition Care and Standards of Professional Practice for RDs give dietitians the rationale for standards, delineate the interaction between the RD and NDTR, and specify quality indicators (14).

The Academy has stated that the RD uses the SOP in conjunction with the Standards of Practice and the Standards of Professional Performance (SOPP) to help assess and make decisions about:

1. Evaluation of practice and performance through self-assessment
2. Reflection on the minimum competence required for a given level of practice and performance
3. Measurement of quality and performance improvement using examples of outcomes

4. Specification of quality indicators for practice and performance
5. Guidance in professional growth and practice development

The Academy has also developed resource tools to assist the RD in this assessment and decision making in their dietetic practice relative to the SOP and SOPP, including a continuing education video series, definitions for Academy terminology, and case study with practice tips (15). The Academy has developed SOPs and SOPPs for numerous practice areas with articles published in the Journal and available to members at the Academy website (Box 1.5).

BOX 1.5

Dietetic Practice Areas with SOP and SOPP

Adult Weight Management

Behavioral Health Care

Clinical Nutrition Management

Diabetes

Diabetes Care

Disordered Eating and Eating Disorders

Education of Dietetics Practitioners

Extended Care Settings

Integrative and Functional Medicine

Intellectual and Developmental Disabilities

Management in Food and Nutrition Services

Nephrology Nutrition

Nutrition Care for Registered Dietitians

Nutrition Care for Dietetic Technicians

Nutrition Support

Pediatrics

Public Health and Community Nutrition

Sports Nutrition

Sustainable, Resilient, and Healthy Food and Water Systems

Oncology Nutrition Care

Code of Ethics

The Academy Board of Directors and CDR developed the Code of Ethics in 1999 and revised the document in 2009 to reflect the values and ethical principles of the organization and its members (16). The 19 principles of this enforceable Code outline obligations, responsibilities, and commitments of dietetics professionals to the people they serve, including the general public, clients, patients, fellow dietitians, other professionals, and the dietetics profession at large; i.e., all within their professional sphere. The Code of Ethics document is contained and fully detailed in the Journal publication (16), and it is currently under revision.

Evidence Analysis Library (EAL)

One of the most important tools available at no charge to Academy members is the Evidence Analysis Library (EAL), which represents an evidence-based approach to nutrition and dietetic research and professional practice. The EAL is an online searchable database of relevant research and evidence-based nutrition practice guidelines. In addition, members can purchase at reduced cost a wide array of toolkits and other resources. The EAL provides the RD with the ability to conduct a literature search for a specific topic, such as nutritionally relevant diseases, nutrients, food constituents, food safety, and methodologies, including nutrition counseling and the nutrition care process.

The advantages of the EAL in comparison to other searchable databases include that the research on a specific topic has been qualitatively assessed and the evidence summarized for the user. In addition, the panel of experts involved in the EAL grade the research based on the strength of the evidence and present conclusions. Also, the EAL provides the RD with recommendations for using the evidence-based information in their professional practice. This tool has been widely recognized with many agencies using it, including the US Food and Drug Administration.

Nutrition Care Process (NCP) Tools

The Nutrition Care Process (NCP) is perhaps one of the most important developments in the dietetics profession. The Academy provides several NCP tools on the website, many of which are offered at no charge to members including presentations on learning the NCP. The Academy also offers an Electronic Health Record Toolkit at no charge to familiarize RDs with how the NCP is used in this type of medical record format.

Members can purchase at reduced cost an online subscription to the eNCPT: *Nutrition Care Process Terminology Reference Manual,* an indispensable tool for RDs in all practice venues, but particularly for those in hospitals, long-term care facilities, and in settings where services are documented in a medical record. The eNCPT includes the most current NCP terminology, definitions, application resources for every term, and a set of matrices for NCP diagnostic statements.

Position Papers and Practice Papers

Additional indispensable tools for Academy members are the publication of position papers and practice papers. Both papers represent critical analyses of current research and data and are developed by health professionals who are leading experts in their fields and on the paper topic. The Academy Positions Committee workgroup is responsible for managing the development of both papers (17). In the case of position papers, at least one of the paper's authors is an Academy member; it includes an abstract, is fully referenced, and represents the Academy's viewpoint on the issue in an effort to promote healthy food choices and improve consumer nutritional status.

The practice paper essentially translates the current science on a topic into practice that the dietetic professional can implement in providing services. The paper may include evidence-based analysis guidelines, implications for the NCP, best practices, the Academy Standards of Practice and Standards of Professional Performance, and other practice tools. The reason for the two different types of papers relates primarily to the practice focus of the practice papers, and the decision to develop practice papers was based on member survey data. The Academy makes both papers available to members at no cost on the Academy's website. They are published in their entirety in the *Journal of the Academy of Nutrition and Dietetics*.

Academy of Nutrition and Dietetics Health Informatics Infrastructure (ANDHII)

The Academy of Nutrition and Dietetics Health Informatics Infrastructure (ANDHII) provides members with a process for tracking outcomes for the dietetics profession in order to prove the effectiveness of nutrition therapy (18). The ANDHII is an online tool that guides RDs through the steps of the NCP and simultaneously helps establish a national quality improvement database that includes patient outcomes. The ANDHII ultimately will promote evidence-based nutrition practice research. After establishing a user identification and password, the RD has available numerous practice resources, such as patient charts, reports, visit summaries, which can all be tailored to the RD's professional practice (19).

In addition to the important long-term goals for the profession and advancing high-quality patient care, the benefits to individual RDs in practice is significant, particularly in light of the current state of potential problems in data collection from electronic health records (EHRs). These problems include lack of uniformity in nutrition terminology—where the NCP standardized nutrition terminology is not in use, which makes monitoring and documentation difficult—and the problems in combining data from varying practice venues.

THE NUTRITION CARE PROCESS

The Nutrition Care Process (NCP), developed by the Academy in 2003, is a systematic approach to providing high-quality nutrition care to patients and clients. The NCP provides RDs with a framework for critical thinking, problem solving and decision making to identify and resolve nutrition-related problems (Box 1.6) (20). In 1605, Francis Bacon described critical thinking as a "desire to seek, patience to doubt, fondness to meditate, slowness to assert, readiness to consider, carefulness to dispose and set in order; and hatred for every kind of imposture." The importance of these two skills is clear in considering the purpose of the NCP—to ensure the consistency and quality of nutrition care and the predictability of outcomes. The NCP is the professional standard in a wide array of venues to provide nutrition services and document the process.

The NCP encompasses four steps: 1) nutrition <u>A</u>ssessment; 2) nutrition <u>D</u>iagnosis; 3) nutrition <u>I</u>ntervention; and 4) nutrition <u>M</u>onitoring and <u>E</u>valuation (which gives rise to the acronym ADIME), both a summary of the NCP and a documentation format. The first two steps, nutrition assessment and nutrition diagnosis, comprise the nutrition problem identification phase, and the last two steps of nutrition intervention and nutrition monitoring and evaluation are the problem-solving phase. The entire NCP must be documented, and depending on the practice setting, this will be a patient's medical record in a hospital, long-term care facility, clinic, or community nutrition client assessment file. The documentation format still varies widely because of the sporadic use nationally of EHRs, although fully electronic records are the national goal.

BOX 1.6

Critical Thinking and Problem Solving

Critical Thinking

"Critical thinking is the intellectually disciplined process of actively and skillfully conceptualizing, applying, analyzing, synthesizing, and/or evaluating information gathered from, or generated by, observation, experience, reflection, reasoning, or communication, as a guide to belief and action."

Problem Solving

"Problem solving is the act of defining a problem; determining the cause of the problem; identifying, prioritizing and selecting alternatives for a solution; and implementing a solution. The four basic steps of problem solving are:

Define the problem
Generate alternative solutions
Evaluate and select an alternative
Implement and follow up on the solution."

Source: The Foundation and Center for Critical Thinking. Available at: http:// www.criticalthinking.org/pages/ defining-critical-thinking/766

Source: ASQ. Learn About Quality. Available at: http://asq.org/learn-about-quality/ problem-solving/overview/overview.html

Step 1: Nutrition Assessment

Nutrition assessment of the patient, client, or resident (Box 1.7) is the first step of the NCP for the delivery of effective nutrition care to identify, diagnose nutrition problems and risks, and plan appropriate interventions to solve nutrition problems (21). Nutrition assessment comprises the collection of comprehensive data covering five domains, analysis of the data beginning with a comparison to appropriate standards, and assessment of nutrition status. The five domains, with examples of relevant data within each domain (but not all-inclusive), consist of the following:

1. **Anthropometric measurements:** Height, weight, body mass index (BMI), weight history, growth pattern indices/percentile ranks (for infants and children), body measures, including fat, muscle, and bone.

2. **Biochemical data and medical tests:** Findings from laboratory tests (blood and urine) and results from diagnostic medical tests and procedures.

3. **Nutrition-focused physical findings:** Findings from a nutrition-focused physical examination performed by dietetic professional, data from medical record regarding muscle and subcutaneous fat, oral health, suck/swallow/breathe ability, and affect.

4. **Client history:** Personal, medical and health (patient and family), and social histories.

5. **Food/Nutrition-related history:** Food and nutrient intake, appetite, diet history (including previous history of therapeutic diets), prescription and over-the-counter medications, dietary supplements and complementary/alternative medicine, food and nutrition knowledge, beliefs and attitudes about food and

nutrition-related topics, physical activity and exercise, and food availability and accessibility (21).

What's in a Name?

It is proper to refer to the people for whom you provide services in the following way, based on the health care setting.

Health Care Setting	Term
Acute care, i.e., hospital; primary care (physician office)	Patient
Long-term care, extended care (nursing home)	Resident
Clinic; private practice; health club	Client

Step 2: Nutrition Diagnosis

Nutrition diagnosis is the second step in the NCP. After assessment, the patient's nutrition-related problems and needs are determined, which form the nutrition diagnosis/diagnoses. The nutrition diagnosis, in turn, is expressed and documented in a specific format: Problem, etiology, signs, and symptoms (PES) (22). Boxes 1.8 and 1.9 provide an example for the PES format and demonstrate how to generate a PES statement for each nutrition diagnosis. Depending on the number of nutrition problems (diagnoses), there may be just one nutrition diagnosis expressed as a PES statement, or there may be more.

Nutrition Diagnosis: Problem/Etiology/Signs

The problem (P) describes alterations in patient nutritional status:

A diagnostic label (qualifier) is an adjective that describes the physiologic response, e.g., altered, impaired, risk of

The etiology (E) refers to cause(s) or contributor(s) to the problem:

It is linked to the problem by the words "related to" (RT)

The signs/symptoms (S) are clusters of subjective and objective factors that provide evidence that a problem exists:

– They also quantify the problem and describe severity

– They are linked to (E) by the words "as evidenced by" (AEB)

BOX 1.9

Writing the Nutrition Diagnosis (ND) Statement

Example for the ND statement format: (P)roblem/(E)tiology/(S)igns/symptoms

Excessive energy intake (P) related to frequent consumption of large portions of high-fat meals (E), as evidenced by:

1. Daily caloric intake exceeding DRI by 500 kcal (S)
2. 2.12-lb weight gain during past 18 months (S)

It is essential that the nutrition assessment supports all components of each PES statement. Each PES statement must be specific, measurable, and most importantly, can be resolved or improved by the RD; i.e., within the RD's scope of practice. The nutrition diagnostic terms are classified according to the following three domains and subclasses:

1. **Intake:** Energy balance; oral or nutrition support intake; fluid intake; bioactive substances; nutrients
2. **Clinical:** Functional; biochemical; weight; malnutrition disorders
3. **Behavioral/environmental:** Knowledge and beliefs; physical activity and function; food safety and access (21)

Step 3: Nutrition Intervention

Nutrition intervention is the third step in the NCP. Interventions target nutrition problems, which are expressed as the nutrition diagnoses, to bring about positive health outcomes for the individual under the RD's care. Most typically, an intervention targets the etiology of the nutrition diagnosis in the PES statement. However, less frequently an intervention can also target the signs and symptoms to minimize their impact. The intervention step comprises two interconnected tasks: planning and implementation.

In planning interventions, the RD prioritizes the nutrition diagnoses as to each problem's severity or importance, and the use of evidenced-based interventions and practice guidelines to establish patient-focused expected outcomes for each of the nutrition diagnoses. Next, the RD begins the implementation of the nutrition intervention and communicates the plan of care to the patient, caregivers, and other members of the health care team (14). The nutrition professionals continue to collect data (which represents the next NCP step of monitoring and evaluating). Based on the responses the patient provides, the nutrition professional refines and creates an appropriate nutrition intervention strategy. The standardized nutrition terminology for nutrition intervention is organized into four domains and associated subclasses (21):

1. **Food and/or nutrient delivery:** Meals and snacks; enteral and parenteral nutrition; supplements; medical food supplements; vitamin and mineral supplements; bioactive substance supplements; feeding assistance; feeding environment; nutrition-related medication management.

2. **Nutrition education:** Initial/brief nutrition education; comprehensive nutrition education.

3. **Nutrition counseling:** Theoretical basis/approach; strategies.

4. **Coordination of nutrition care by nutrition professional:** Collaboration and referral of care during nutrition care; discharge and transfer of nutrition care to new setting or provider.

Step 4: Nutrition Monitoring and Evaluation

The final step in the NCP is monitoring and evaluation. This is a critical component of the NCP because it "identifies important measures of patient/client outcomes relevant to the nutrition diagnosis and intervention, and describes how best to measure and evaluate these outcomes"

(21). During this step, the patient's status is re-examined by gathering new data (monitoring) and assessing to see how it compares to previous status, expected outcomes, and established standards (evaluation).

This fourth step helps to determine whether the patient is meeting the nutrition intervention goals or desired outcomes. The domains and standardized nutrition terminology used in monitoring/evaluation are the same as those used in nutrition assessment, except for client history. There is no client history domain in this step, because there are no nutrition care outcomes associated with client history.

1. Anthropometric measurements
2. Biochemical data
3. Food and nutrition-related history
4. Nutrition-focused physical findings

In determining indicators for monitoring and evaluation, the RD considers the appropriateness of an indicator and reference standards. In addition, the RD identifies the baseline values for indicators in order to measure outcomes, potential obstacles, and reasons for any variation from the expected planned outcomes. It is also important for the RD to discriminate between short-term and long-term outcomes. As an example, for the typical short hospital stay after a mild myocardial infarction, it is not reasonable to expect to observe reductions in elevated serum cholesterol levels and adherence to the therapeutic diet. Serum cholesterol levels generally will take six to eight weeks to be affected by a dietary change, and sustained behavior change can only assessed over a significant period of time.

NUTRITION CARE PROCESS PROBLEM SOLVING MATRIX

A key feature of the NCP is the focus on a critical-thinking and problem-solving approach inherent in the NCP model. The NCP Problem Solving Matrix (PSM) (Tables 1.1–1.5) provides the reader with a step-by-step guide through the process to facilitate these important aspects of the NCP. In addition to serving as a guide to the NCP steps, the PSM is a tool for data collection, calculations, analysis, and development of the nutrition diagnosis PES statements. The next chapters

TABLE 1.1 Problem Solving Matrix—Assessment

1.0 Assessment

♦*Collect assessment data from:* Review of the medical record & interview of the patient

♦*Analyze collected data:* Use nutrition equations & standard lab parameters

Assessment Data Categories	Collect Data Fill in the date collected from MR and interview	Analyze Data Calculate BMI, IBW, %UBW, %wt change, etc.; identify abnormal labs
Anthropometric	Data collected	Analyze data (BMI, IBW, %UBW, %wt change, etc.)
Weight/Height		
Biochemical Data, Medical Test, Procedures	**Data collected**	**Analyze data (identify any abnormal lab values)**
VPS: albumin, RBP, transferrin, prealbumin, TLC (moderated by inflammation/stress)		
Lipids: TC, HDL, LDL, ratio, TG		
Dx/Disease-related (CVD, DM, GI, liver, renal)		

(Continued)

TABLE 1.1 Problem Solving Matrix—Assessment (*Continued*)

Nutrition-Focused Physical Findings	Data collected from NFPE and History & Physical (Review of Systems)	Analyze data (identify any physical findings that are outside the normal parameters)
Physical appearance (muscle wasting, fat loss, edema, skin, hair, nails, etc.)		
Physical function (hand grip)		
Functional Problems (GI, etc.)	□N □V □D □C Oral motor: □ Intact □ Dysphagia □ Difficulty chewing □ Other:	

History		Data collected
Food / Nutrition: Food intake, appetite, wt history, physical activity, cultural, religious, food allergy & intolerances, medications, supplements, food availability		
Client History: Medical: nutritionally relevant Dx		
Social History: Lives alone, support, occupation, income, education level, program participation		

(*Continued*)

TABLE 1.1 Problem Solving Matrix—Assessment (*Continued*)

Determine/Estimate Nutrient Needs	Estimated Nutrient Needs (Nutrition Prescription)
Energy needs: Use range equation, Mifflin, Harris-Benedict, etc. (consider activity and stress or disease-specific factors)	
Protein needs: Use facility intake standards (consider disease-specific needs)	
Fluid needs: Use facility intake standards (consider disease-specific needs)	

TABLE 1.2.0 Problem Solving Matrix—Diagnosis

2.0 Diagnosis

• *Compare analyzed data to standards:* Use the data from 1.0 Assessment to identify all potential nutrition concerns; analyze each concern by comparing it to all others listed and looking for correlations that verify only nutritionally relevant concerns; then determine if those can be resolved by the RD and list nutrition diagnoses.

Data Categories	**A. Identify & list all potential nutrition concerns (any abnormal parameters)**	**B. Analyze potential concerns as they relate to each other to determine if actual concerns exist; list only actual, nutritionally relevant current concerns** (for ex: Is low BMI d/t decreased appetite or does hx show the patient's BMI has always been low?)	**C. Determine if concerns listed in column B can be resolved by the RD, and then list all possible Nutrition Diagnoses for each domain** (Intake, Clinical, Behavior-Environmental)
Anthropometric			
Biochemical, Test, Procedures			
NFPE Findings			

(Continued)

TABLE 1.2.0 Problem Solving Matrix—Diagnosis

History		
(Appetite/intake, knowledge & behavior, any other relevant history)		
Current intake/Diet Rx status	Can patient meet EEN? Y/N	Is diet Rx tolerated? Y/N

TABLE 1.2.1 Problem Solving Matrix—Diagnosis in PES Format

2.1 Diagnosis in PES format

♦ Describe all identified concerns from 2.0 C. as Nutrition Diagnoses in PES format

Nutrition diagnosis or problem (P)	Etiology (E)	Signs and/or Symptoms (S)
	related to	*as evidenced by*
	related to	*as evidenced by*
	related to	*as evidenced by*
	related to	*as evidenced by*

Determine Nutrition Status

From the Nutrition Diagnoses, identify the patient's Nutrition Status

1. **Normal**
2. **Mildly compromised**
3. **Moderately compromised**
4. **Severely compromised**

TABLE 1.3: Problem Solving Matrix—Nutrition Prescription / Interventions

3.0 Nutrition Prescription / Interventions

♦ PGIE Model For Planning (Problem/Goal/Intervention/Evidence)

Nutrition Prescription:	Current Diet Order:	Estimated Needs for Energy:	Estimated Needs for Protein:
Nutrition Diagnoses	**Goal / Expected Outcome**	**Intervention/s**	**Evidence-Based Rationale**
Nutrition Diagnoses are those problems identified from the assessment section and written in PES format	Goal represents what the problem will look like when it is resolved (the ideal)	The Prescription is the estimated nutrient needs and Intervention is what to do to reach the goal (these are the plan components); Interventions usually target the etiology of the ND problem	Rationale is the "why" of the plan; it must be **"Evidence-Based"** Use ADA Evidence Analysis Library

TABLE 1.4 Problem Solving Matrix—Nutrition Monitoring and Evaluation

4.0 Nutrition Monitoring and Evaluation

◆ **Select indicators that evaluate Interventions directed at signs/symptoms; Indicate time frame for reassessment**

Nutrition Dx in PES format	Intervention/s	Selected Indicators	Criteria Specify measurable patient-centered goals and time frame (days/wks/mos)

TABLE 1.5 Problem Solving Matrix—Documentation in ADIME Format

5.0 ADIME Documentation for Medical Record

ASSESSMENT

Anthropometric Measurements

Biochemical Data

Nutrition-Focused Physical Findings

Client History / Medical History

Food and Nutrition History / Medications

DIAGNOSIS

TABLE 1.5 Problem Solving Matrix—Documentation in ADIME Format

INTERVENTION

Nutrition Prescription

Intervention/s

MONITORING/EVALUATION

cover each step of the NCP using a patient case study as a special feature at the end of each chapter, 'Our Case Study of Patient SB' (Table 1.6). For each NCP step in the subsequent chapters, the relevant section of the PSM for the patient case study will also be included.

Put It into Practice: Develop a Learning Assessment Portfolio

Objective
Develop a Learning Assessment Portfolio (LAP), which will enable you to 1) determine your preferred learning style; 2) assess skills needed for selected area of dietetics for your future career; 3) evaluate performance through all stages of a dietetics program; 4) collect examples of your work for presentation to potential employers; and 5) plan for continuing education to lead to completion of the CDR Professional Development Portfolio (PDP).

Overview
Complete an initial learning-styles assessment to determine your preferred method of learning. In addition, review ACEND's Knowledge (KRDN) and Competency Statements (CRDN) needed for dietetic practice. As you go forward in your dietetic program, you assess their own knowledge and skills relative to the KRDNs and CRDNs and collect samples of your work to include in the portfolio.

LAP Description
Use the following format to set up your LAP, ideally in a professional looking three-ring binder with tabbed sections.

Section	Description
Section 1: Learning Styles	People tend to have a preferred style of learning, and knowing your learning style can enhance your learning. The Index of Learning Styles (ILS) is a validated tool to determine your learning style preferences based on four dimensions (active/reflective, sensing/intuitive, visual/verbal, and sequential/global) developed by Richard M. Felder:

http://educationdesignsinc.com/

1. "Learning Styles and Strategies," an article that provides background on learning styles:

    http://www4.ncsu.edu/unity/lockers/ users/f/felder/public//ILSdir/styles.pdf

2. Index of Learning Styles (ILS), the online survey:

    https://www.webtools.ncsu.edu/ learningstyles/

Section 2: Learning Style and Strategies	Using the content from the article "Learning Styles and Strategies" and the results of your ILS, write a one-page summary entitled "Learning Style and Strategies." The summary should include an assessment of your learning style and strategies for how you can optimize your learning and performance.
Section 3: Areas of Interest in the Dietetic Profession	Write a one-page summary, "Areas of Interest in Dietetics," to describe your areas of interest in the field of dietetics. Include the type of position you will most likely pursue and where you would like to work upon completing the program. If you are not sure, include the areas that you would like to learn more about during the program and why.
Section 4: Learning Needs	Write a one-page summary, "Learning Needs," based on your areas of interest in dietetics, and your review of the ACEND (CRDNs and KRDNs). Identify the areas in which you are strong and those which represent your continued learning needs.

Section 5: Performance Evaluation Tracking	Track your performance on projects, assignments, and exams, and continually update as you progress through your dietetic program. Include the names of the projects, dates of completion, and grades.
Section 6: Performance Analysis	Write a one-page summary, "Performance Analysis," based on your performance evaluation tracking that describes your progress as you move forward in your program and toward meeting your learning needs. Summarize your learning experiences, progress, and continued areas of learning needs.
Section 7: Plan	Write a one-page summary, "Plan," using the "Performance Analysis" that outlines a plan for next semester based on your achievements and areas which need to be strengthened.
Section 8: Examples of Work	Add examples of work to your portfolio as you progress through your program.
Section 9: Final Assessment of Learning Needs	When you've completed your dietetic program, reassess your learning needs in a comparison to the ACEND KRDNs and CRDNs. The expectation is that after program completion, you have achieved competency in all of these standards.
Section 10: Résumé	Develop a professional résumé. If you haven't done this in the past, use online resources to develop a résumé.

Section 11: CDR Professional Development Portfolio	Log on to the CDR website at http://www.cdrnet.org
	Click on "About CDR"
	Click on "Professional Development Portfolio" (PDP)
	This will guide you through the development of your PDP; once completed, print your plan and include in your LAP.

To Sum It Up

1. The profession of dietetics has existed for many years, and the professional association was established in 1917 with 39 members. Today, the Academy of Nutrition and Dietetics has over 100,000 members.

2. The designations of "RD" and "RDN" are equivalent credentials for Registered Dietitians/Nutritionists and identify nutrition professionals who have met the educational, experiential, and examination requirements of the Academy's educational and credentialing arms, ACEND and CDR.

3. The Academy offers numerous professional standards and tools to assist RDs in maintaining the highest professional standard possible. These include Standards of Practice (SOP), Standards of Professional Performance (SOPP), Code of Ethics, and the Evidence Analysis Library.

4. The NCP is a systematic approach to high-quality nutrition care that facilitates the RD's provision of services in a variety of practice settings.

5. The four steps of the NCP are nutrition assessment, nutrition diagnosis, nutrition intervention, and monitoring and evaluation. The NCP culminates in documentation of nutrition care in the ADIME format.

6. Subsequent chapters will use the NCP Problem Solving Matrix and the case study of SB to illustrate each step of the NCP and guide the reader toward a comprehensive understanding of the NCP.

Check for Understanding

1. The Academy of Nutrition and Dietetics "Standards of Practice and Standards of Professional Performance" are used
   a. by dietitians to plan their continuing education
   b. by employers to determine equitable pay for dietitians
   c. for planning college courses in related sciences
   d. by accrediting agencies to regulate dietetic practice

2. In the correct order, what are the steps in the nutrition care process?
   a. plan development, assessment of data, implement plan, evaluate
   b. nutrition assessment, diagnosis, intervention, monitoring, and evaluation
   c. implement plan, interview patient, gather data from medical record, assess, evaluate
   d. evaluation of subjective data, assess objective data, develop plan, implement

3. Three of the five components of initial eligibility for Dietetic Registration include:
   a. BS degree, supervised practice, examination
   b. MS degree, dietetic internship, maintenance fees
   c. ADA-approved coursework, supervised practice, continuing education
   d. BS degree, dietetic internship, credits toward graduate degree

4. The monitoring and evaluation phase of the nutrition care process refers to
   a. the RD checking on the effectiveness of the implemented plan
   b. the physician requesting that a new diet order be implemented
   c. the nurse requesting a diet instruction for a patient who can't follow the diet order
   d. reinterpretation of original medical orders

5. The main purpose of ACEND's Knowledge (KRDN) and Competencies for Nutrition and Dietetics (CRDN) is to

   a. ensure dietetic program graduates meet educational standards for entry-level practice

   b. allow RDs to assess their current and ongoing learning needs for professional practice

   c. promote the collective knowledge of the field of nutrition and dietetics to the public

   d. provide other health care professionals with an knowledge of the RD's scope of practice

Answers in Appendix B

References

1. Academy of Nutrition and Dietetics. Academy History. Available at: http://www.eatrightpro.org/resources/about-us/academy-vision-and-mission/academy-history. Accessed June 8, 2017.

2. Academy of Nutrition and Dietetics. Scope of Practice. Academy Definition of Terms. Available at: http://www.eatrightpro.org/~/media/eatrightpro%20files/practice/scope%20standards%20of%20practice/academydefinitionoftermslist.ashx. Accessed June 7, 2017.

3. Baylor University. History of Military Dietitians. Available at: http://www.baylor.edu/graduate/nutrition/index.php?id=68073. Accessed June 8, 2017.

4. Rogers, D. (2016). Compensation and benefits survey. *J Acad Nutr Diet, 116*(3): 370–388.

5. Academy of Nutrition and Dietetics, Commission on Dietetic Registration. Visioning Report Moving Forward—A Vision for the Continuum of Dietetics Education, Credentialing and Practice. Available at: https://www.cdrnet.org/vault/2459/web/files/10369.pdf. Accessed June 13, 2017.

6. Academy of Nutrition and Dietetics. 2017 Standards and Templates. Available at: http://www.eatrightpro.org/resources/acend/accreditation-standards-fees-and-policies/2017-standards. Accessed June 20, 2017.

7. Griswold, K., Rogers, D., Sauer, K. L., et al. (2016). Entry-Level Dietetics Practice Today: Results from the 2015 Commission on Dietetic Registration Entry-Level Dietetics Practice Audit. *J Acad Nutr Diet, 116*(10): 1632–1684.

8. Commission on Dietetic Registration. (2017). Registration Examination for Dietitians: Handbook for Candidates. Available at: http://www.pearsonvue.com/cdr/cdr_rd_handbook.pdf. Accessed January 12, 2018.

9. Commission on Dietetic Registration. Registered Dietitian Examination—Test Specifications. Available at: https://www.cdrnet.org/vault/2459/web/files/RDTestSpecs2017.pdf. Accessed June 20, 2017.

10. Academy of Nutrition and Dietetics. Summary of Licensure Statutes by State. Available at: http://www.eatrightpro.org/resource/advocacy/quality-health-care/consumer-protection-and-licensure/summary-of-licensure-statutes-by-state. Accessed June 16, 2017.

11. Academy of Nutrition and Dietetics: Scope of Practice for the Dietetic Technician, Registered. (2013). *J Acad Nutr Diet*; *113*(6): S346–355.

12. Academy of Nutrition and Dietetics. Member Benefits. Available at: http://www.eatrightpro.org/resources/membership/member-benefits. Accessed June 20, 2017.

13. Academy of Nutrition and Dietetics: Scope of Practice for the Registered Dietitian.

Academy Quality Management Committee and Scope of Practice Subcommittee of Quality Management Committee. (2013). *J Acad Nutr Diet*, *113*(6): S17–28.

14. Academy of Nutrition and Dietetics: Revised 2017 Standards of Practice in Nutrition Care and Standards of Professional Performance for Registered Dietitians. (2018). *J Acad Nutr Diet*, *118*(1): 132–140.e15.

15. Academy of Nutrition and Dietetics. Scope of Practice. Available at: http://www.eatrightpro.org/resources/practice/quality-management/scope-of-practice. Accessed June 21, 2017.

16. American Dietetic Association. American Dietetic Association/Commission on Dietetic Registration code of ethics for the profession of dietetics and process for consideration of ethics issues. (2009). *J Am Diet Assoc*, *109*(8):1461–1467.

17. Academy of Nutrition and Dietetics. Position and Practice Papers. Available at: http://www.eatrightpro.org/resources/practice/position-and-practice-papers. Accessed June 26, 2017.

18. Academy of Nutrition and Dietetics. ANDHII. Available at: http://www.eatrightpro.org/resources/research/projects-tools-and-initiatives/andhii. Accessed June 26, 2017.

19. Academy of Nutrition and Dietetics Health Informatics Infrastructure. Help and Training Center. Available at: https://www.andhii.org/info/. Accessed June 26, 2017.

20. Lacey, K., & Pritchett, E. (2003). Nutrition Care Process and Model: ADA adopts road map to quality care and outcomes management. *J Am Diet Assoc*, *103*: 1061–1071.

21. Academy of Nutrition and Dietetics. (2018). Abridged Nutrition Care Process Terminology (NCPT) Reference Manual: Standardized Terminology for the Nutrition Care Process.

22. Writing Group of the Nutrition Care Process/Standardized Language Committee. Nutrition Care Process and Model Part II: Using the International Dietetics and Nutrition Terminology to Document the Nutrition Care Process. (2008). *J Am Diet Assoc*, *108*(8): 1287–1293.

NCP PROBLEM SOLVING MATRIX: A CRITICAL THINKING AND PROBLEM SOLVING APPROACH

Table 1.6 Our Case Study of Patient SB

Admission Sheet				
Name	**LOS**	**Age**	**Sex**	**Marital Status**	**Race/Ethnicity**
SB	2	68	M	Married	Arab

Primary Language	**Interpreter Needed**	**Next of Kin**	**Attending**
English	No	Wife	Wayne, K., MD

Allergies	**Chief Complaint**	**Admitting Diagnosis**
Shellfish	RT leg and foot pain	RT Diabetic Foot Ulcer-Cellulitis

Patient History

Medical and Surgical History	**Social History**	**Weight History**	
T2DM GERD HTN Peripheral Neuropathy Foot ulcer x 1 yr	**Smoking Status**: Current smoker; 2 packs/day for 40 years **Alcohol Use**: 1 drink/day Drug Use: None **Residence**: Lives with wife	3 months ago	106.5 kg
		1 year	106.5 kg

RN Admission Assessment

Height	**Weight**	**BMI**	**A&O**	**Glasgow**	**Braden**
190.5 cm Pt Estimate	106.5 kg Standing scale	29.3	To person x 3 To place x 3	15	17

Skin Integrity	**Malnutrition Universal Screening Tool**	
RT foot ulcer s/p debridement and wound vac placement	Decrease in appetite or intake? (Yes = 1, No = 0)	0
	Weight loss >10 lb in 3 months? (Yes = 1, No = 0)	0
	BMI score (<18.5 = 2, 18.5-20.0 = 1, >20.0 = 0)	0
	Total Score (2 or more triggers dietitian consult)	0

Table 1.6 Our Case Study of Patient SB

Active Orders

Consults	Nursing
CONSULT TO PHYSCIAN—candidate for proximal amputation right foot CONSULT TO PHYSCIAN—*diabetic foot ulcer* CONSULT TO PHYSCIAN— CONSULT DIETITIAN—nutritional needs for wound healing and diabetic diet education WOUND/OSTOMY/CONTINENCE NURSE—*wound vac left foot* PT EVAL/TREATMENT	ALTERNATIVE SPLINT AND/OR FOAM BOOTS WITH SCDs GLUCOSE, POINT OF CARE WOUND VAC ONGOING WOUND CARE MEASURE WEIGHT—*on admission*

Laboratory/Imaging	Medications/Infusions
CULTURE, BLOOD CULTURE, WOUND DEEP CULTURE, TISSUE COMPLETE BLOOD COUNT W DIFF COMPREHENSIVE METABOLIC PANEL	Carvedilol—oral Cefazolin—*intravenous* Heparin injection—*subcutaneous* Insulin lispro—*subcutaneous* Linagliptin—*oral* Lisinopril—*oral* Acetaminophen—*PRN* Simvastatin (Zocor)—*oral*

DIET: Diabetic 1600–1800

Physician H & P

History of Present Illness: Patient is a 68-year-old male who presents with chronic diabetic ulcer on his right foot that is worsening. Patient speaks English, is a current smoker. He denies fever, chills, chest pain, nausea, and vomiting.

Temp	BP	Heart Rate	Resp	SpO2	O2 (L/min)
36.4°C	139/85 mmHg	94	20	94%	RA

Review of Systems and Physical Exam

Constitutional	HEENT	Neck
Awake and alert; no distress	Normal	Normal
Pulmonary/Chest	Cardiovascular	Gastrointestinal
Clear to auscultation	Regular rate and rhythm	No masses felt; non-tender

(Continued)

Table 1.6 Our Case Study of Patient SB

Extremities	Skin	Neurological
No edema	Diabetic ulcer to right foot	No focal motor deficits

Assessment	Plan
Diabetic foot ulcer Diabetes mellitus, type 2 Suspected lower extremity peripheral vascular disease	Wound care; infectious disease consulted Ulcer debridement and wound vac placement Wound and blood cultures Continue antibiotics Dietitian consulted for wound healing recommendations and diabetic diet instruction

K. Wayne, MD

Flowsheets

Date	Hospital Day 1			Hospital Day 2		
Time	0800	1200	1600	0800	1200	
Meal Intake	100%	100%	100%	100%	100%	

Outputs

Urine Occurrences	1	2	1	1		
Stool Occurrences				1		
Negative Pressure Wound Therapy	Right foot, placed at 1 at 1120					

Edema

RUE	None			None		
LUE	None			None		
RLE	None			None		
LLE	None			None		

Laboratory Results

	Ref. Range	Day 1 0845
WBC	3.5–10.1 bil/L	22.1 (H)
Sodium	135–145 mmol/L	136

Table 1.6 Our Case Study of Patient SB		
Potassium	3.5–5.2 mmol/L	4.6
Glucose	60–99 mg/dL	208 (H)
BUN	8–22 mg/dL	29 (H)
Creatinine	0.60–1.40 mg/dL	1.19
GFR Non-African American	>59 mL/min/1.73m2	61
GFR African American	>59 mL/min/1.73m2	71
HbA1c	4.0–5.6%	7.5 (H)
Estimated Average Glucose		162
Glucose, Point of Care		
Day 1 1412	Day 1 1738	Day 2 0712
207 (H)	139 (H)	176 (H)

Dietitian Interview and Physical

Your patient speaks English and his wife is at bedside.

Appetite and intake: "My appetite is good, maybe too good! It was just as good before coming here, and I am eating all my meals. I could use more food! I've had diabetes for about 10 years, and I have cholesterol (I take pills for it), but I don't pay too much attention to what I eat; I never talked to anyone about diet. I eat everything my wife cooks."

Weight loss and UBW: "I don't weigh myself, but my clothes fit the same as a few years ago."

Food allergies: "Shellfish."

Cultural or religious food preference: "I am Muslim, but pork is the only food I don't eat."

Difficulty chewing or swallowing: "No."

Nausea, vomiting, constipation, or diarrhea: "No, but I get acid a lot, so I take two calcium tablets every day."

Preferences: "I eat all the traditional Lebanese foods, and I like meat and chicken; I have one or two pitas a day, and I like to put butter on it. We have rice every day. I also really like my potato chips, so I eat those every night! *Wife:* "I use olive oil to cook" every meal."

Musculoskeletal Depletion: None

Subcutaneous Fat Depletion: None

You talk to his nurse.

"Pt's wife has brought food every day, looks like lots of rice and pitas, and several desserts. They don't appear to be considering sugar or counting carbohydrates."

(Continued)

Table 1.6 Our Case Study of Patient SB

Typical Daily Intake / Food Frequency

Food Category	Specific Type/Preparation	Frequency	Amount
Meat / Fish / Poultry	No pork, shellfish	Daily	Unsure
Dairy: Milk, Cheese, Yogurt	Only whole milk	Daily	1 cup
Eggs		Twice/week	2
Starch (bread, grain, cereal)	Pita, rice, wheat flakes cereal	Usually daily	1 lge pita; 2 cups cereal; 2 cups rice
Vegetables	Spinach, broccoli (sautéed in oil)	3 to 4/week	1 cup
Fruits	Only juice, usually orange	Daily	1 cup
Sugars, Sweets / Desserts	Chocolate chip cookies, donut, baklava (one of these types/day)	Daily	2 cookies, 1 donut, 2-inch square baklava
Snack Foods (salted)	Potato chips	Daily	2 cups
Fats	Olive oil (for food prep), butter (on pita)		
Beverages: Coffee, Tea, Soda	Coffee (with cream)	Daily	3 cups
Alcohol	None		

CHAPTER 2

Nutrition Assessment

DATA GATHERING FROM THE MEDICAL RECORD AND DETERMINING NUTRIENT NEEDS

Nancy J. Park, MS, RDN-AP, CNSC

LEARNING OBJECTIVES

By the end of the chapter, the reader will be able to

- Identify the differences between a nutrition screen and nutrition assessment, and the individuals responsible for both
- Identify the five assessment domains in the Nutrition Care Process, as well as the types of data collected in each domain during a nutrition assessment
- Describe the process for finding nutrition-related data in the electronic medical record
- Determine the nutrient needs of a patient using evidence-based predictive equations

NUTRITION SCREENING AND ASSESSMENT: AN OVERVIEW

A team effort is necessary to gather all the information needed to determine a patient's nutritional status and level of risk. The nutritional screening and assessment of hospitalized patients is paramount, given the statistics on numbers of patients with malnutrition. For example, patients requiring medical or surgical care may be at risk for becoming malnourished during their inpatient stay. Other patients may present with some degree of nutrition compromise, varying from mild to severe.

Nutritional status is impacted by a myriad of factors, including environmental, physical, and psychosocial. Factors such as appetite, unplanned weight loss or gain, polypharmacy, income, literacy, quality and quantity of food intake, socialization at mealtimes, functional status, frequent hospitalizations, and acute or chronic illness all play a role in nutritional health. Understanding the patient's underlying nutritional status, as well as accounting for current disease processes and treatments, will direct how much energy, protein, and fluid (macronutrients) the patient will require for healing and repletion. Categorizing the information gathered into specific criteria will help define if the patient is at risk of malnutrition, or may already have some degree of malnutrition. Nutrition assessment is the first step in the Nutrition Care Process (NCP), while estimating needs provides a goal toward which the patient, dietitian, and other members of the health care team can work to achieve through the development of the nutrition care plan (1).

Appropriate assessment of nutrition risk has evolved over the past 40–50 years. Malnutrition in hospitalized patients was brought sharply into focus when C. E. Butterworth's article, "The Skeleton in the Hospital Closet," was published in 1974 (2). This landmark commentary on malnutrition was considered to be eye-opening at the time, yet in the span of nearly a half-century, there still has not been a universally accepted definition or widespread understanding of the implications of this condition. Current scrutiny of health care costs has further demonstrated the economic impact of malnutrition on health systems. Based on these facts, the Joint Commission on Accreditation of Healthcare Organizations (JCAHO) created a mandate specifying the screening and assessment of all hospitalized patients, and this mandate has been in place since 1995 (3).

Efforts have been made to develop meaningful and more universal nutrition screening and assessment tools. While health care professionals such as physicians and nurses have a role in identifying malnutrition, dietitians pull together all the pieces and are uniquely positioned to not only identify, but put forward action plans for treating malnutrition. Firstly, all patients should be screened for nutritional risk utilizing a standardized tool, and secondly, the dietitian should be consulted for further investigation and diagnosis.

Screening for Nutrition Risk and Malnutrition in Hospitalized Patients

Screening is used as a preliminary process to identify patients who are at risk of malnutrition. As implied in the name, a screen is a short set of standardized questions designed to differentiate problems with diet or nutrition. Timeliness is a key factor to the success of nutrition screening, and the process needs to be performed within 24 hours of admission, as required by JCAHO (3). The majority of nutrition screenings are completed by nurses as part of their initial intake and assessment of the patient. Nutrition and dietetic technicians, registered (NDTRs) are also often involved in the nutrition screening of patients. While the task of screening is typically assigned to nurses and technicians, dietitians can also perform screenings; however, this is typically reserved for higher-risk areas, such as oncology and intensive care.

The nutrition screen sorts out those patients needing referral to a dietitian for further assessment and treatment. Many of the questions asked in the screening tool are similar to those used by the dietitian when assessing the patient; the difference being that assessment takes the questioning further to provide more explicit and in-depth information into understanding the patient's degree of, or risk for, malnutrition. Typical areas addressed in a nutrition screen include, but are not limited to:

- Weight changes (particularly unintentional weight loss)
- Appetite status, feeding abilities/difficulties, use of adaptive feeding devices
- Presence of pressure ulcers and severity
- Current diet; use of enteral or parenteral nutrition.

Screening processes have evolved in response to the call for earlier and more consistent identification of nutrition risk. There are many malnutrition screening tools available, and a list of some of the more common ones is provided in Table 2.1 (4–7). Each tool has pros and cons; some are more complicated than others, thereby taking more time to complete. Others are designed for the community, primary care, or residential living settings. One of the best tools designed for hospitalized patients is the Malnutrition Screening Tool (MST), designed by Ferguson et al. (8) and detailed in Box 2.1. This short questionnaire (only three questions) is quick and easy to complete, rendering it useful for busy nurses. The MST has been shown to be both specific and sensitive for identifying patients with malnutrition and has a high inter-rater reliability. A score of 2 or greater will trigger a nutrition assessment.

TABLE 2.1 Malnutrition Screening Tools for Use in Hospitalized Patients

Name/Year	Primary Author	Users	Complexity	Validated?
Malnutrition Screening Tool (MST) – 1999	Ferguson, M., et al.	Nurses, technicians, dietitians, physicians, patients, patients' families	Simple	Yes
Malnutrition Universal Screening Tool (MUST) – 2003	Malnutrition Advisory Group of BAPEN – (British Association for Parenteral and Enteral Nutrition)	Nurses, technicians, dietitians, physicians	Complex	Yes
Nutritional Risk Screening (NRS) – 2002	Kondrup, J., et al.	Nurses, technicians, dietitians, physicians	Simple	Yes
Mini Nutritional Assessment (MNA) – 1990			Complex	Yes – focuses more on geriatric population

Name/Year	Primary Author	Users	Complexity	Validated?
Short Nutritional Assessment Questionnaire© (SNAQ) – 2005	Kruizenga, H. M., et al.	Nurses, dietitians	Simple	Yes
Subjective Global Assessment (SGA) – 1987	Detsky, A. S., et al.	Physicians, nurses, dietitians	Simple	Yes – more of an assessment than screening tool

Data from references 4–7:

(i) Dietitian/Nutritionists from the Nutrition Education Materials Online, "NEMO," Team Disclaimer: http://www.health.qld.gov.au/masters/copyright.asp. Validated malnutrition screening and assessment tools: comparison guide. Reviewed May 2017. https://www.health.qld.gov.au/__data/assets/pdf_file/0021/152454/hphe_scrn_tools.pdf. Accessed February 17, 2018.

(ii) Skipper, A., Ferguson, M., Thompson, K., et al. (2012). Nutrition screening tools: An analysis of the evidence. J Parenter Enteral Nutr, 36(3): 292–298.

(iii) Neelmaat, F., Meijers, J., Van Ballegooijen, H., et al. (2011). J Clin Nurs, 20(15–16): 2144–2152.4

(iv) Anthony, P. S. (2005). Nutrition screening tools for hospitalized patients. *Nutr Clin Pract*, 23(4): 373–382.

BOX 2.1

Malnutrition Screening Tool (MST)

Have you lost weight without trying?

No	0
Unsure	2

If yes, how much weight have you lost? (in kilograms)

1–5	1
6–10	2
11–15	3
>15	4
Unsure	2

Have you been eating poorly because of a decreased appetite?

No	0
Yes	2

Total

Data from reference 8: Ferguson, M., Capra, S., Bauer, J., et al. (1999). Development of a valid and reliable malnutrition screening tool for adult acute hospital patients. *Nutrition*, 15(6): 458–464.

Even with the development of easy-to-use screening tools, the crucial process of nutrition screening may be overlooked. Steps may be taken in the hospital setting to ensure nurses do not skip over this task. Educating the nursing staff on the importance of identifying malnourished patients may help with compliance. Appropriate use of the MST, with generation of an automatic referral to dietitians for those meeting established criteria, can get the ball rolling early on in the hospital stay. Many health care professionals, even those with an interest in nutrition, remain unaware of the steps involved in the nutrition care of patients, and opportunity exists for more education and institutionalization of the NCP (8).

BOX 2.2

How to Develop a Facility-Targeted Malnutrition Risk Screen

Many institutions have been inspired by the nutrition screening tools that have been developed, and have modified the published formats to be specific to their settings. Depending on your area of practice, university versus community hospital versus residential living care, etc., the screening tool may be modified to capture patients and create automatic referrals to dietitians for assessment.

Questions to consider when deciding upon a tool for selection include:

- Who will be performing the screen, and in what section of the EMR should it be located?

- How long does it take to perform the screen? (It should be quick and easy to complete.)
- Is the screen applicable to your patient population?
- What criteria will be included as part of the screen, and how will it be scored?

Dietitians need to be involved in the development of the form so that they can ensure all the correct parameters are being evaluated. The scoring system that is created should be stringent enough to identify all patients that need to be seen by the dietitian, but not too stringent so that too many patients are being identified for referral that may not actually need it. Modifications may be made to create a prioritization system for decisions on which patients to see first. All dietitians should be aware of the screening tool at their facility and work together will all members of the health care team to identify nutritionally at-risk patients early in their hospitalization.

Nutrition Assessment

Nutrition assessment, as mentioned in Chapter 1, is the first step in the NCP (1). Patients/clients are identified as needing nutrition assessment through nutrition screening, referral from other health care providers, or through identification by the dietitian. During this step, the dietitian gathers data and information from the medical record, patient interview, and communication with the health care team to determine the nutrition status of the patient, identify nutritional problems and risks, and to plan interventions and further nutrition care. Collected data is analyzed and interpreted by comparing to evidence-based standards whenever possible. The nutrition assessment step of the NCP consists of five assessment domains (1):

1. Anthropometric measurements
2. Biochemical data, medical tests, and procedures
3. Nutrition-focused physical findings
4. Client history
5. Food/nutrition-related history

All of the domains will be covered in this chapter, except for nutrition-focused physical findings domain, which is covered fully in Chapter 4. The majority of data collected by the RD will come from the patient's medical record. The patient interview, another significant source of information for the assessment, will be covered in detail in Chapter 3. Before going into details about what data is collected in each of the assessment domains, a discussion of the medical record is important.

MEDICAL RECORD

The medical record (MR) is the primary communication device utilized by the health care team to discuss and provide documentation on the patient's medical condition and treatment. It is a continuous written account of the patient's health care experience and a compilation of data regarding patient history, assessment, diagnosis, intervention, treatment, and therapy. The MR is a legal document, and care must be taken to ensure patient confidentiality when utilizing this document (9).

Most MRs in hospitals and other health care organizations are now electronic. The National Alliance for Health Information Technology categorizes electronic medical information into three types of records (10):

- **Electronic Medical Record (EMR):** The EMR is the digital version of a paper medical chart. This is a record of all the health-related information that is collected, gathered, and managed by one health care organization, such as a hospital. When a patient is admitted to a facility for the first time, an EMR is created for that patient, and all information relating to diagnosis and treatment, from the entire health care team, is kept in this digital file.

- **Electronic Health Record (EHR):** The EHR is similar to the EMR, except that the information in this record is shared across more than one health care organization. Primary care doctors, specialists, laboratories, pharmacies, hospitals, and other organizations can all contribute to and access the information in this record.

- **Personal Health Record (PHR):** The PHR contains the same type of information as the EHR (diagnoses, immunizations, family medical history, medications, etc.), but is designed to be accessed and managed by the individual patient. Patients can use PHRs to manage their own health care information from many different sources.

When completing a nutrition assessment, dietitians will utilize the EMR for the patient at the facility where they are working. Dozens of EMR software systems are available, and use depends on which system the organization has purchased. Some top systems include eClinicalWorks®, McKesson®, Cerner®, Allscripts®, athenahealth®, GE Healthcare®, and Epic®.

Electronic Medical Record (EMR)

During the nutrition assessment, the RD will collect both objective and subjective data. Subjective data is obtained from the patient and their family members during the patient interview (see Chapter 3). The objective data is provided by health care professionals and can be found in the EMR. Objective data includes physical findings, vital signs, laboratory or diagnostic testing results, height and weight data, etc. Depending on the type of documentation format used in the EMR, the data can be found in various sections. There are two different formats typically used in medical records: the problem-oriented and source-oriented medical record.

Problem-Oriented Medical Record

The problem-oriented medical record (POMR) was developed in the 1970s by a physician, Lawrence L. Weed (11). This type of medical record documentation is organized by the creation of a patient problem list and the subsequent treatment of those problems. The basic components of the POMR include Data Base (history, physical exam and lab data), Complete Problem List (a numbered list of all patient problems), Initial Plans, Daily Progress Notes, and Final Progress Note or Discharge Summary.

The POMR format uses the subjective, objective, assessment, plan (SOAP) note format for the progress note section (11). See Table 2.2 for an explanation of the SOAP note components. This type of medical record format is still used today, but with the advent of the EMR, the POMR is used less frequently.

TABLE 2.2 SOAP Note Documentation

Section	Data That Can Be Included
Subjective	Narrative describing the patient's current condition, including areas such as onset, severity, factors affecting the condition, symptoms, any treatment received.
Objective	Includes objective, traceable, or verifiable facts about the patient's status, including results from laboratory tests or medical procedures, physical exam findings, anthropometric measurements, vital signs.
Assessment	The physician's medical diagnoses.
Plan	What the health care team will do to treat the patient, including ordering labs, procedures or medications, education, and referrals to other providers or specialists.

Data from reference 11: Weed, L. L. (March 14, 1968). "Medical records that guide and teach." N Eng J Med, 278(11): 593–600.

Source-Oriented Medical Record

The source-oriented medical record (SOMR) is organized by subject matter, with all information categorized into sections based on the type of information. Sections may include orders, history and physical, nursing notes, laboratory, diagnostic testing and procedures, medications, flowsheets, and progress notes (a narrative account of the patient's progress on a daily basis) (12). The data is entered into each section by the "source" or the individual or service that is providing the information. The SOMR is kept in reverse chronological order, with the latest or most recent information at the top or beginning of the section. The SOMR is the most typical documentation format in the electronic version of medical records.

Navigating the Electronic Medical Record— Where Should the Dietitian Begin?

The Electronic Medical Record (EMR) is here to stay! The original intent of US legislation was to institute electronic documentation and records that were meaningful. While these ideas have been emerging over the past 40 years, the American Recovery and Reinvestment Act (ARRA) provided both incentives and penalties for health systems to convert from paper charts to EMR by 2014. As this initial deadline has come and gone, the EMR continues to evolve. Hospitals in urban settings, teaching institutions, and hospitals of greater size are generally more likely to have EMRs (13). The Nutrition Care Process (NCP) is ideally suited for EMR documentation and can be easily adapted. One study showed an advantage in capturing nutrition-related diagnoses using the EMR (14). Depending on the facility where you work, the dietitians may work from a nutrition template. This template typically will be set up to take the dietitian through all the necessary background information, as well as the ADIME (NCP documentation that stands for assessment, documentation, intervention, monitoring, & evaluation) and PES (problem, etiology, signs/symptoms) statements. Becoming accustomed to the template will help the dietitian be expeditious in gathering the necessary data. It will also familiarize the dietitian to the information that is "pulled in" from other areas of the EMR.

As previously mentioned, there are dozens of EMR software programs available for use. Due to this, the category names and locations of information in each system may vary. The categories, section names, and terminology used below are meant to be general and not specific to any one EMR software program.

Step 1: History and Physical

The patient's History and Physical, or H & P, is typically taken by a medical student, intern, resident, fellow, or mid-level provider. It not only contains the patient's past medical, surgical, family, and social history, it contains pertinent information surrounding the patient's chief complaints. Often these complaints are the main reason the patient will seek medical attention. Key items for dietitians to search for include weight loss, poor appetite, changes in eating habits, nausea, vomiting, diarrhea, food insecurity, alcohol intake, and illicit drug use. Other items include use of specialized nutrition therapies, such as enteral or parenteral nutrition therapy, or modified diets, fad diets, oral nutrition supplements, or other vitamin, mineral, or herbal supplements. Oftentimes, medical personnel will obtain information on nutritionally relevant pieces of information, such as weight loss, but not include this information on the patient's problem list or diagnoses. Careful review of the H & P—with attention to nutrition prescriptions—is paramount to making an accurate nutrition diagnosis and developing a care plan. The EMR provides the advantage of having items "pull through" from one part of the EMR to another. Additionally, tests and procedures will be listed in a chronological time line, which can facilitate assessment and appropriate nutrition interventions.

Step 2: Medications

Medications are typically listed in the EMR as the Medication Administration Record, or "MAR." Medications are also listed in the patient orders, report summaries, and MAR summaries. It is important to review all patient medications, including frequency and dosing, as medications may have interactions with nutrients. Additionally, medications may cause adverse symptoms that impair nutrient intake. Some examples include nausea, altered taste, drowsiness, or lethargy. The timing of medication is imperative in the dosing of enteral feedings, particularly when feedings need to be held for optimal blood levels of medications, such as Dilantin (phenytoin), or Coumadin (warfarin). The patient's medication list and route of medications can be important for patients receiving enteral or parenteral nutrition therapy. Certain medications should not be given via the enteral route, and medication compatibilities with parenteral nutrition are imperative to patient safety. Medication allergies are generally well marked, as adverse drug reactions can be fatal. More recently, allergy lists include foods and food ingredients, as well as environmental allergens. Allergies may also be listed in the EMR chart header, found at the top of each patient chart.

Step 3: Input and Output Flowcharts

Most EMRs have a graphic section for nursing documentation of all patient intake and output, or "I's and O's." Intake lists typically include all oral, intravenous fluid, enteral, parenteral, and medications given intravenously as drips. Output lists typically include urine, stool, tubes (such as nasogastric tubes), and drains, as well as dialysis treatments. These are listed over a 24-hour period. Advantages to the EMR include continuous and automatic tallying of intake and output, thereby reducing chance of nursing error with calculations. This is helpful to dietitians when obtaining information surrounding amounts of nutrition support therapy received, as well as fluid balance.

Input and output records are typically the responsibility of the nursing staff. Nurses and Patient Care Technicians record information on hourly, per-shift, or per-day intervals. Nutrition orders for enteral nutrition are typically ordered on an hourly basis, for example, "60 mL/hr." Yet, feedings are often held for procedures, medications, nursing care, or respiratory therapies. To understand the quantity of enteral feeding received versus prescribed, dietitians must review input records closely. This information is only as good as the data entered. With the EMR, it is simple to scroll back to the admission date and glean data on enteral or parenteral infusions. Newer trends in provision of and documentation of enteral feeding include volume-based feedings. Policies and procedures surrounding this method of feeding provision allow the nurse to increase the rate of tube feeding to better meet the patient's needs.

Step 4: Flowsheets

Flowsheets are a large section containing various subheadings. These subheadings include the patient's Vital Signs, Laboratory Data, Radiology Reports, and Assessments.

Vital Signs: Usually, the patient's height and weight will be listed under vital signs. Again, an advantage to the EMR includes calculation of the patient's ideal body weight (IBW) for height, and body mass index (BMI). Historical weight data may be found if previous admissions to the hospital and health system are searched within the EMR. Vital signs are of importance in the intensive care unit setting. Items such as blood pressure and mean arterial pressure (MAP) help assess blood flow to the gastrointestinal tract. This then determines when to provide or withhold enteral nutrition. An elevated white blood cell count and systemic inflammatory response syndrome (SIRS) criteria are found in the information provided in the Vital Signs section of the flowsheets. These pieces of data may be utilized in the determination of nutrition diagnoses.

The patient's weight in an EMR is of critical importance. Patient body weights are used not only for assessing the patient's overall health and well-being and nutrition indices, but are also used for the dosing of certain weight-based medications and other medical treatments, like dialysis. While an accurate weight is essential, it is often difficult to capture. That said, while documented weight over time in the EMR is an excellent tool, the dietitian should always obtain a weight history from the patient. Human error in charting or differences in the scales used may render the information useless. Also, the EMR can calculate the IBW based on height. If the height is entered incorrectly, the IBW will be calculated incorrectly. If the patient is unable to provide this information, it should be obtained from a family member or significant other. Even if the weight seems reasonable, the dietitian should confirm this with the patient or reliable source. Additionally, an order may be placed to have the patient weighed and recorded in the EMR. Weights may be obtained daily, as in renal or heart failure patients, or weekly, as in trauma or nutrition support patients. Many patients lose weight while hospitalized. Having a baseline weight and periodic actual weights thereafter help to provide accurate nutritional diagnoses and direction for the nutrition care plan.

Laboratory Data: Laboratory Data are generally viewed when the dietitian performs an initial assessment and upon reassessment. The EMR will list laboratory data typically by date; however, an advantage with the EMR is that this can be rearranged as needed to view laboratory data over time. For example, blood glucose levels, or hemoglobin A1c levels can be trended over a hospitalization or over several years. This may give the dietitian information to shape and tailor an individualized nutrition care plan. Additionally, monitoring protein levels over time may assist the dietitian in determining if more protein is needed for the patient. Some dietitians, such as those in nutrition support, will utilize flowsheets to monitor daily laboratory values to make recommendations pertaining to the patient's nutrition support therapy.

Radiology Reports: Radiology reports may contain information useful to how to provide nutrition support to the patient and/or determining the nutrition diagnosis. Firstly, determining appropriate enteral and parenteral access may be found in this section via chest or abdominal X-rays. Knowledge of when and where tubes and lines are placed and located is essential to determining the nutrition therapy prescription, and also for patient safety. Radiology reports can include data supporting the nutrition diagnosis; for example, inflammatory changes of an organ, or studies showing leaks or obstructions of the gastrointestinal tract.

Assessments: Assessments is a catch-all category that takes the reviewer through the patient's condition, head to toe, system by system. This section is valuable particularly to body systems relating to nutrition therapy, particularly the gastrointestinal (GI) tract. The EMR will contain data on GI symptoms (pain, nausea, vomiting, diarrhea), bowel sounds, bowel movements (frequency, consistency), presence of abdominal drains, ostomies, fistulas, and related output. Enteral tube placement and location will also be noted in this section. Other findings in the assessment include skin condition, frequently noted as "integumentary." Pressure ulcers are linked with poor nutritional status. The location, size, and quantity of skin abnormalities are essential. Sometimes the EMR will have a separate section for pressure ulcer and Wound, Ostomy Care Nurse (WOCN) documentation. Color pictures occasionally will be uploaded to this section to document the progression of healing. Again, this plays a key role in determining the amount of energy, protein, fluid, vitamins, and minerals a patient may need. In the intensive care unit, the assessment section will include information on the patient's respiratory and ventilator status. This includes ventilator settings and minute volume. This information may be utilized in determining energy needs if indirect calorimetry or Penn State Equations are employed for determining energy needs (see determining nutrient needs later in this chapter). If the facility has a template for nutritional assessment, the calculations for resting energy expenditure and other validated equations may be in place.

Step 5: Activity Log

The activity log is a list of all the charting activity that has taken place in the EMR in 24-hour increments. The category name will likely be different with various EMR software programs, with some calling this section "Form Browser," "Patient Encounters," or "Patient Activity Summary." Regardless of the name, all the non-physician or mid-level staff members' charting can be found here. An important section for the RD to review in the activity log is the nursing admission assessment. Within this assessment you will typically find the Nutrition Screen. The dietitian can review that screen to see why the nutrition consult was triggered. This can also serve as an auditing tool for compliance, as nutrition risk screening within 24 hours of admission is a requirement of the JCAHO. All nursing interventions will be listed here, often including various subheadings. Enteral tube placements and calorie count information is provided in this section.

Step 6: Orders

The Orders section of the EMR is self-explanatory. This is the list of orders to be carried out by various hospital staff personnel, including nursing, pharmacy, nutrition, and other ancillary staff. Orders are categorized into sections and subsections. It is possible to tell what and when tests and procedures are ordered, changes to medications, and the diet the patient is on, as well as consultations to other staff personnel. Items included under the dietitian's purview are typically nutrition assessments, calorie counts, and nutrition education.

Consults to all hospital staff will usually be under the Consult subsection. Special instructions, or "pick-list" items, may be included for further clarification as to why the dietitian is consulted. For example, consults may be ordered for "tube feedings," "TPN," or "diabetic diet." The date, time, and type of order can help the dietitian prioritize the patient workload for each day. Consults to dietitians for medical nutrition therapies and related items may be placed by physicians or mid-level providers, known as CPOE, or Computer Physician Order Entry. However, the EMR also has the technical capabilities to automatically generate orders or consults. This is where nutrition screening comes into play. Completion of the Nutrition Screen by the nurse within 24 hours of admission to the hospital will generate a consult to the dietitian if the patient meets the criteria. The JCAHO has mandated nutrition screening using a validated tool within 24 hours of admission to the hospital. While there are many validated tools available, these can be modified to meet specific institutional needs. Some screening tools will not only generate a consult but will also create a "risk" score. This risk score will help the dietitian prioritize who is seen and when. As everyone in the hospital needs to eat, "Diet" is another subsection under "Orders." In addition to the diet order, oral nutrition supplements and enteral feedings are listed in this area.

Ordering of diets is not as simple as it sounds. Each institution may have different names not only for diets, but for texture modifications, modular additives, and even enteral feedings (generic versus brand name). Physicians and mid-level providers often have little to no training on diets and diet planning, so the ordering of diets in the acute care setting can be tricky. There can also be legal ramifications, particularly surrounding dysphagia diets and patient safety. The dietitian must be aware of recommendations for diet consistency. Furthermore, busy physicians may have their own standard "go-to" diet orders, such as the "cardiac diet," which may be too restrictive and not individualized to the patient's needs. Liberalization of the diet may be more appropriate, especially if the patient has a poor appetite. With enteral feedings, oftentimes what is ordered is not always what is received. Many enteral feeding containers look the same, and the nurse may hang a formula they think is correct, but is not what is ordered.

It is wishful thinking on the part of the dietitian to believe the information available in the EMR precludes a visit to the patient at the bedside. Orders should always be double-checked and updated to reflect the appropriate recommendations to best meet the patient's needs. Timely order entry and frequent review are essential to ensure patients receive the food and nourishment they desire, as the diet office is obligated to send the most restrictive order. If the physician verbally tells the patient, "You can have some crackers and juice" but does not remove the NPO order, the patient will not receive the food items.

Step 7: Consultations and Progress Notes

The consultation section will include assessments and recommendations from specialty physicians and surgeons, and possibly from specialty groups such as Palliative Care or Nutrition Support Teams.

This information is listed by the specialty—e.g., Oncology or Cardiology—and the date the consult was completed. Consultations help guide the care the patient is receiving and can shed light on the overall goals of care.

Progress Notes are categorized by specialty heading as well. These are charted daily and listed chronologically. Formatting may be similar to the SOAP note, from paper chart days, or other templates and formats can be utilized. Other items listed in this section may include dictated operative procedures. Some specialty groups may have separate sections. This may include Radiology or highly specialized Cardiology reports. Typically, Consultations and Progress Notes are reserved for physicians and mid-level providers. Information from other ancillary and rehabilitation personnel is found in separate sections of the EMR.

Step 8: Documentation from Ancillary, Rehabilitation, Case Management, Social Work, and Wound Care

All non-physician documentation is found under separate categories, and many of these specialty areas will have their own templates and electronic forms for documentation. In health systems and hospitals that do not have a separate section for nutrition, the nutrition documentation will be found in the ancillary section. Speech Language Pathology and Occupational and Physical Therapy are typically found under "Rehabilitation." Case Management and Social Work may be combined together. Wound care, due to the increasing risk burden associated with pressure ulcers, may have its own subheading. Depending on how the nutrition documentation template is set up at a particular institution, the wound care information may flow into the nutrition assessment template. Understanding where to glean particular information from each section takes some time.

May hospitals and health systems are beginning to upload photographs of wounds to create a powerful "visual" progress note. What better way to show improvement since it is well known that a picture is worth a thousand words? Ideas for future documentation of malnutrition may include photographs of the patient, keying into areas of muscle wasting, fat loss, or other areas where micronutrient deficiencies may be noted. Serial photographs at regular intervals can provide excellent documentation as to how the nutrition care plan's goals are met, or whether they need revision and continued follow-up.

Step 9: Discharge Documentation

The most important piece in this section for dietitians will be transfer information to alternate care facilities. Phone numbers and contact personnel from the facilities will be listed here. This is helpful when communication needs to take place. Examples would include discussing goals of care in a challenging patient who requires ongoing nutrition support therapy, or finding out what the enteral formula was for a patient prior to admission.

The EMR is evolving and emerging as the standard of care for medical documentation. Dietitians using the EMR for the first time may find things overwhelming and not be sure where to begin. Take some time to go through the EMR, section by section, as this will help you see how the EMR is organized. Delve into each section to see what each category contains and how it is subdivided. It may be helpful to start with the documentation template your facility utilizes. Review the template to see what information is provided (automatically pulled in from other areas of the EMR) and what needs to be filled in by you. Familiarize yourself where key and pertinent information is found in the EMR to help save time. As you establish your own workflow, documentation should become easier. While documentation is legally binding and key to communication between medical and other hospital personnel, the EMR does not preclude dietitians from face-to-face interaction with patients.

ANTHROPOMETRIC ASSESSMENT

Accurate determination of a patient's height, weight and weight history, or weight change over time is crucial to determining nutrition risk. A patient's height and weight are two of the most important factors in describing the patient's degree of malnutrition and in estimating macronutrient needs. The guidelines for defining malnutrition list percent weight loss as a major factor in determining malnutrition risk, and as a predictive factor for increased morbidity and mortality (15). Therefore, the collection of anthropometric data and its analysis by the dietitian are an essential part of the nutrition assessment.

Measurement of Height

Most clinicians will verbally ask a patient their height based on the patient's recall. Most facilities will have a height and weight entered into the medical record, and these can usually be found in the Vital Signs or History and Physical section of the chart. However, when possible, measurement of height and weight should take place. Measurement of weight can take place on a standing scale or bed scale. Height is recorded in centimeters (cm) and weight in kilograms (kg). See Box 2.3 for instructions on measuring height.

BOX 2.3

Procedure for Measuring Height on the Floor or a Standing Scale

- Have the patient stand as straight as possible, heels together, and against a flat surface or on a scale, without shoes.
- For scales with yardstick attachments, have the patient stand erect with head, shoulder blades, buttocks, and heels touching the vertical yardstick (or flat surface if the patient is not on a scale).
- The patient should be looking straight ahead, without tipping the head up or down.
- Using the built-in measuring device, lower the horizontal bar gently atop the patient's head.
- For patients standing on the floor, use a ruler or tongue depressor, and gently lay this atop the patient's head to line up with the centimeter (cm) mark.
- Measured to the nearest 0.1 cm.
- Note and record the measurement.

An estimation of height is necessary for patients who are confined to bed or a wheelchair, have curvature of the spine or contractures, paralysis, or are otherwise unable to stand for an actual height measurement (16). Alternate methods to estimate height include arm span and knee-height (17, 18). A quick search of research articles will produce numerous studies that show that both methods provide a close approximation of actual body height. See Box 2.4 and Box 2.5 for the procedures for measuring arm span and knee height, and Table 2.3 for knee height calculations.

BOX 2.4

Measurement of Height Using the Arm-Span Method

- *Note: Always check with nursing staff prior to moving patients*
- Extend out both arms at shoulder level (90-degree angle), with palms facing forward.
- Using a tape measure, measure the distance from the longest fingertip of one hand to the longest fingertip of the other hand (for most individuals, this is the middle finger).
- Do not include fingernails in the measurement.
- For patients who are unable to stand, attempt to have them as flat as possible in the bed.
- Note and record the centimeter marking as measurement of height.

BOX 2.5

Measurement of Height Using the Knee-Height Method

- *Note–always check with nursing staff prior to moving patients*
- Knee height is measured using a sliding broad-blade caliper.
- Patient should be in the supine position or sitting with the knee at a 90-degree angle.
- Place one blade of the caliper under the heel of the foot and the other on the anterior surface of the thigh.
- The shaft of the caliper should be held parallel to the long bone of the lower leg, and pressure applied to compress the tissue.

- Record the measurement to the nearest .01 cm.

- Height (in cm) is calculated using the equations in Table 2.3.

Data from references 17 & 18:

(i) Lee, R. D., & Nieman, D. C. (2013). *Nutritional Assessment*, 6th ed. New York, NY: McGraw-Hill.

(ii) Chumlea, W. C., Guo, S. S., & Steinbaugh, M. L. Prediction of stature from knee height for black and white adults and children with application to mobility-impaired or handicapped persons. *Journal of the American Dietetic Association, 94*(12): 1385–1391.

TABLE 2.3 Equations for Estimating Stature from Knee Height

Age	Equation	Error
White Males		
6–18	2.22 (Knee Height) + 40.54	+/- 8.42 cm
18–60	1.88 (Knee Height) + 71.85	+/- 7.94 cm
> 60	2.08 (Knee Height) + 59.01	+/-7.84 cm
Black Males		
6–18	2.18 (Knee Height) + 39.60	+/- 9.16 cm
18–60	1.79 (Knee Height) + 73.42	+/- 7.2 cm
> 60	1.37 (Knee Height) + 95.79	+/-8.44 cm
White Females		
6–18	2.14 (Knee Height) + 43.21	+/- 7.8 cm
18–60	1.87 (Knee Height) + 70.25 − (0.17 age)	+/- 7.2 cm
> 60	1.91 (Knee Height) + 75.00 − (0.06 age)	+/- 8.82 cm
Black Females		
6–18	2.02 (Knee Height) + 46.59	+/- 8.78 cm
18–60	1.86 (Knee Height) + 68.10 − (0.06 age)	+/- 7.2 cm
> 60	1.96 (Knee Height) + 58.72	+/-16.5 cm

Evaluating Body Weight

After the patient's height and weight are obtained, the nutrition assessment involves interpreting or evaluating the patient's weight. The use of the Hamwi Method for calculating ideal body weight serves as a reference to a normal body weight. Adjustments should also be used for frame size, amputations, and spinal cord injuries. Other calculations that can be used to evaluate body weight include the percent of the patient's ideal and usual body weights, percent of weight loss or change, and body mass index.

Body weight relative to height is a frequently used measurement to determine risk of morbidity and mortality. Although there is limited published research on their validity, many ideal body weight (IBW) equations and height/weight tables are used to assess an individual's nutrition status by comparing actual body weight to IBW standards in various settings (19). One common method frequently use in the United States is the Hamwi Method (20), shown in Box 2.6. Adjustments to the IBW should be made for all patients according to frame size to account for differences in body build (muscularity, bone thickness, and body proportions) (21). Frame size can be determined by measuring wrist circumference (Table 2.4), which is a quick and easy method, or using elbow breadth (Table 2.5), which is more complex, but tends to provide a more accurate estimate of frame size (22). In addition, adjustments for amputations (Table 2.6) and spinal cord injuries (Box 2.7) should be made when applicable (23, 24).

BOX 2.6

The Hamwi Method for Calculating Ideal Body Weight

For	**Females**	**Males**
Medium Frame Size*	Allow 100 pounds for the first 5 feet of height, plus 5 pounds for every inch > 5 feet Subtract 2.5 pounds for each inch < 5 feet	Allow 106 pounds for the first 5 feet of height, plus 6 pounds for every inch > 5 feet Subtract 2.5 pounds for each inch < 5 feet

* IBW by the Hamwi method is used for individuals with an average or medium size body frame. For those with small or large frames, subtract (small) or add (large) 10% to the calculated IBW.
Data from reference 20: Hamwi, G J. Changing dietary concepts. In T. S. Danowski (Ed.), *Diabetes mellitus: Diagnosis and treatment*, Vol. 1, (pp. 73–78). New York, NY: American Diabetes Association, Inc.

TABLE 2.4 Estimating Frame Size Using Wrist Circumference

Method: Measure the wrist circumference just distal to the styloid process at the wrist crease of the left hand, in inches, using a tape measure. Compare the measurement to the values below.

Male Wrist Measurements

		Height >5'5"
	Small	5.5"–6.5"
	Medium	6.5"–7.5"
	Large	>7.5"

Female Wrist Measurements

	Height <5'2"	Height 5'2"–5'5"	Height >5'5"
Small	<5.5"	<6.0"	<6.25"
Medium	5.5"–5.75"	6.0"–6.25"	6.25"–6.5"
Large	>5.75"	>6.25"	>6.5"

Date from reference 21: U.S. National Library of Medicine (NLM). Calculating body frame size. Available at: http://www.nlm.nih.gov/medlineplus/ency/imagepages/17182.htm. Accessed March 19, 2018.

TABLE 2.5 Estimating Frame Size Using Elbow Breadth

Method:
- Subject should stand, if possible, and extend the arm forward so that it is horizontal and parallel to the ground.
- Turn palm so that it is facing up, and bend elbow so that the forearm is at a 90-degree angle to the ground.
- Measure the distance between the two prominent bones on either side of the elbow (the epicondyles of the humerus). This measurement can be taken with a ruler or tape measure, but using commercially available calipers is preferable.
- Compare the measurement to the values below.

Female Elbow Measurements for Medium Frame*

Height	Elbow Breadth
4'10"–4'11"	2 1/4"–2 1/2"

5'0"–5'3"	2 1/4"–2 1/2"
5'4"–5'7"	2 3/8"–2 5/8"
5'8"–5'11"	2 3/8"–2 5/8"
6'0"–6'4"	2 1/2"–2 3/4"

Male Elbow Measurements for Medium Frame*

Height	**Elbow Breadth**
5'2"–5'3"	2 1/2"–2 7/8"
5'4"–5'7"	2 5/"–2 7/8"
5'8"–5'11"	2 3/4"–3"
6'0"–6'3"	2 ¾"–3 1/8"
6'4"–6'7"	2 7/8"–3 1/4"

*If elbow breadth is less than those in the table for a specific height, subject is small framed, and if elbow breadth is greater, subject is large framed.

Data from references 17 & 22:

(i) Lee, R. D., & Nieman, D. C. (2013). *Nutritional assessment*, 6th ed. (pp. 179–180). New York, NY: McGraw-Hill.

(ii) National Health and Nutrition Examination Survey III. Body measurements (anthropometry). Available at: https://wwwn.cdc.gov/Nchs/Data/Nhanes3/Manuals/anthro.pdf. Accessed April 1, 2018.

TABLE 2.6 Amputation Adjustments for Estimating Ideal Body Weight

For patients with amputations, estimation of IBW should be adjusted with the following equation using the factors below:

$$\frac{100 - \% \text{ amputation}}{100} \times \text{IBM for original height}$$

Percentage Body Weight Contributed by Body Part

Hand	0.7%
Forearm and hand (below elbow)	2.3%
Entire arm	5.0%
Foot	1.5%

(*Continued*)

Lower leg and foot (below knee)	5.9%
Entire leg	16.0%

Data from reference 23: Osterkamp, L. K. (1995). Current perspective on assessment of human body proportions of relevance to amputees. *J Am Dietetic Assoc, 95*: 215–218.

BOX 2.7

Spinal Cord Injury Adjustment

- **Paraplegia:** Subtract 5% to 10% from IBW
- **Quadriplegia:** Subtract 10% to 15% from IBW

Data from reference 24: Academy of Nutrition and Dietetics, Evidence Analysis Library. (2009). *Spinal cord injury: Assessment of body composition: Estimation of ideal body weight.* Available at https://www.andeal.org/. Accessed April 1, 2018.

Several other equations that can be used in body weight evaluation are percent IBW, percent usual body weight (UBW), and percent weight change (or loss), which are included in Box 2.8 (25). Table 2.7 shows how both percent IBW and UBW can be used to estimate nutrition risk.

BOX 2.8

Percent Ideal Body Weight, Percent Usual Body Weight, and Percent Weight Loss

$$\text{Percent IBW} = \frac{\text{Actual Weight}}{\text{Ideal Body Weight}} \times 100$$

$$\text{Percent UBW} = \frac{\text{Actual Weight}}{\text{Usual Body Weight}} \times 100$$

$$\text{Percent Weight Change (or loss)} = \frac{(\text{Usual Weight} - \text{Actual Weight})}{\text{Usual Weight}} \times 100$$

Data from reference 25: Blackburn, G. L., Bistrian, B. R., Maini, B. S., et al. (1977). Nutritional and metabolic assessment of the hospitalized patient. *J Parenter Enteral Nutr, 1*: 11–22.

TABLE 2.7 Interpreting % IBW and % UBW

% IBW	Nutritional Risk	% UBW
>120	Obesity	—
110–120	Overweight	—
90–109	Not at risk	—
80–89	Mild	85–95
70–79	Moderate	75–84
<70	Severe	<75

Data from reference 25: Blackburn, G. L., Bistrian, B. R., Maini, B. S., et al. (1977). Nutritional and metabolic assessment of the hospitalized patient. *J Parenter Enteral Nutr, 1*: 11–22.

As mentioned previously, percent weight loss is a major factor for determining nutrition risk and for predicting morbidity and mortality (15). It is important for clinicians to understand that even severely obese patients can be malnourished, as determined by percent of weight loss over time. Weight loss can occur as a harbinger of an underlying disease, such as cancer. It can also occur over time in relation to a chronic disease, such as cardiac (congestive heart failure), or pulmonary failure (chronic obstructive pulmonary disease), or AIDS. Weight loss may be an inevitable result of acute traumatic illness (accidents or burns), or elective surgeries, due to the accelerated inflammatory response.

Regardless of the cause, the amount and time frame of weight loss and possible causes must be reported by the patient or significant others. If this information is not available firsthand, or the patient is unsure of the amount of weight loss, review of previous admissions can provide information. Once percentage of weight loss has been calculated, use Table 2.8 to assess the significance of the change (26).

TABLE 2.8 Interpreting Unintentional Weight Changes

Time Frame	Significant Weight Loss	Severe Weight Loss
1 week	1%–2%	>2%
1 month	5%	>5%
3 months	7.5%	>7.5%
6 months	10%	>10%

Data from reference 26: Evan, A. & Gupta, R. Approach to the patient with unintentional weight loss. Available at: https://www.uptodate.com/contents/approach-to-the-patient-with-unintentional-weight-loss. Accessed April 3. 2018.

Finally, body mass index (BMI) is a direct calculation based on height and weight, regardless of gender, and can be used to identify individuals at both ends of the weight spectrum. Interpretation of BMI is important, as it is incorrect to automatically assume that a patient with a high BMI is well nourished. An obese patient who has had an unexpected weight loss may be at risk for malnutrition. Conversely, BMI can also be used to assess the severity of obesity. This is why it is vital to consider all components when completing a sound nutrition assessment.

BMI does have limitations, and factors such as age, sex, ethnicity, and muscle mass can influence the relationship between BMI and body fat (27, 28). In addition, the presence of edema should be considered when interpreting BMI results. For every liter of excess body fluid, weight is increased by 1 kilogram. Rapid increases or losses of weight should be judiciously interpreted and correlated with increasing or decreasing fluid retention (29). See Table 2.9 for classifications of body weight based on BMI.

TABLE 2.9 Classification of Weight by Body Mass Index

$$BMI = \frac{\text{weight (kg)}}{\text{height (m}^2)} \quad \text{or} \quad BMI = \frac{\text{weight (lb)}}{\text{height (in}^2)}$$

BMI (kg/m²)	Weight Status	Obesity Class
<18.5	Underweight	
18.5–24.9	Normal	
25.0–29.9	Overweight	
30.0–34.9	Obesity	I
35.0–39.9	Obesity	II
>40.0	Extreme obesity	III

A BMI of <18.5 in adults ages 18–65 or <23 in adults over 65 years is a flag that the weight is less than normal when performing the nutrition assessment.

Data from references 27 & 28:

(i) National Institutes of Health Clinical Guidelines on the identification, evaluation, and treatment of overweight and obesity in adults: The Evidence Report. (1998). Available at: http://www.ncbi.nlm.nih.gov/books/bv.fcgi?rid=obesity. Accessed March 28, 2018.

(ii) Centers for Disease Control and Prevention, Division of Nutrition, Physical Activity, and Obesity. Available at: http://www.cdc.gov/healthyweight/assessing/bmi/adult_bmi/About adult BMI. Accessed March 28, 2018.

BIOCHEMICAL DATA, MEDICAL TESTS, AND PROCEDURES

Laboratory data is used during a nutrition assessment to determine what is happening inside the patient's body. Blood and urine samples can be used to determine if a patient has any nutrition deficiencies or excesses that may affect their nutrition status. The concepts of sensitivity and specificity are important in laboratory assays. Sensitivity indicates the degree to which the test for a particular blood or urine component is accurate in determining the amount of that component in the sample. Specificity refers to how precise the test is in measuring a particular substance in a sample (30).

When interpreting laboratory data, it is important to consider some basic concepts. No single test is diagnostic on its own; serial testing that measures changes in lab results is typically more valid than a single lab result that can be taken out of context of a patient's clinical status. There can be daily variations for certain tests, which validates the need for serial measurement. Finally, some components (such as nutrients) that are being measured may be altered by comorbid conditions, diseases, medications, and hydration status.

One particular condition that can skew laboratory (lab) data is hydration status. Both dehydration (hypovolemia) and overhydration (hypervolemia) can affect lab results. Dehydration can occur due to lack of fluid intake, or from fluid loss for various reasons, including excessive vomiting or diarrhea, fever, excessive sweating, excessive urination, or the use of certain medications such as diuretics. With dehydration, lab values can be increased from normal levels due to hemoconcentration from too little fluid in the bloodstream. On the other hand, overhydration is typically caused by too much fluid intake from either drinking too much water or from overuse of intravenous (IV) fluids. Overhydration can also result from the body retaining more fluid than is necessary due to conditions such as congestive heart failure, liver or kidney problems, uncontrolled diabetes or the use of certain drugs. Lab values that are most commonly affected by hydration status include albumin, electrolytes, blood urea nitrogen (BUN), creatinine, and hemoglobin and hematocrit. Hydration status of the patient should be evaluated before interpreting lab values during the nutrition assessment.

Appendix E gives a listing of common lab measurements that are relevant to nutrition assessment, as well as a listing of test panels that are disease or organ specific, that have significance to the RD. Below is additional biochemical information of importance to the RD regarding protein status and anemias.

Protein Status

Historically, dietitians used both visceral protein and somatic protein status as an important part of the nutrition assessment in acute care settings. Somatic protein refers to skeletal muscle, while visceral protein refers to nonmuscular proteins, such as those that make up organs and other proteins found in the blood. The three major hepatic proteins used to assess visceral protein status are albumin, transferrin, and prealbumin (Table 2.10) (31, 32). However, these proteins, referred to as negative acute-phase proteins (APP), also reflect the body's physiologic response to stress, including infections, surgery, injuries, and trauma (33). Protein synthesis is profoundly altered during the stress response. The liver diverts synthesis from negative APPs to produce more positive acute-phase reactant proteins, all in response to systemic inflammation, which is the hallmark of the stress response. Albumin is especially affected, with reduced synthesis, increased degradation, and transcapillary leakage (34).

In addition to acute stress, inflammation is also present at low levels in the background of chronic diseases, such as heart disease, diabetes, and cancer. Due to this decrease in the negative APPs in the presence of inflammation, it has become clear that using albumin and prealbumin to determine protein status is of little use in the acute care setting where the majority of patients have either acute stress or chronic comorbid conditions. Increased levels of positive APPs, including C-reactive protein (CRP), can be used to identify patients who might be at nutritional risk because of acute or chronic health conditions that contribute to inflammation. Albumin can be used in other settings, since extensive research has shown that hypoalbuminemia is an important predictor of morbidity and mortality among subsets of patients, such as those with burns, pressure ulcers, severe sepsis, cancer, renal disease, and surgical patients (35–38).

Lymphocytes are an important part of the immune system, and it is well known that malnutrition can detrimentally affect immune function. Total lymphocyte count (TLC), the clinical measure of immune function, can indicate malnutrition when levels are decreased (31, 32) (Table 2.11).

TABLE 2.10 Visceral Protein Parameters

Protein	Normal Range	Implications & Considerations
Albumin	3.5–5.0 g/dL	Low when visceral protein is depleted; 17–20 days; low in liver disease, malabsorption syndromes, protein-losing nephropathies, ascites, burns, overhydration, inflammation; elevated in dehydration

(Continued)

Protein	Normal Range	Implications & Considerations
Fibronectin	220–400 mg/dL	Low when visceral protein is depleted; half-life 15 hrs; low in inflammation, injury; affected by coagulation factors
Prealbumin	15–36 mg/dL	Low when visceral protein is depleted; half-life 1.9 days; low in liver disease, burns, inflammation; elevated in nephrotic syndrome, chronic kidney disease, pregnancy, Hodgkin's lymphoma
Retinol binding protein	3–6 mg/dL	Low when visceral protein is depleted; half-life 12 hrs; low in chronic pancreatitis or carcinoma, cystic fibrosis, intestinal malabsorption, chronic liver diseases, vitamin A deficiency; elevated in renal failure
Transferrin	188–341 mg/dL	Low when visceral protein is depleted (only if iron status is normal); half-life 8–10 days; low in chronic infection, malignancy; elevated in late pregnancy, use of oral contraceptives, viral hepatitis

Data from references 31 & 32:

(i) Pagana, K. D. (2014). *Mosby's manual of diagnostic and laboratory tests*, 5th ed. St. Louis, MO: Elsevier Mosby.

(ii) U.S. National Library of Medicine, Medline Plus. Laboratory Tests. Available at: https://www.nlm.nih.gov/medlineplus/laboratorytests.html. Accessed February 1, 2018.

TABLE 2.11 Total Lymphocyte Count and Visceral Protein Status

Formula: TLC = % of lymphocytes × No. of WBCs (10^3)

TLC values in cells/mL^3	Interpretation
> 1500	Normal
1,200–1,500	Mild degree of depletion
800–1,199	Moderate degree of depletion
<800	Severe degree of depletion

Affected by: Injury, viral infection, radiation therapy, surgery, chemotherapy, and other immunosuppressive medications. TLC may not be reliable indicator of malnutrition in the elderly

TLC, total lymphocyte count; WBC, white blood cells.

Data from references 31 & 32:

(i) Pagana, K. D. (2014). *Mosby's manual of diagnostic and laboratory tests*, 5th ed. St. Louis, MO: Elsevier Mosby.

(ii) U.S. National Library of Medicine, Medline Plus. Laboratory Tests. Available at: https://www.nlm.nih.gov/medlineplus/laboratorytests.html. Accessed February 1, 2018.

The somatic protein compartment is typically assessed using anthropometric measurements, such as mid-arm circumference, but it can also be measured biochemically through creatinine excretion and nitrogen balance. Creatinine is a catabolic product of creatine phosphate, a compound needed in muscular contraction. It is excreted at a constant daily rate proportional to muscle mass, and using creatinine levels to calculate creatinine height index can help to determine protein depletion severity; however, this testing is rarely done in the clinical setting.

In a healthy adult, nitrogen is typically in balance, meaning excretion is equal to intake (with intake coming from dietary protein). When protein catabolism exceeds anabolism, a person is in negative nitrogen balance (NB), which occurs in malnutrition (39). Conversely, when anabolism exceeds catabolism, this signifies a positive NB, which happens during growth phases, such as in children and during pregnancy. To measure NB, a 24-hour urine sample must be collected, as well as a measurement of protein intake during the same period. This limits the routine use of NB in the clinical setting; however, it is more commonly used in critical care, particularly with patients receiving nutrition support. Table 2.12 lists the measurement specifics and equations used to measure NB.

TABLE 2.12 Nitrogen Balance

Monitor and calculate dietary intake of protein (PRO) for 24 hrs; then convert dietary protein intake to nitrogen intake with the equation below:

$$\text{Nitrogen} = \frac{\text{PRO intake}}{6.25\text{g nitrogen}}$$

- Collect 24-hr urine; obtain urinary urea nitrogen (UUN) from the lab

- Nitrogen Balance = Nitrogen intake − (UUN + 3[a])

- Interpretation: Adults are normally in nitrogen balance (0); pregnant women and children (growth states) are in positive balance; negative balance may suggest malnutrition

[a] Insensible losses.

Data from reference 39: Dickerson, R. Using nitrogen balance in clinical practice. (December 2005). *Hospital Pharmacy, 40*(12): 1081–1085. Wolters Kluwer, Inc.

Nutritionally related anemias can be identified by analyzing hematologic parameters (Table 2.13). Several of these parameters may also be affected by compromised visceral protein status.

TABLE 2.13 Hematologic Parameters Related to Anemia

Constituent	Normal Range	Implications & Considerations
Erythrocyte protoporphyrin	<5 µg/dL RBCs	High in later stages of iron deficiency anemia
Ferritin	Males: 18.0–350 ng/mL Females: 15–49 yrs: 12.0–156 ng/mL >49 yrs: 18.0–204 ng/mL	Low in early deficiency state in the presence of depleted iron stores
Folate, red blood cell content	95 ng/mL	Low in later stages of folate deficiency anemia
Folate, serum	1.9 ng/mL	Low as folate deficiency progresses

Constituent	Normal Range	Implications & Considerations
Hematocrit	Males: 41%–50% Females: 35%–46%	Low in anemia; represents percentage of red blood cells in total blood volume
Hemoglobin	Males: 14.0–17.2 g/dL Females: 12.0–15.6 g/dL	Low in anemia; represents total amount of hemoglobin in red blood cells
Mean corpuscular hemoglobin concentration	32–36 g/dL	Low in iron deficiency anemia hypochromic); normal in B12 and folate deficiency (normochromic); represents hemoglobin (pigmentation) contained in an average red blood cell
Red blood cell count	Male: $4.4 - 5.8 \times 10^6$ µL Female: $3.9 - 5.2 \times 10^6$ µL	Low in anemia; the number of red blood cells in sample
Transferrin	188–341 mg/dL	High in iron-deficiency anemia as transport of iron increases
Vitamin B12	200–800 pg/mL	Low in B12 deficiency

Data from references 31 & 32:

(i) Pagana, K. D. (2014). *Mosby's manual of diagnostic and laboratory tests*, 5th ed. St. Louis, MO: Elsevier Mosby.

(ii) U.S. National Library of Medicine, Medline Plus. Laboratory Tests. Available at: https://www.nlm.nih.gov/medlineplus/laboratorytests.html. Accessed February 1, 2018.

CLIENT HISTORY AND FOOD/NUTRITION-RELATED HISTORY

Patient History

A comprehensive patient history is an important component of a complete nutrition assessment. The main types of history that should be obtained include health or medical, medications, personal, and food and nutrition. Sources for this information can include the medical record, the patient, and their significant others.

The health or medical history identifies conditions, diseases, and other factors that can place a client at risk of malnutrition due to their effect on food intake, appetite, and the ability to obtain and prepare foods. The patient's current and past medical diagnoses may have significant nutritional relevance and should always be considered in the nutrition assessment (Box 2.9). Additional factors to consider include the disease/condition's duration and severity, the presence of other physiologic stressors the patient may be experiencing, and the patient's genetics and age, which all have the potential to alter nutritional status.

BOX 2.9

Diseases or Conditions with Nutritional Relevance

AIDS-HIV	Hepatitis
Alcohol and/or drug abuse	Hypertension
Cachexia	Inflammatory bowel disease
Cancer	Malabsorption
Celiac disease	Malnutrition
Cerebrovascular accident	Multiple sclerosis
Chronic obstructive pulmonary disease	Nephrotic syndrome
Cirrhosis	Neutropenia
Coronary heart disease (MI)	Obesity
Crohn's disease	Pancreatitis
Dehydration	Parkinson's disease
Diabetes	Peritonitis
Dysphagia	Pressure ulcers
Eating disorders	Renal failure
Gastrointestinal bleeding	Sepsis
Hepatic encephalopathy	Tuberculosis

The medication history identifies all prescribed medications, over-the-counter (OTC) medications, and dietary supplements that can affect nutrient needs or alter nutritional status, or result in food-drug interactions (see Appendix G for a listing of nutritionally relevant medications and food-drug interactions). Personal history includes any psychosocial and lifestyle patterns that may affect the patient's nutrient needs, influence their diet and food choices, or limit nutrition therapy options. Table 2.14 lists general information for all categories of history in addition to specific information to collect from the patient or the medical record.

TABLE 2.14 Patient History Categories

History Category	Specific Information
Health/Medical	
Current health status and diagnoses	Date of first diagnosis
	Previous education on diagnosis
Previous medical history and health status	Specific family members affected by nutritionally relevant disease and onset age
Family history	Recent diagnostic procedures requiring NPO status
Surgical history	Difficulty chewing (state of dentition) or swallowing
	Chronic gastrointestinal problems (diarrhea, constipation, nausea, vomiting)
Medications	
Prescription medications	Use of multiple medications
OTC meds	Duration of medication use
Dietary supplements (nutrient, herbal, essential nutrients)	Frequency of use (chronic or as needed)
	Changes in sense of smell or taste related to medications
Illegal drugs	Previous education on potential interactions
Personal	
Age	Income
Gender	Use of or eligibility for government programs
Cultural/ethnic identity	Communication barriers
Occupation/economic status	Cognitive function
Role in family	Smoking
Educational level	Ability to perform daily functions
Motivational level	Person responsible for grocery shopping, meal preparation

(*Continued*)

History Category	Specific Information
	Access to transportation
	Recent loss of spouse
Food and Nutrition/Diet	
Food intake	Food intolerances or allergies
Eating habits and patterns	Appetite (current and prior to admission)
	Weight history (recent weight loss in particular)
	Physical handicaps affecting food preparation or intake
	Typical daily intake (types and amounts of foods and beverages consumed)
	Meal pattern
	Religious dietary restrictions
Lifestyle patterns	Ethnic dietary habits
	Alcohol consumption
	Frequency of dining out; types
	Exercise, physical activity (type and frequency)
	Attitude regarding diet and health
	Previous diet instruction (location, year, topic)
	Interest in diet instruction or outpatient counseling
	Stage of change/readiness to learn

Food and Nutrition History

A food and nutrition history (FANH) is the analysis of a patient's dietary practices, food consumption patterns, and the knowledge and attitudes they have regarding their diet. A comprehensive FANH may not be possible with all patients in the acute care setting; however, components of the history are vital in nutrition assessment, so it's important for the clinical RD to obtain as much information as possible. The goal of a FANH is to identify nutrient intake and possible deficiencies, the reasons for potential food and nutrition problems, and all dietary factors important in generating the nutrition diagnosis and subsequent intervention. Data that is collected during the FANH typically includes: food intake, eating habits and patterns, food allergies and intolerances, nutrition knowledge, food availability, weight history, physical activity and exercise patterns, physiologic factors that affect eating (such as chewing ability or the fit of dentures), psychosocial factors that affect eating (environment, culture, religion, etc.), and lifestyle patterns related to nutrition and health.

There are several methods and techniques that the dietitian can use to obtain a patient's food intake history, but it's important to use those that are practical to the setting. In acute or extended care, the Typical Daily Intake (TDI) (Table 2.15) and simplified Food Frequency (FF) are the most commonly used methods (Table 2.16). The TDI focuses on a typical day's eating pattern, beginning with the first meal of the day. For example, the dietitian may ask, "What is the first thing you would normally eat or drink when you get up in the morning?" It's best not to label meals as "breakfast, lunch, and dinner" in the questioning so as not to lead the patient in their responses. Questions should also inquire as to the quantity of food eaten, when and where eating takes place, as well as food preparation methods.

An FF is used to determine the foods the patient eats, and then compares them to an established guideline to determine if there are any food groups or specific nutrients missing from the normal diet. This can either be a comprehensive or simplified process. A simplified FF questionnaire is advantageous because it's a quick method for determining whether the patient avoids any major category of food, and it can be used as a cross-reference to the TDI. The Dietary Guidelines for Americans or the Dietary Reference Intakes are typically the standards used for comparison. A simplified evaluation form of general aspects of diet can also be used to collect food intake data (Table 2.17).

In addition to asking patients about food intake, in the clinical setting, a calorie count can also be ordered to obtain actual amounts of food eaten by the patient during meals and snacks. Each facility has its own protocol for calorie counts, but typically the RD will order the calorie count, and then nursing or hospital aides will assist by documenting the amount of food eaten by the patient. Kitchen personnel, such as those who pick up the trays after meals, may also assist by documenting plate waste for the patient. The RD will then analyze the data and determine the amount of calories consumed.

TABLE 2.15 Typical Daily Intake Form

Meal Timing	Food Item	Amount	Where Eaten

TABLE 2.16 Food Frequency Form

Food Item/Group	Amount/Day	Amount/Week
Milk or other dairy products (yogurt, cheese)		
Meat, poultry, eggs		
Fish		
Nuts, legumes, and legume products		
Fruits		
Vegetables		
Starches (breads, cereals, grains)		
Fats, added (oils, margarine, salad dressing)		
Snack foods (chips, pretzels, crackers)		
Desserts/sweets		
Dining out:		
Fast food		
Restaurant dining		
Beverages:		
Alcohol		
Coffee, tea		
Carbonated beverages		
Fruit juices		

TABLE 2.17 Evaluation of Dietary Intake

Group	Servings/Day	Recommended	Adequate/Excess
Dairy			
Protein			
Fruit			
Vegetable			
Starch			
Fat/sweets			
Overall Diet Adequacy: ____yes ____no			
Specific Nutrients:			
Deficit of: ____kcals ____PRO[a] ____fiber ____Vit A ____Vit C ____Fe ____ Ca ____Other			
Excess of: ____kcals ____Fat ____SFA ____Chol ____Sugar ____ Alcohol ____Na			
Other:			
Summary:			

[a]PRO, protein; Fe, iron; Ca, calcium; SFA, saturated fatty acid; Chol, cholesterol; NA, sodium.

ESTIMATING NUTRIENT NEEDS

Since ancient Grecian times, people have been interested in how the body works, and how food is utilized as fuel for the body. In the last two centuries, science has expanded our understanding of the rudiments of metabolism. Lavoisier is considered the "father of modern chemistry," and his work shed light on respiration and heat exchange, or as we now know it, metabolism. The study of gas and heat exchange led to the development of Direct Calorimetry. In the early 20th century, Cuthbertson's study on the impact of critical illness is still used in modern-day medicine (40). Continued efforts to quantify energy metabolism based on gas exchange led to the development of indirect calorimetry (IC). Indirect calorimetry, while considered the most accurate method of determining energy needs in critical illness, is not always available in clinical settings. Therefore, predictive equations have been developed that calculate resting metabolic rate (RMR) and closely approximate the results from IC.

Estimating Energy Needs Using Predictive Equations—Noncritical Care

Energy is provided to the body in the form of carbohydrate and fat, with protein sometimes being used as a source of energy. Adequate energy intake is needed to preserve body systems. With too little energy intake, or at times when body catabolism is high, weight loss occurs. When energy intake exceeds expenditure, weight gain occurs.

There are over 200 published predictive equations for estimating energy needs, with researchers attempting to develop equations intended to estimate energy expenditure as accurately as possible. One of the first was the Harris-Benedict (HB) equation in 1919 (41, 42) (Box 2.10). Although not seen as frequently today, this equation is still used in some clinical settings. Since HB only estimates the resting metabolic rate (RMR), once RMR has been calculated, the total energy expenditure (TEE) would need to be estimated using a combination of activity and stress factors. Stress factors are used for hospitalized patients in a hypermetabolic state due to disease, infection, or trauma. The clinician's judgment should be used to determine the appropriate activity and/or stress factor to use to estimate TEE with the HB equation.

BOX 2.10

Harris-Benedict Equation

Females: BEE = 655.1 + 9.6W + 1.9H − 4.7A

Males: BEE = 66.5 + 13.8W + 5.0H − 6.8A

W = weight in kilograms (use of actual vs. ideal vs. adjusted body weight is determined by the clinician*); H = height in centimeters; A = age in years.

*The Evidence Analysis Library does report that the Harris-Benedict equation was most accurate when used with actual body weight (42).

Data from reference 41: Harris, J. A., & Benedict, F. G. (1919). *A biometric study of metabolism in man.* Publication No. 279. Washington, DC: Carnegie Institute.

Another equation that has grown in popularity is the Mifflin-St. Jeor (MSJ) equation (43) (Box 2.11). The Academy of Nutrition and Dietetics Evidence Based Library rates the MSJ equation as the most accurate predictive equation in both the nonobese and obese non-critically ill population (44). In addition, a review by Frankenfield et al. shows the MSJ to be the most reliable out of four of the most commonly used predictive equations in clinical practice, with the MSJ predicting RMR within 10% of that measured by IC, with the smallest margin of error (45–47). As with HB, the MSJ only calculates RMR, so a patient activity level must be applied to calculate the patient's TEE. See Table 2.18 for activity and stress factors that can be used with both the HB and MSJ equations.

BOX 2.11

Mifflin-St. Jeor Equation

Female: Energy Expenditure = 10W + 6.25H − 5A) - 161
Male: Energy Expenditure = 10W + 6.25H − 5A + 5

W = actual weight in kilograms (regardless of BMI); H = height in centimeters; A = age in years.

Data from references 43 & 44:

(i) Mifflin, M. D., St. Jeor, S. T., Hill, L. A., et al. (1990). A new predictive equation for resting energy expenditure in healthy individuals. *Am J Clin Nutr, 51*:241–247.

(ii.) Dougherty, D., Bankhead, R., Kushner, R., Mirtallo, J., & Winkler, M. (1995). Nutrition care given new importance in JCAHO standards. *Nutr Clin Pract, 10*(2)(suppl): 57s–62s.

TABLE 2.18 Activity and Stress Factors for Determining Total Energy Expenditure

Patient Activity Levels	Factors
Confined to bed	1.2
Ambulatory, out of bed	1.3
Seated work, little or no strenuous leisure activity	1.6–1.7
Strenuous work or highly active leisure	2.0–2.4

Stress Conditions	Factors
Burns	
≤20% BSA	1.5
20%–40% BSA	1.8
>40% BSA (use max. of 60% TBSA)	1.8–2.0
Infection	
Mild	1.2
Moderate	1.4
Severe	1.8
Starvation	0.85
Surgery	
Minor	1.1
Major	1.2
Trauma	
Skeletal	1.2
Blunt	1.35
Closed head injury	1.4
BSA, body surface area.	

Date from references 41–45:

(i) Harris, J. A., & Benedict, F. G. (1919). *A biometric study of metabolism in man*. Publication No. 279. Washington, DC: Carnegie Institute.

(ii) Academy of Nutrition and Dietetics, Evidence Analysis Library. (2005). Energy Expenditure: Evidence Analysis: Harris-Benedict. Available at: http://www.eatrightpro.org/resources/research/evidence-based-resources/evidence-analysis-library. Accessed April 2, 2018.

(iii) Mifflin, M. D., St. Joer, S. T., Hill, L. A., et al. (1990). A new predictive equation for resting energy expenditure in healthy individuals. *Am J Clin Nutr, 51*: 241–247.

(iv) Dougherty, D., Bankhead, R., Kushner, R., Mirtallo, J., & Winkler, M. (1995). Nutrition care given new importance in JCAHO standards. *Nutr Clin Pract, 10*(2)(suppl): 57s–62s.

(v) Academy of Nutrition and Dietetics, Evidence Analysis Library. (2006). Energy Expenditure: Evidence Analysis: Estimating RMR with prediction equations. Available at: http://www.eatrightpro.org/resources/research/evidence-based-resources/evidence-analysis-library. Accessed April 4, 2018.

Finally, a frequently used, fast and easy method for estimating energy needs is using kilocalories per kilogram of body weight, with the reference weight as actual or ideal body weight, based on the clinician's judgment (Table 2.19) (49, 50).

TABLE 2.19 Energy Requirements Based on Kilocalories per Kilogram of Body Weight

Condition	Energy Requirement (kcal/kg)
Normal	25–30
Stress, mild	30–35
Stress, moderate to severe	35–45

Data from references 49 & 50:

(i) Escott-Stump, S. (2015). *Nutrition and diagnosis-related care*, 8th ed. Philadelphia, PA: Wolters Kluwer.

(ii) McClave, S. A., et al. (2009). Guidelines for the provision and assessment of nutrition support therapy in the adult critically ill patient: Society of Critical Care Medicine and American Society for Parenteral and Enteral Nutrition (A.S.P.E.N.). *JPEN J Parenter Enteral Nutr, 33*: 277–316.

Estimating Energy Needs—Critical Care

When available in the clinical setting, indirect calorimetry (IC) is considered the gold standard for measuring RMR. IC is the measurement of inspired oxygen and expired carbon dioxide, as measured in volume exchanged. These numbers are used to calculate resting energy expenditure (REE) and to determine the patient's respiratory quotient (RQ). The numbers are then entered into the abbreviated Weir equation, to obtain the calorie requirement of the patient. IC equipment is expensive to obtain and maintain and is often not available to perform the study. Also, there are circumstances when IC may be inaccurate, such as multisystem trauma and sepsis, rendering IC not as useful (50).

The Academy's Evidence Analysis Library (EAL) recommends that if indirect calorimetry is not available to determine energy requirements for critically ill patients, then the Penn State University equations, which were specifically designed for this population, have the best prediction accuracy (51). For the purposes of energy expenditure estimates, critically ill patients are defined as those requiring mechanical ventilation, or life support. For nonobese, ventilator-dependent, critically ill patients of any age, and for obese, ventilator-dependent, critically ill patients < 60 years of age, the EAL recommends using the Penn State equation [PSU(2003b)]. Concerns were raised that the PSU(2003b) equation overestimated requirements for older, obese patients, which led to a modification to the equation in 2010. For obese, ventilator-dependent, critically ill patients > 60 years of age, the Modified Penn State equation [PSU(2010)] has better accuracy (45, 46, 50). See Box 2.12 for both of the Penn State equations.

BOX 2.12

The Penn State Equations: Penn State (2003b) and Modified Penn State (2010)

Penn State (2003b): (use with nonobese any age, obese <60 years of age)
$$RMR = MSJ(0.96) + V_E(31) + T_{max}(167) - 6212$$

Modified Penn State (2010): (use with obese >60 years of age)
$$RMR = MSJ (0.71) + V_E(64) + T_{max}(85) - 3085$$

VE = expired minute ventilation in L/min; T_{max} = maximum body temperature in previous 24 hrs in degrees Celsius; MSJ = Mifflin-St. Jeor Equation Determining energy requirements for non–ventilator-dependent, critically ill patients can be done by modifying the MSJ equation by a factor of 1.25, although accuracy rates for this method are only around 50%.

Permissive Underfeeding in the Adult Critically Ill Patient

As the percentage of Americans who are overweight and obese has increased, estimating the energy needs of these patients becomes important. The 2016 guidelines from the Society for Critical Care Medicine (SCCM) and the American Society for Parenteral and Enteral Nutrition (ASPEN) provide recommendations for providing energy to class 1 obese patients (BMI >30), and up to class 3 obese patients (BMI >40). The recommendations are 11–14 calories per kilogram of actual body weight, or 22–25 calories per kilogram of IBW. Currently, there are no validated studies for energy recommendations for patients with a BMI > 45 (46).

Estimating Protein Needs

Intake of protein is needed to maintain body structures, for muscle growth and repletion, and for cell functions. Proteins play a major role in hormones, cellular transport and detoxification, maintenance of fluid and acid-base balance, and immunity. Protein is also a source of energy. Evidence-based guidelines for protein provision is lacking in the primary literature. Oftentimes the amounts used by dietitians are not referenced, but anecdotal. Ferrie et al. did an expansive literature review of articles from 1950 to 2011 pertaining to the estimation of protein needs (52). They found the studies too heterogeneous to do a meta-analysis. The review was prompted by the fact most protein ranges for hospitalized patients are not referenced, even those widely used as standards. These ranges for protein needs are provided in grams per kilogram of body weight (Table 2.20). The 2016 ASPEN/SCCM guidelines for the assessment and provision of nutrition support therapy in the adult patient also make recommendations for protein and energy needs, particularly in the obese critically ill patient (49).

TABLE 2.20 Estimated Protein Needs for Hospitalized Patients

Category	Grams protein/kg IBW
Healthy Men and Women	0.8
- Pregnant women	+ 0.43 (third trimester)
- Lactating women	+ 0.35
Elderly hospitalized patient	1.0–1.2
- Malnourished, pressure ulcers	1.2–1.5
- Malnourished with glomerular filtration rate 30–60 mL/min	1.1
General Surgery	1.5
- Gastrointestinal Surgery	1.7
- Intestinal failure	1.5–2.0
Gastroenterology	
- Pancreatitis	1.0–1.5
Renal Failure	
CKD stages 3, 4, 5—not dialyzed	0.75–1.0
Hemodialysis—stable	1.2–1.4
- Acute illness	≥ 1.2
Peritoneal dialysis—stable	≥ 1.2
- Acute illness	≥ 1.3
- Peritonitis	1.5
Conservative management—CKD Stage 5	0.6–0.8
Post-transplant—first four weeks	>1.4
Post-transplant—long-term; women	0.75
men	0.84
Liver Disease	1.2–1.5
Oncology; general	− 1.2
- radiotherapy	1.2
- head and neck cancer	1.0–1.5
- cancer cachexia	1.4
HIV—stable	1.2–1.5
- Acute illness	1.2–1.6

Category	Grams protein/kg IBW
Head Trauma	1.5
General Trauma and Burns	1.5–2.0
Burns > 15% Body Surface Area (BSA)	1.0–1.5
- 15–30% BSA	1.5
- > 30% BSA	1.5–2.0
- > 50% BSA	2.0–2.3
- Rehabilitation phase	1.7–2.0
Critical illness	1.2–2.0
Continuous renal replacement therapy	≥ 2.0
Sepsis	1.2–2.3
Obese critically ill with permissive underfeeding	
BMI 30–40	≥ 2.0
BMI > 40	≥ 2.5

Data from references 52 & 53:

(i) Ferrie, S., Rand, S., & Palmer, S. (2013). Back to basics: Estimating protein requirements for adult hospitalized patients: A systematic review of randomized controlled trials. *Food and Nutrition Sciences, 4*: 201–214. http://dx.doi.org/10.4236/fns.2013.42028. Accessed February 18, 2018.

(ii) Hydration Evidence-Analysis Project. (2007). Academy of Nutrition and Dietetics Evidence Analysis Library. Academy of Nutrition and Dietetics. Available at: https://www.andeal.org/. Accessed February 18, 2018.

Estimating Fluid Needs

Methods for estimating fluid requirements for the normal person are typically based on kilocalorie intake, body weight, or age (53). According to the Academy of Nutrition and Dietetics Evidence Analysis Library, actual body weight (ABW) should be used to calculate the fluid needs of adult patients. Exceptions to using ABW include patients who have severe edema or ascites where fluid retention is increasing the weight. In these instances, use IBW. See Table 2.21 for methods of estimating fluid needs. Patients with heart failure, pulmonary failure, liver disease, lymphedema, and/or end-stage renal disease may need fluid restriction as part of the medical management of these disease states.

TABLE 2.21 Calculations for Fluid Requirements in Adults

Recommended Daily Allowance (RDA)	1 milliliter per kilocalorie
Disease Management Method	< 25 mL/kg for renal, cardiac disease, and fluid overload 35 mL/kg for draining infected wounds
Age Method	18–55 years old: 30–35 mL/kg 55–65 years old: 30 mL/kg Greater than 65 years old: 25 mL/kg
Weight Method:	First 10 kg: 100 mL/kg/day Second 10 kg: 50 mL/kg/day Each additional kg: 20 mL/kg (< 50 years) 15 mL/kg (> 50 years)

Data from reference 53: Hydration Evidence-Analysis Project. (2007). Academy of Nutrition and Dietetics Evidence Analysis Library. Academy of Nutrition and Dietetics. Available at: http://www.andevidencelibrary.com. Accessed February 18, 2018.

Put It into Practice: Estimate Your Nutrient Needs

- Using the equations in the Estimating Needs: Noncritical Care section of this chapter, estimate your energy needs using the Harris-Benedict, Mifflin-St. Jeor, and kilocalorie per kilogram methods. How do the three methods compare? You can also estimate your protein and fluid needs as well.

- As an extra step, calculate your daily intake for one day or even two or three days, and compare this to your estimated needs. How close is your caloric and protein intake to your estimated needs? You can find free food trackers online or on your phone with mobile apps. Do a quick Internet search or search the apps on your phone for a free tracking tool (use keywords "diet tracker" or "food journal" for your search).

To Sum It Up

1. The nutritional screening and assessment of hospitalized patients is paramount, given the statistics on numbers of patients with malnutrition. Screening is a preliminary process that identifies patients that need further care from the dietitian, based on data such as weight changes, appetite, skin integrity, and dentition. Through nutrition assessment, the dietitian plays a vital role in the treatment of the patient by identifying nutrition problems and providing a plan of care, using the Nutrition Care Process (NCP).

2. As the first step in the NCP, nutrition assessment is the data-gathering phase, covering the five domains of Anthropometric data, Biochemical data, medical tests and procedure, Nutrition-Focused Physical Exam, Client History, and Food and Nutrition History.

3. The medical record is the primary communication device utilized by the health care team to discuss and provide documentation on the patient's medical condition and treatment. With the advent of the electronic medical record (EMR), access to data has become faster and easier, allowing for more accurate care.

4. Accurately estimating a patient's nutrient needs is an important part of the nutrition assessment. Indirect calorimetry is the ideal method, but when it is not available, predictive equations can be used to calculate requirements for energy. In addition, protein and fluid needs are estimated using various evidence-based equations.

Check for Understanding

1. The first step in the Nutrition Care Process is
   a. data gathering
   b. the diet order
   c. nutrition screening
   d. nutrition assessment

2. The type of record used in a hospital to document the care of the patient at that facility is called the
   a. personal health record (PHR)
   b. electronic health record (EHR)
   c. electronic medical record (EMR)
   d. electronic chart system (ECS)

3. The section of the patient's chart where you would find a record of the amounts of IV fluids, enteral or parenteral nutrition, or IV medications given to a patient would be the
   a. history & physical
   b. intake & output flowchart
   c. activity log
   d. nutrition assessment documentation

4. The nutrition assessment domain where you would find detailed information on the patient's dietary practices would be the
   a. client history
   b. anthropometric
   c. nutrition-focused physical exam
   d. food and nutrition history

5. Which predictive equations does the Academy's Evidence Analysis Library rate as the most accurate predictive equation in both the nonobese and obese noncritically ill?
   a. Mifflin-St. Jeor
   b. Harris-Benedict
   c. Penn State (2003b)
   d. Kilocalories per kilogram

Answers in Appendix B

References

1. Academy of Nutrition and Dietetics. Nutrition Terminology Reference Manual (eNCPT): Dietetics Language for Nutrition Care. http://www.ncpro.org. Accessed March 12, 2018.

2. Butterworth, C. E. (April 1974). The skeleton in the hospital closet. *Nutrition Today*, 9(2):4–8.

3. Joint Commission on Accreditation of Healthcare Organizations. (2009). *Comprehensive accreditation manual for hospitals: The official handbook*. Oakbrook Terrace, IL: Joint Commission Resources. PC.01.02.01, PC 01.02.03.

4. Dietitian/Nutritionists from the Nutrition Education Materials Online, "NEMO," Team Disclaimer: http://www.health.qld.gov.au/masters/copyright.asp. Validated malnutrition screening and assessment tools: Comparison guide. Reviewed May 2017. https://www.health.qld.gov.au/__data/assets/pdf_file/0021/152454/hphe_scrn_tools.pdf. Accessed February 17, 2018.

5. Skipper, A., Ferguson, M., Thompson, K., et al. (2012). Nutrition screening tools: An analysis of the evidence. *J Parenter Enteral Nutr, 36*(3): 292–298.

6. Neelmaat, F., Meijers, J., Van Ballegooijen, H. et al. (2011). *J Clin Nurs, 20*(15–16): 2144–2152.4.

7. Anthony, P. S. (2005). Nutrition screening tools for hospitalized patients. *Nutr Clin Pract, 23*(4): 373–382.

8. Ferguson, M., Capra, S., Bauer, J., et al. (1999). Development of a valid and reliable malnutrition screening tool for adult acute hospital patients. *Nutrition, 15*(6): 458–464.

9. AHIMA EHR Practice Council. Developing a Legal Health Record Policy. (October 2007). *Journal of AHIMA* 78, no. 9: 93–97. Available online in the AHIMA Body of Knowledge at www.ahima.org.

10. The National Alliance for Health Information Technology Report to the Office of the National Coordinator for Health Information Technology (Department of Health and Human Services) on Defining Key Health Information Technology Terms, April 28, 2008. Available at http://www.himss.org/national-alliance-health-information-technology-report-office-national-coordinator-health. Accessed April 10, 2018.

11. Weed, L. L. (March 14, 1968). Medical records that guide and teach. *New Eng J Med, 278*(11): 593–600.

12. Post, A., & Harrison J. (2006). Data Acquisition Behaviors during Inpatient Results Review: Implications for Problem-Oriented Data Displays. AMIA Annual Symposium Proceedings, 2006: 644–648.

13. Jha, A. K., DesRoches, C. M., Campbell, E. G., et al. (2009). Use of electronic health records in U.S. hospitals. *N Engl J Med, 360*: 1628–1638. doi:10.1056/NEJMsa0900592 (Accessed April 16, 2018).

14. Rossi, M., Campbell, K. L., & Ferguson, M. (2014). Implementation of the nutrition care process and international dietetics and nutrition terminology in a single-center hemodialysis unit: Comparing paper vs. electronic records. *J Acad Nutr Diet, 114*(1): 124–130. doi:10.1015/j.jand.2013.07.033 epub 2013 Oct 22. (Accessed April 16, 2018).

15. White, J. V., Guenter, P., Jensen, G., Malone, A., & Schofield, M. (May 2012). Academy Malnutrition Work Group; A.S.P.E.N. Malnutrition Task Force; A.S.P.E.N. Board of Directors. Consensus statement: Academy of Nutrition and Dietetics and American Society for Parenteral and Enteral Nutrition: Characteristics recommended for the identification and documentation of adult malnutrition (undernutrition). *JPEN J Parenter Enteral Nutr, 36*(3): 275–283.

16. Estimating height in bedridden patients. Available at: http://www.rxkinetics. com/height_estimate.html. Accessed March 18, 2018.

17. Lee, R. D., & Nieman, D. C. (2013). *Nutritional Assessment*, 6th ed. New York, NY: McGraw-Hill.

18. Chumlea, W. C., Guo, S. S., & Steinbaugh, M. L. Prediction of stature from knee height for black and white adults and children with application to mobility-impaired or handicapped persons. *Journal of the American Dietetic Association, 94*(12): 1385–1391.

19. Shah, B., Sucher, K., & Hollenbeck, C. B. (2006). Comparison of ideal body weight equations and published height-weight tables with body mass index tables for healthy adults in the United States. *Nutr in Clin Pract, 21*: 312–319.

20. Hamwi, G. J. (1964). Changing dietary concepts. In T. S. Danowski (Ed.), *Diabetes mellitus: Diagnosis and treatment*, Vol. 1 (pp. 73–78). New York, NY: American Diabetes Association, Inc.

21. U.S. National Library of Medicine (NLM). Calculating body frame size. Available at: http://www.nlm.nih.gov/medlineplus/ency/imagepages/17182. htm. Accessed March 19, 2018.

22. National Health and Nutrition Examination Survey III. Body measurements (anthropometry). Available at: https://wwwn.cdc.gov/Nchs/Data/Nhanes3/ Manuals/anthro.pdf. Accessed April 1, 2018.

23. Osterkamp, L. K. (1995). Current perspective on assessment of human body proportions of relevance to amputees. *J Am Dietetic Assoc, 95*: 215–218.

24. Academy of Nutrition and Dietetics, Evidence Analysis Library. (2009). Spinal cord injury: Assessment of body composition: Estimation of ideal body weight. Available at: https://www.andeal.org/. Accessed April 1, 2018.

25. Blackburn, G. L., Bistrian, B. R., Maini, B. S., et al. (1977). Nutritional and metabolic assessment of the hospitalized patient. *J Parenter Enteral Nutr, 1*:11–22.

26. Evan, A. T., & Gupta, R. Approach to the patient with unintentional weight loss. Available at: https://www.uptodate.com/contents/approach-to-the-patient-with-unintentional-weight-loss. Accessed April 3, 2018.

27. National Institutes of Health Clinical Guidelines on the identification, evaluation, and treatment of overweight and obesity in adults: The Evidence Report. (1998). Available at: http://www.ncbi.nlm.nih.gov/books/bv.fcgi?rid=obesity. Accessed March 28, 2018.

28. Centers for Disease Control and Prevention, Division of Nutrition, Physical Activity, and Obesity. Available at: http://www.cdc.gov/healthyweight/assessing/ bmi/adult_bmi/About adult BMI. Accessed March 28, 2018.

29. Patel, V., Romano, M., Corkins, M. R., et al. (2014). Nutrition screening and assessment in hospitalized patients: A survey of current practice in the United States. *Nutr Clin Pract, 29*(4): 483–490.

30. Saah, A. J., & Hoover, D. R. (January 1, 1997). "Sensitivity" and "specificity" reconsidered: The meaning of these terms in analytical and diagnostic settings. *Ann Intern Med, 126*(1): 91–94.

31. Pagana, K. D. (2014). *Mosby's manual of diagnostic and laboratory tests*, 5th ed. St. Louis, MO: Elsevier Mosby.

32. U.S. National Library of Medicine, Medline Plus. Laboratory Tests. Available at: https://www.nlm.nih.gov/medlineplus/laboratorytests.html. Accessed February 1, 2018.

33. Academy of Nutrition and Dietetics. Nutrition Care Manual. https://www.nutritioncaremanual.org. Accessed March 16, 2018.

34. Huckleberry, Y. Nutritional support and the surgical patient. (2004). *Am J Health Syst Pharm, 61*(7). Available at: http://www.medscape.com/viewarticle/474066_6. Accessed December 16, 2015.

35. Aguayo-Becea, O. A., Torres-Garibay, C., Macia-Amerzxua, M. D., et al. (July 2013). Serum albumin level as a risk factor for mortality in burn patients. *Clinics, 6*(7): 90–945.

36. Lin, M. Y., Liu, W. Y., Tolan, A. M., et al. (October 2011). Preoperative serum albumin but not prealbumin is an excellent predictor of postoperative complications and mortality in patients with gastrointestinal cancer. *Am Surg, 77*(10): 1286–1289.

37. Peralta, R. Hypoalbuminemia. Available at: http://emedicine.medscape.com/article/166724-overview#a6. Accessed December 15, 2015.

38. Eljaiek, R., & Dubois, M. J. (June 7, 2012). Hypoalbuminemia in the first 24 hours of admission with organ dysfunction in burned patients. *Burns , 39*(1): 113–118.

39. Dickerson, R. (December 2005). Using nitrogen balance in clinical practice. *Hospital Pharmacy, 40*(12): 1081–1885. Wolters Kluwer, Inc.

40. Lawson, C. M., Chandler, A. L., Bollig, R., et al. (2014). *Introduction to metabolism.* In K. A. Davis & S. H. Rosenbaum (Eds.), *Surgical metabolism: The metabolic care of the surgical patient* (pp. 1–22). New York, NY: Springer.

41. Harris, J. A., & Benedict, F. G. (1919). *A biometric study of metabolism in man.* Publication No. 279. Washington, DC: Carnegie Institute.

42. Academy of Nutrition and Dietetics, Evidence Analysis Library. Energy Expenditure: Evidence Analysis: Harris-Benedict. (2005). Available at: http://www.eatrightpro.org/resources/research/evidence-based-resources/evidence-analysis-library. Accessed April 2, 2018.

43. Mifflin, M. D., St. Joer, S. T., Hill, L. A., et al. (1990). A new predictive equation for resting energy expenditure in healthy individuals. *Am J Clin Nutr, 51*: 241–247.

44. Dougherty, D., Bankhead, R., Kushner, R., Mirtallo, J., & Winkler, M. (1995). Nutrition care given new importance in JCAHO standards. *Nutr Clin Pract, 10*(2)(suppl): 57s–62s.

45. Academy of Nutrition and Dietetics, Evidence Analysis Library. Energy Expenditure: Evidence Analysis: Estimating RMR with prediction equations. (2006). Available at: http://www.eatrightpro.org/resources/research/evidence-based-resources/evidence-analysis-library. Accessed April 4, 2018.

46. Frankenfield, D., Ashcraft, C., & Galvan, D. (2013). Prediction of resting metabolic rate in critically ill patients at the extremes of body mass index. *J Parenter Enteral Nutr, 37*(3): 361–367.

47. Frankenfield, D. C., Omert, L. A., Badellino, M. M., et al. (1994). Correlation between measured energy expenditure and clinically obtained variables in trauma and septic patients. *J Parenter Enteral Nutr, 18*: 398–403.

48. Frankenfield, D., Roth-Yousey, L., & Compher, C. (2005). Comparison of predictive equations for resting metabolic rate in healthy nonobese and obese adults: A systematic review. *J Am Diet Assoc , 105*(5): 775–789.

49. Escott-Stump, S. (2015). *Nutrition and diagnosis-related care*, 8th ed. Philadelphia, PA: Wolters Kluwer.

50. McClave, S. A., et al. (2009). Guidelines for the provision and assessment of nutrition support therapy in the adult critically ill patient: Society of Critical Care Medicine and American Society for Parenteral and Enteral Nutrition (A.S.P.E.N.). *JPEN J Parenter Enteral Nutr, 33*: 277–316.

51. Academy of Nutrition and Dietetics, Evidence Analysis Library. (2012). Critical illness: Critical illness guidelines: Determination of resting metabolic rate. 2012. Available at: http://www.eatrightpro.org/resources/research/evidence-based-resources/evidence-analysis-library. Accessed April 4, 2018.

52. Ferrie, S., Rand, S., & Palmer, S. (2013). Back to basics: Estimating protein requirements for adult hospitalized patients: A systematic review of randomized controlled trials. *Food and Nutrition Sciences, 4*:201–214. http://dx.doi.org/10.4236/fns.2013.42028. Accessed February 18, 2018.

53. Hydration Evidence-Analysis Project. (2007). Academy of Nutrition and Dietetics Evidence Analysis Library. Academy of Nutrition and Dietetics. Available at: http://www.andevidencelibrary.com. Accessed February 18, 2018.

OUR CASE STUDY OF PATIENT SB: GATHERING ANTHROPOMETRIC, BIOCHEMICAL, AND HISTORICAL DATA

The nutrition assessment of a patient begins with a thorough review of the medical record (MR). The RD collects pertinent data from all areas of the MR, including admission information, nursing notes and assessments, physician progress notes, assessments and orders, and biochemical and other test results. This information is then analyzed in subsequent steps of the assessment process and is used to determine the nutritional status of the patient. Nutrient needs are also calculated using predictive equations, or indirect calorimetry, if available.

Our Case Study of Patient SB					
Admission Sheet					
Name	**LOS**	**Age**	**Sex**	**Marital Status**	**Race/Ethnicity**
SB	2	68	M	Married	Arab
Primary Language	**Interpreter Needed**		**Next of Kin**		**Attending**
English	No		Wife		Wayne, K., MD

Our Case Study of Patient SB

Allergies	Chief Complaint	Admitting Diagnosis
Shellfish	RT leg and foot pain	RT Diabetic Foot Ulcer—Cellulitis

Patient History

Medical and Surgical History	Social History	Weight History		
T2DM GERD HTN Peripheral Neuropathy Foot ulcer x 1 yr	**Smoking Status**: Current smoker; 2 packs/day for 40 years **Alcohol Use**: 1 drink/day **Drug Use**: None **Residence**: Lives with wife	3 months ago	106.5 kg	
		1 year	106.5 kg	

Nursing Admission Assessment

Height	Weight	BMI	A&O	Glasgow	Braden
190.5 cm Pt Estimate	106.5 kg Standing scale	29.3	To person x 3 To place x 3	15	17

Skin Integrity	Malnutrition Universal Screening Tool	
RT foot ulcer s/p debridement and wound vac placement	Decrease in appetite or intake? (Yes = 1, No = 0)	0
	Weight loss >10 lb in 3 months? (Yes = 1, No = 0)	0
	BMI score (<18.5 = 2, 18.5–20.0 = 1, >20.0 = 0)	0
	Total Score (2 or more triggers dietitian consult)	0

Active Orders

Consults	Nursing

Our Case Study of Patient SB

CONSULT TO PHYSCIAN—*candidate for proximal amputation right foot* CONSULT TO PHYSCIAN—*diabetic foot ulcer* CONSULT TO PHYSCIAN— CONSULT DIETITIAN—*nutritional needs for wound healing and diabetic diet education* WOUND/OSTOMY/CONTINENCE NURSE—*wound vac left foot* PT EVAL/TREATMENT	ALTERNATIVE SPLINT AND/OR FOAM BOOTS WITH SCDs GLUCOSE, POINT OF CARE WOUND VAC ONGOING WOUND CARE MEASURE WEIGHT—*on admission*

Laboratory/Imaging	**Medications/Infusions**
CULTURE, BLOOD CULTURE, WOUND DEEP CULTURE, TISSUE COMPLETE BLOOD COUNT W DIFF COMPREHENSIVE METABOLIC PANEL	Carvedilol—*oral* Cefazolin—*intravenous* Heparin injection—*subcutaneous* Insulin lispro—*subcutaneous* Linagliptin—*oral* Lisinopril—*oral* Acetaminophen—*PRN* Simvastatin (Zocor)—*oral*

DIET: Diabetic 1600–1800

Physician H & P

History of Present Illness: Patient is a 68-year-old male who presents with chronic diabetic ulcer on his right foot that is worsening. Patient speaks English, is a current smoker. He denies fever, chills, chest pain, nausea, and vomiting.

Temp	BP	Heart Rate	Resp	SpO2	O2 (L/min)
36.4°C	139/85 mmHg	94	20	94%	RA

Review of Systems and Physical Exam

Constitutional	HEENT	Neck
Awake and alert; no distress	Normal	Normal
Pulmonary/Chest	**Cardiovascular**	**Gastrointestinal**
Clear to auscultation	Regular rate and rhythm	No masses felt; non-tender
Extremities	**Skin**	**Neurological**

Our Case Study of Patient SB

No edema	Diabetic ulcer to right foot	No focal motor deficits

Assessment	Plan
Diabetic foot ulcer Diabetes mellitus, type 2 Suspected lower extremity peripheral vascular disease	Wound care, and infectious disease consulted Ulcer debridement and wound vac placement Wound and blood cultures Continue antibiotics Dietitian consulted for wound healing recommendations and diabetic diet instruction

K. Wayne, MD

Flowsheets

Date	Hospital Day 1			Hospital Day 2		
Time	**0800**	**1200**	**1600**	**0800**	**1200**	
Meal Intake	100%	100%	100%	100%	100%	

Outputs

Urine Occurrences	1	2	1	1		
Stool Occurrences				1		
Negative Pressure Wound Therapy	Right foot, placed at 1 at 11:20					

Edema

RUE	None			None		
LUE	None			None		
RLE	None			None		
LLE	None			None		

Laboratory Results

	Ref. Range	Day 1 0845
WBC	3.5–10.1 bil/L	22.1 (H)
Sodium	135–145 mmol/L	136

Our Case Study of Patient SB		
Potassium	3.5–5.2 mmol/L	4.6
Glucose	60–99 mg/dL	208 (H)
BUN	8–22 mg/dL	29 (H)
Creatinine	0.60–1.40 mg/dL	1.19
GFR Non-African American	>59 mL/min/1.73m2	61
GFR African American	>59 mL/min/1.73m2	71
HbA1c	4.0-5.6%	7.5 (H)
Estimated Average Glucose		162
Glucose, Point of Care		
Day 1 1412	**Day 1 1738**	**Day 2 0712**
207 (H)	139 (H)	176 (H)

Problem Solving Matrix Assessment for SB Case Study

Step: Collection of data from the medical record and determining nutrient needs

1.0 Assessment

♦*Collect assessment data from*: Review of the medical record & patient interview

♦*Analyze collected data:* Use nutrition equations & standard lab parameters

Assessment Data Categories	*Collect Data* Fill-in the date collected from MR and interview	*Analyze Data* Calculate BMI, IBW, %UBW, %wt change, etc.; identify abnormal labs
Anthropometric	**Data collected**	**Analyze data (BMI, IBW, %UBW, %wt change, etc.)**
Weight/Height	Ht: 190.5cm (Pt estimate); Wt: 106.5 kg (actual)	
Biochemical Data, Medical Test, Procedures	**Data collected**	**Analyze data (identify any abnormal lab values)**

VPS: albumin, RBP, transferrin, prealbumin, TLC (moderated by inflammation/ stress)		
Lipids: TC, HDL, LDL, ratio, TG		
Dx/Disease-related (CVD, DM, GI, liver, renal)	Glu 208 (H); HbA1c-7.5% (H); Na 136; Cr 1.19; GFR-61	
Nutrition-Focused Physical Findings	**Data collected from NFPE and History & Physical (Review of Systems)**	**Analyze data (identify any physical findings that are outside the normal parameters)**
Physical appearance (muscle wasting, fat loss, edema, skin, hair, nails, etc.)		
Physical function (hand grip)		
Functional Problems (GI, etc.)	☐N ☐V ☐D ☐C Oral motor: ☐ Intact ☐ Dysphagia ☐ Difficulty chewing ☐ Other:	

History	**Data collected**
Food/Nutrition: Food intake, appetite, wt history, physical activity, cultural, religious, food allergy & intolerances, medications, supplements, food availability	
Client History: Medical; nutritionally relevant Dx	T2DM, HTN, GERD (uses OTC calcium CO3), peripheral neuropathy, foot ulcer x 1yr
Social History: Lives alone, support, occupation, income, education level, program participation	Positive for tobacco; denies ETOH, drug use; lives w/wife (wife cooks); owns bookstore
Determine/Estimate Nutrient Needs	**Estimated Nutrient Needs (Nutrition Prescription)**
Energy needs: Use range equation, Mifflin, Harris-Benedict, etc. (consider activity and stress or disease-specific factors)	2380 cal

Protein needs: Use facility intake standards (consider disease-specific needs)	93–112 g
Fluid needs: Use facility intake standards (consider disease-specific needs)	2380 ml

CHAPTER 3

Nutrition Assessment

DATA GATHERING FROM THE PATIENT USING COMMUNICATION AND INTERVIEWING SKILLS

Deanne K. Kelleher, MS, RDN

LEARNING OBJECTIVES

By the end of the chapter, the reader will be able to

- List the types of communication used in dietary interviews
- Discuss how communication impacts the relationship between the dietitian and patient
- Describe the difference between verbal and nonverbal communication
- Explain potential verbal and nonverbal communication distractors
- Summarize the communication skills necessary for completing a dietary interview
- Identify the key components in a dietary interview
- Compare and contrast various dietary intake methods

Communication is essential in establishing a trusting relationship with a patient from the first meeting during the assessment portion of the Nutrition Care Process. This is an active skill that requires both ears and eyes to monitor verbal and nonverbal communication (1). Dietitians must be aware of how they communicate, both verbally and nonverbally, in order to build rapport with the patient. DeNegri and colleagues report the following five outcomes are the result of effective communication in health care (2):

1. The patient discloses enough information about the illness to lead to an accurate diagnosis.
2. The provider, in consultation with the patient, selects a medically appropriate treatment acceptable to the patient.
3. The patient understands his/her condition and the prescribed treatment regimen.
4. The provider and client establish a positive rapport.
5. The patient and provider are both committed to fulfilling their responsibilities during treatment and follow-up care.

These outcomes support that a trusting relationship is key to obtaining the necessary information to complete a thorough assessment and progress to an accurate diagnosis and creation of a strong evidence-based intervention. In order to adequately prepare for patient interactions, such as the initial interview and the implementation of nutrition education, it is essential to have knowledge of communication models, verbal and nonverbal communication, and listening skills.

COMMUNICATION SKILLS

Communication Models

Strong communication skills are essential in the patient relationship and lead to an increase in patient satisfaction (3, 4). The more a dietitian understands how to communicate with patients, the more effective the nutrition care process becomes. Having a conversation in the health care setting is more complex than one would think at first glance. Communicating with a patient is like a game of chess. The dietitian makes a calculated move and watches for cues from the patient to determine whether it was the right move, and then anxiously awaits the patient's move while considering how her/his own next move will be impacted by the patient's move. This exchange continues while becoming more complex with each move. A number of communication models have been proposed to describe the components that influence communication between dietitian and patient.

Figure 3.1 depicts how each of the components interact and has been adapted from a variety of communication models to reflect the dietitian/patient communication chain (5-9). The dietitian is the sender of the message and is impacted by many things, including her own culture, communication skills, knowledge, attitudes, nutrition point of view, and credibility. The dietitian encodes the message with understandable wording and gestures. The message itself is the content of the interview or counseling session and needs to be clear and concise. The message then is decoded (interpreted) by the receiver. The patient is the receiver and needs to be the central focus of the entire process, as seen in the patient-centered approach (5). The patient as the receiver is influenced by his own knowledge, attitudes, and culture as the message is interpreted. Before the decoding can occur, the element of noise can potentially complicate and interfere with the message being delivered. Noise may come in many forms, including:

- Environmental noise: actual noise that is distracting to the interview
- Semantic noise, or the meaning of words. For example, when the dietitian mentions a "cup," she may mean that to be eight fluid ounces, where the patient may interpret a cup to mean their favorite cup at home, which actually holds 16 fluid ounces
- Cultural noise, either through word meaning or different value of nonverbal cues
- Psychological noise: patient/client fears

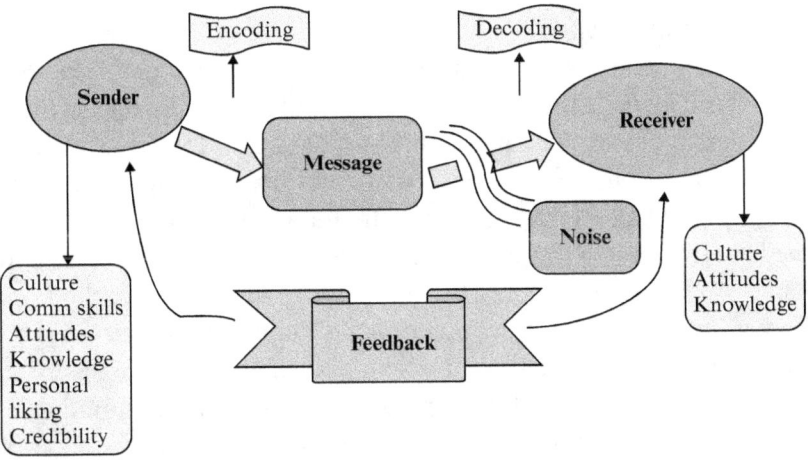

FIGURE 3.1 The Communication Chain

The communication cycle is not complete without feedback. Feedback can exist in the form of reflective listening and interpretation of nonverbal cues. The dietitian is the leader of the conversation, continually evaluating the feedback before proceeding further in the process.

Types of Communication

Communication is not only conveyed by spoken words, but also vocal tone and nonverbal cues. Communication experts may disagree on the exact breakdown between verbal and nonverbal communication and vocal tone, (10, 11) but what is clear is that the majority of communication is relayed nonverbally. Nonverbal cues help form judgments even before the first word is spoken. Dietitians need to be skilled in synchronizing their verbal and nonverbal communication when assessing patients and throughout the entire Nutrition Care Process. Bavelas and Chovil argue that these are intertwined in communication and cannot be separated in what they term the integrated message model (12). While nonverbal communication accounts for the majority of communication in an interaction, the words used are just as important, and if not chosen deliberately, a breakdown in the patient-clinician relationship can occur at the level of the message in the communication model.

Verbal Communication

Word choice matters when crafting a message for a patient. Research indicates that while the majority of the population reads at an eighth-grade reading level, 20% are at a fifth-grade level or lower (13). This is an important consideration not only for written materials but also for interviewing and counseling. If the dietitian is using complex words, medical terminology, and acronyms, the patient may not understand what is being said and may be too embarrassed to let the dietitian know that she does not understand. This could devastate the relationship from the beginning. For example, if the dietitian has been consulted to see a patient for hypertension, the dietitian should refer to hypertension as high blood pressure instead. The education level of a patient does not equate to health and nutrition literacy (14). The dietitian should go into the session with the assumption that the patient does not have nutrition or health knowledge (15). Even if a patient has a family member that appears to have medical/nutrition knowledge, the dietitian should still refrain from the use of jargon with the patient, who may not share the same level of knowledge in this area. To help bridge the gap and improve health literacy, the Centers for Disease Control and Prevention and the National Institutes of Health have created tools for health care providers on using plain language. This includes not only more complex medical terms but also other words to modify for improved understanding. For example, instead of asking a patient, *"What have you consumed over the last 24 hours?"* the dietitian should reframe the question to ask, *"What have you had to eat and drink over the last 24 hours?"* Plain language alternatives for common nutrition terms are outlined in Table 3.1.

TABLE 3.1 Plain Language for Common Nutrition Terminology (16, 17)

Term	Plain Language
Overconsume	Eat too much
Lipids	Fat
Cardiovascular	Heart
Adequate	Enough
Approximate	About
Benefit	Help
Demonstrate	Show
Minimize	Decrease
Portion	Part

In addition to word choice, is also important for the interviewer to use proper grammar to make the message clear. This is a professional interaction, and the dietitian needs to convey confidence to the patient to gain their respect as the expert in nutrition. Delivering clear, concise messages helps build the relationship between the patient and dietitian.

Vocal Tone

The dietitian's use of plain language and proper grammar in the interview is one aspect, but the tone in which the words are communicated is equally important. Vocal tone accounts for a portion of nonverbal communication according to Mehrabian (10), while others describe vocal tone as paralanguage (18, 19). There are four different vocal tone categories:

- Voice Quality refers to the pitch, rhythm, loudness, accent and tone of the voice (19, 20).
- Vocal Characteristics, such as laughing, yawning, whispering, groaning, or coughing, can disrupt the flow of the conversation.
- Vocal Segregates can inhibit the conversation and include the use of *um*, *uh*, *ah*, and silent pauses.
- Voice Qualifiers place emphasis on different words and include intensity (overloud or over-soft), pitch height, and extent.

If the tone of the message is not clear, the receiver may interpret the sender as not being interested or sincere. The tone used needs to match the words being said, or this also contributes to a potential disconnect. If a dietitian uses an excited and animated tone when talking about a patient's serious health condition, they may be confused and question the authenticity of the dietitian during a stressful time in their life.

Nonverbal Communication

There are many ways we speak with others without using words. Tone, or paralanguage, is just one example of nonverbal communication. Kinesics and proxemics represent other nonverbal cues. Kinesics includes movements like hand gestures, facial expression, and eye contact. Proxemics includes awareness of spatial relationships, touching, and posture. Wertheim proposes five roles that nonverbal cues take on during the counseling session: repetition, contradiction, substitution, complementing, and accenting (21). These roles illustrate the robust *impact nonverbals have on the session. It is important to remember that nonverbal communications are not universal and that culture defines the norms. The dietitian needs to be educated and aware of how culture impacts nonverbal cues. Direct eye contact is a sign of respect and understanding in the United States, but direct eye contact in East Asian countries is a sign of aggression (22).

Kinesics

Birdwhistell first defined kinesics and its impact on communication (11). Kinesics encompasses how the body expresses itself through the eyes, facial expressions, and arm and body movements. The dietitian is cognizant of her own kinesics while monitoring those of the patient during the interview. Eyes can convey interest, aggression, displeasure, and understanding of the conversation. The dietitian maintains eye contact with a client with regular breaks to create comfort and trust, unless the patient's culture or condition does not allow that. Culture alone does not define differences in eye contact. Individuals on the autism spectrum may not be comfortable with eye contact during a conversation, so the dietitian needs to keep this in mind when evaluating the patient's nonverbal signals (23).

Even without words, mood is conveyed on the face by more than just eyes. A neutral facial expression keeps the conversation moving forward while making the patient feel comfortable. The dietitian should maintain a slight smile to be welcoming but not too big where it is not perceived as genuine. Awareness of how one's face appears at rest helps to unknowingly violate kinesics. Is the mouth neutral, slightly turned up, or slightly turned down to appear to be frowning? An interviewer with a normally downturned mouth should be conscious of this and be mindful to keep a slight smile at all times. A simple head nod shows interest and engagement in the conversation; however, overuse of the head nod is a distractor. Communication also happens when the eyebrows are raised or the eyes are widened. These cues can communicate shock and surprise and thus may confuse the sender or receiver. Equally important is the dietitian's monitoring of the facial expressions of the patient and addressing emotions displayed with reflective listening.

Hand gestures are used to emphasize a point. Sometimes a simple gesture like hand or foot tapping can derail the communication since it is relaying boredom or wanting the other person to speak faster. The folding of arms across the body shows disinterest and impatience.

Pointing as a gesture should be avoided, as it can make another person feel uncomfortable or be misinterpreted, depending on culture. While the interviewer takes notes during the interview, she should be careful not to twirl or tap the writing utensil, as that also is a sign of disinterest.

Proxemics

Proxemics differs from kinesics since it primarily involves spatial relations. This space can be physical, environmental, or cultural. The physical distance between the dietitian and patient can make a difference in the comfort for the interview. Hall defined space as intimate (0–18 inches), personal (1.5 to 5 feet), and social (5 to 7 feet) (24). The dietitian should respect a patient's intimate space and stay within the personal space zone. Distance can increase comfort while not having distracting objects exist between the sender and receiver. For example, avoiding large tables or desks between the patient and interviewer can aid in the communication exchange. Standing over a patient in a clinical setting instead of getting down to the patient's level can be perceived as a power position and can lead to a decrease in patient openness and willingness to participate in the encounter. The posture of the interviewer is also important, with the goal to lean forward without slouching. Touch, or invasion of the intimate space, during a patient interview would not be appropriate unless in situations to demonstrate empathy with the permission of the patient. The dietitian needs to be mindful of her/his own proxemics.

The verbal message being relayed by the interviewer must be synchronized with the nonverbal message. When they are not in line with each other, the sending of mixed messages can be the result. When the verbal message is one of concern and the nonverbal cues are overly pleasant, the receiver may not understand what the intended message should be. The mismatch of cues may be a sign of anxiety or discomfort. Another example of this disconnect is when a patient tells the dietitian he has had no problems following the gluten-free diet for their celiac disease, while looking around the room and picking his/her fingernails. The dietitian may sense that there are problems with the patient following the gluten-free diet and that they will have to investigate further with proper interview techniques to be discussed later in this chapter.

LISTENING SKILLS

Listening can be defined as a passive skill of hearing what the sender is saying. Listening for an effective interview requires the process of active listening. Active listening is not only hearing the message but showing interest with nonverbal cues. Reflective listening is a form of active listening that should be employed during the diet interview. With reflective listening, the dietitian is paraphrasing what the patient said to make sure they heard them correctly. Neglecting reflective listening is what leads to incorrect assumptions.

Reflective listening also requires showing empathy to the patient. Empathy is defined by Merriam-Webster as "the action of understanding, being aware of, being sensitive to, and vicariously experiencing the feelings, thoughts, and experience of another of either the past or present without having the feelings, thoughts, and experience fully communicated in an objectively explicit manner" (25). Empathy can be exhibited during the interview with secondary questions, a simple nonverbal cue like a head nod, or a touch to the shoulder or arm (26).

Showing empathy is not telling the person that "I know exactly how you feel," since each person experiences life based on their own values and beliefs, and no two situations are exactly the same. The process of listening also involves the use of silence to process what is being asked or said. The dietitian does not need to feel that she has to be talking at all times. Allow the patient to think about responses, and do not lead or rescue them when there is silence. This demonstrates that you are truly interested and listening to what they have to add.

THE PATIENT INTERVIEW

A strong understanding of the nuances of communication is essential to complete a thorough interview that leads to the patient trusting the dietitian. The purpose of the interview is very pointed in that the dietitian is gathering the necessary information in order to accurately assess, diagnose, and intervene. This is not intended to be a casual conversation. The interview may be exclusively with the patient or include significant others/caregivers, depending on the situation. The setting of the interview may also vary between a private office, a clinic exam room, a hospital room, and others. Each setting offers different challenges that the dietitian needs to be aware of, such as privacy. The structure of the patient interview includes the preparation, greeting, information gathering, then closing and next steps.

Interview Preparation

Chapter 2 illustrated how to gather the necessary data from the medical record. For the interview, the dietitian should thoroughly review the patient's medical information and start to piece together the patient story. After analyzing the data, the dietitian must identify gaps to build the interview questions, in addition to verifying information in the patient's own words. The questions will help identify various pieces of information, including

- the patient's overall knowledge of reason for the consult; was it patient initiated, health care team initiated, or identified via a screening tool?
- eating patterns
- relationship with food
- health habits
- food security
- dietary supplement use
- dietary intake and past dieting
- medication adherence, and
- overall motivation.

It is crucial to be aware of one's own bias about weight, food, and nutrition in order to be nonjudgmental. The dietitian should consider the patient's ability to communicate and provide an accurate history. A surrogate source of information is suggested to be present for children and patients with cognitive deficits, such as head injuries, dementia, cognitive impairment, and some brain tumors. The dietitian can also find information on a patient's cognition prior to the interview via medical record notes or reviewing the neurological examination results of the patient physical. The neurological examination will include "alert and oriented" information by a numerical value of 0 to 4. A patient who is neurologically intact will be stated to be "alert and oriented times four," which refers to person, place, time, and situation. Regardless of whether the patient can provide additional information, the dietitian should always visually assess the patient via the nutrition-focused physical examination (NFPE). The better prepared the dietitian is, the less anxiety there is for the encounter (27).

Setting the Stage

Maintaining confidentiality throughout the interview is essential to build trust and rapport. This starts with the location of the interview, which may be a private office with a door, or a health care facility with multiple patients in the same room. In the latter, the closing of the curtain between patients is often done but does not provide complete privacy, so the patient may be less open to share information. Another protection of privacy involves including the support people that accompany the patient or are in a patient room. The dietitian needs to demonstrate respect by asking who is attending the interview with the patient. These individuals can aid in the dietitian's understanding of who is supporting—or may be deterring—the patient. The patient should approve of having others present during the interview before moving forward. The next step is to make sure the patient is comfortable. Temperature and seating arrangements are key for patient comfort. Allowing the patient to choose his seat in the interview will increase the comfort level. Additionally, eliminating any physical barriers between the patient and dietitian will help to create an ideal environment for open discussion.

The interview encounter begins with a handshake and greeting. The handshake allows the dietitian to judge grip strength, nail quality, and skin integrity, which aids in the NFPE in the clinical setting. A warm greeting sets the tone of the interview. As the dietitian greets the patient, she should ask if the patient prefers to be called by title and surname (e.g., Mrs. Smith) or by their first name. The dietitian should introduce herself and explain her role on the health care team. During all interactions, nonverbal cues should be actively monitored to judge the patient's comfort level. Once the greeting is complete, a brief discussion can take place to break the ice and put the patient at ease, but the dietitian should maintain control of the conversation so that the introductory conversations do not take up excessive time (27).

Throughout the interview, body positioning and cues are important for the clinician. The use of the acronym **SOLER** is a way to remember how to keep the patient engaged:

- **S**itting squarely.
- Having an **O**pen posture.
- **L**eaning toward the client.
- Maintaining good **E**ye contact.
- Being **R**elaxed in their presence (28).

After the greeting portion, the dietitian should determine exactly what the patient wants to accomplish from the visit. Since the visit may have been requested by a physician via a consult, or the patient is being seen as part of the facility's standards of care instead of being patient-initiated, it is important to establish the reason for the visit. Next, the dietitian states the visit expectations and time frame. The patient should be asked to verify that he has the required amount of time available for the visit. If he does not, the visit can be rescheduled or broken into two sessions. The guidelines of the visit should also be reviewed with the patient; for example, asking them to turn off the television to limit the distraction or to turn off their cell phone, but also respecting if it needs to be left on for an emergency. The interview then moves on to the questions to complete the assessment.

Questions

The objective of the interview is to help the patient to open up and talk about his health and nutrition habits. In order to facilitate conversation, **open-ended questions** should be used; the dietitian should avoid **closed-ended questions**. An example of an open-ended question is, "*What was the first thing you had to eat or drink after waking up?*" instead of the closed-ended question, "*Did you eat or drink anything after waking up?*" A series of open-ended questions helps move the conversation along and prompts the dietitian to ask more probing questions. At times the dietitian will use closed-ended questions to verify information such as, "*Do you take any vitamin or mineral supplements?*" following up with the open-ended question, "*Tell me about the supplements you take.*"

Leading questions can derail the trust and rapport between patient and dietitian. These are questions that prompt or encourage a specific answer and may cause patients to feel pressure to answer the question with what they think they should say rather than a truthful response. Some examples of leading questions are, "*What did you eat for breakfast?*" and "*How much water did you drink today?*" The message the patient receives is that the dietitian expects them to eat breakfast and drink water, so even if they didn't, they may include this information. While those question examples are open-ended, they potentially make the client feel the dietitian is not open to hearing about their own nutrition habits.

There are multiple types of questions the dietitian can utilize to obtain the most information possible from the patient. Starting with a **primary question** leads to additional **probing questions**, referred to as **secondary questions**. After asking the patient about a meal (the primary question), the dietitian needs to follow up with probing/secondary questions to obtain the further details. For example, if a patient reports eating chicken at lunch, the secondary questions would include probing about:

- the type of chicken (breast, leg, thigh, wing)
- the presence of skin on the chicken
- the preparation method (frying, pan-frying, baking, boiling, broiling, etc.)
- use of oil and seasoning in cooking and prior to eating
- portion size.

Accurate dietary assessment relies on a thorough use of primary and probing/secondary questions.

The initial interview also includes questions that help assess a patient's nutrition knowledge and behaviors. These are distinct questions that can delineate what a patient knows (knowledge) and what they practice (behavior). The dietitian may ask a patient who is on dialysis, "*What foods are high in potassium?*" to assess the patient's overall knowledge about potassium-containing foods, but should also ask, "*Which foods do you eat that contain potassium?*" to get at patient behavior regarding potassium intake. If a patient indicates a habit that may contradict their medical condition, the interviewer may be tempted to ask why that habit exists. This is not done to scold the patient but to understand their reasoning as to why they decided to do so. The use of **"why" questions** is not recommended, as it can make the patient feel defensive and can affect the relationship the dietitian is attempting to build. Instead of asking a patient "why," the question should be rephrased to ask "what" led to that behavior.

Diet Interview

Once the stage has been set for the interview with the expectations and goals clearly communicated, and the patient made as comfortable as possible, it is now time to move to the body of the full diet interview. This portion focuses on the dietary aspects of the food and nutrition history component of nutrition assessment, and it includes the patient's nutrition behaviors, dietary intake influencers, and actual intake. The diet history allows a detailed insight into a person's diet over a longer period of time, as it not only examines recent intake but previous intake and habits. Missing an area of the history leaves the dietitian unable to make an appropriate assessment of dietary habits.

The food and nutrition history provides the dietitian with details of what the patient has done in the past, his knowledge, and success/failure with making dietary changes. These questions should include past history of following any special diets, including allergen elimination, weight loss, self-prescribed, fad or athletic performance, or those relating to a chronic health condition. Secondary questions should be included to determine:

- who recommended the diet
- how the patient received/obtained information on the diet—written information provided versus Internet searches
- how long the patient has/had followed the diet
- if the patient met with a dietitian regarding this diet in the past
- if the diet is working for the patient or if it worked in the past
- if the patient stopped following the diet, what was the reason

For patients who have altered their dietary intake in the past, the dietitian can elicit information on their motivation and ability to incorporate changes into their lifestyle. This will also help determine potential roadblocks to the patient following current or future nutrition recommendations. These roadblocks could arise in the form of lack of support systems, financial reasons, or overall stress levels. Other habit history questions may include weight (gain and loss) and growth history, appetite history, physical activity habits, drug and alcohol intake, smoking history, medication history and compliance, and past medical history. The dietitian may include other questions depending on the specific reason for the visit, such as asking the patient about their calcium/vitamin D intake when being seen for osteoporosis prevention or treatment.

Food and health behavior questions are designed to obtain information on the patterns of eating and any habits that may alter total intake. These questions should focus on:

- Meal patterns (number daily, timing, skipping, usual meal sizes)
- Meal location (in front of TV or other media, at a table, with others, at a desk, on the run)
- Food likes/dislikes
- Food allergies/intolerances
- Oral health (dentures—do they fit, tooth decay)
- Chewing and swallowing disorders
- Social activities with food (religious activities, clubs, sporting activities, parties)
- Shopping (who does the shopping, who has a say in food brought into the home, stores, farmers' markets)
- Cooking (skills, available equipment, ingredient availability—staples)
- Physical condition (ability to move around living space, open jars/cans, feed self)
- Housing arrangement (refrigeration, use of stove/oven/hot plate/microwave)
- Transportation (easy access to stores, walk versus drive versus public transportation)

- Food security (do they receive any public assistance programs—SNAP, WIC, free/reduced school meals, etc., do they run out of food at the end of the month, use emergency food sources, skip meals because of lack of food)
- Eating out (fast food, cafeteria, fast-casual, sit-down)
- Food rules (must clean the plate, food can't touch, food is comfort)
- Snacking
- Sleep habits (hours of sleep, eating/drinking in middle of night, food at bedside)
- Work schedule (part time, full time, day/night shift, break/lunch break)
- Religious/cultural practices (fasting, feasting, food avoidance)
- Support systems (friends, family)
- Literacy (reading level, preferred language for written materials)
- Attitudes and belief about health (they have control over their habits, health happens to them and they cannot control medical conditions)
- Bingeing/purging
- Laxative use, diet aids
- Dietary supplements (type, frequency, recommended by)
- Appetite and absorption inhibitors (occurrence and frequency of nausea, vomiting, diarrhea, constipation)

The dietitian can provide the patient with a diet history questionnaire to complete in advance of the visit to save time. To help create a personalized plan and demonstrate interest in the answers and time it took to complete, the dietitian reviews the questionnaire and verifies answers by asking secondary questions based on the responses. Each of these question areas adds to the overall story of the patient's relationship with food and will help the dietitian choose the most appropriate counseling strategy and intervention.

Diet History

There are a number of ways a dietitian can assess a patient's diet. The decision on which tool to use depends upon the purpose and information needed. The dietitian has a number of dietary assessment tools available, including a 24-hour recall, typical daily intake, food record, food frequency questionnaire, and diet screener. Each of the tools will be reviewed, and the dietitian will determine how they can be used in the patient interview.

24-Hour Recall

The first method in a patient interview is the 24-hour recall. This provides a snapshot of intake but may not represent the usual pattern for the patient. This form of assessment can be analyzed in a variety of ways, such as macro and micronutrient intake, comparison with DRI, MyPlate servings, or diet quality using the Healthy Eating Index (www.cnpp.usda.gov/healthyeatingindex). The assessment is chosen based on goals of the interview. This method places a heavy burden on the interviewer and the patient. The 24-hour recall will be advantageous for those with lower literacy but difficult for those with memory issues (29).

The art of conducting a successful 24-recall is a skill every dietitian should have in their toolbox. The USDA Multiple Pass Method is a standardized way to administer a 24-hour recall. While this method is typically used in large population studies, it is a convenient way to learn the workings of the 24-hour recall tool. The steps for this method are outlined in Box 3.1.

BOX 3.1

USDA Multiple Pass Approach (30)

1 Quick list (a list of all foods and beverages consumed over the last 24 hours)

2 Forgotten foods (items missed, such as snacks, condiments, sweets, beverages)

3 Time and occasion (time consumed and what the patient calls the meal/snack)

4 Details (preparation methods, brands, portions, and review)

5 Final probe (walk the patient through the day for anything missed)

The dietitian may not have adequate time to complete this approach by following each individual step, so they can be merged particularly for the clinical setting. The patient should not be interrupted during the development of the quick list in order to keep the flow of communication and improve memory recall. The 24-hour recall usually covers the time span of midnight to midnight but can be modified from waking up to 24 hours later. A full explanation of the procedure is recommended prior to starting. For example, "Let's talk about what you had to eat or drink over the last 24 hours. First, I will ask you what you ate and drank from when you woke up yesterday to 24 hours after that time. After that, I will ask you details about these foods and beverages. What was the first thing you had to eat or drink after waking up?" This is the time when open-ended questions should be used. Probing/secondary questions are often used for food and beverage details.

The accuracy of the recall is enhanced with the use of portion estimation tools. The setting of the interview will guide what type of interview tools can be used. The dietitian can use 3-D food models, 2-D food models, common items (baseball or fist for one cup, tennis ball or handful for a half cup, deck of cards or a woman's palm for three ounces of protein), and household measurements (plates, bowls, cups, measuring cups) to assist in determining the portion the patient consumed. Sometimes patients may feel compelled to believe that they should be eating the portion on the food models. The dietitian prefaces this by asking how much of the portion they consumed. Review of foods and beverages includes questions about foods that often go together but avoiding the use of leading questions. Instead of asking *"Did you have ketchup with the French fries?"* rephrase the question to *"What did you add to the French fries?"* This will allow the patient to disclose if they used cheese or sour cream with the fries instead of ketchup. The use of nonverbal cues that do not reflect emotion (e.g., "poker face") is vital for a reduced bias recall. The patient will be seeking approval or disapproval from the dietitian during the process, so it is important to remain neutral so as to not influence further information.

Typical Daily Intake: The typical daily intake (TDI) method is a modification of the 24-hour recall. This approach is very helpful in a clinical setting, since the previous 24 hours may not be an accurate reflection of the patient's usual intake due to their hospitalization. The procedures to complete a TDI are the same as a 24-hour recall, simply replacing the terminology/time frame of "the last 24 hours" with "what you typically eat on a daily basis." The dietitian can then determine how many days per week the patient eats in a specific manner and how it differs on other days.

Food Record

A food record is the result of documenting all food/drink a patient has consumed over a period of time. The log may be written or aided by the use of technology, such as using a computer program (like Supertracker) or an app (like MyFitness Pal) to keep track of food and beverages. A three-day food record is considered the gold standard in full dietary assessments, and includes two weekdays and one weekend day (31). The patient should be instructed how to complete the log, including the time food/beverages were consumed, food/beverage, brand, form, preparation, portion, where consumed, and overall feelings while eating (if desired). This assessment method shifts the burden from the dietitian to the patient. Food records are better for those with memory issues, as they can write down their intake at the time of the meal occasion. These records can help the dietitian visualize the patient's eating pattern and validate the diet history and/or food frequency questionnaire. Food records do require literacy, and the reported intake may not be their usual, since they are writing it down. People are known to alter their habits because of that alone (29).

Food Frequency Questionnaire

Food frequency questionnaires (FFQs) collect food and beverage intake over a period of time and can include lists of food with or without portions consumed. For tools that include portions, the patient will need to have a portion estimation tool to use in determining actual portion size. The data obtained from the FFQ provides an average intake over time and not exact amounts of macro/micronutrients. There are validated FFQ tools available that are used in large studies, such as the Gladys Block FFQ and the Willet FFQ, which contain 60–100+ food items. These may not be practical to complete in a dietary interview, so shortened versions may be helpful. The dietitian will need to determine, based on the client's needs, what foods to focus on in the FFQ if a shortened version is created. FFQs have advantages like being relatively quick to complete and review, and can also be provided to the patient prior to the visit. On the other hand, FFQs do require literacy, are not typically specific to cultural food patterns, and may lead to over- and underestimation of foods eaten (29).

Diet Screener

Diet screeners are another quick and reliable way to assess patient compliance to prescribed diets. One common diet screener is the **MEDFICTS** for patients with cardiovascular disease that have been prescribed the Therapeutic Lifestyle Changes (TLC) diet. This two-page tool reviews the intake of *M*eats, *E*ggs, *D*airy, *F*ried foods, fat *I*n baked goods, *C*onvenience foods, fats added at the *T*able, and *S*nacks (32). The patient will complete this form, which includes how often he eats the food and the portion. The dietitian then scores the tool, which will provide confirmation of compliance or noncompliance to the diet. The benefit of diet screeners in a clinical setting is that with a new diagnosis, the results will highlight areas of focus for the patient. For those patients following the TLC diet prior to the appointment, the results will give the dietitian a measure of compliance that could lead to further questions about what is working or not working for the patient.

Interview Reflection

The diet interview may be the end point of the interaction between the dietitian and patient in a clinical setting where the dietitian creates an intervention that may be implemented by another member of the medical team. The interview may also be the midpoint of the inter-action, like in an outpatient visit, when the dietitian moves from the interview into a counseling session. Throughout the entire interaction the dietitian demonstrates active listening to ensure the message being heard by the clinician is actually what the patient is conveying. To end the interview, the dietitian summarizes the information learned and asks the patient if there is anything else they wish to share regarding their health habits. This allows the patient an opportunity to add information he feels is pertinent that may not have been conveyed during the interview. To end the interview, the dietitian will provide the next steps to the patient, which may be scheduling a subsequent visit for counseling and education, or, if time permits, moving directly into the counseling portion and allowing time for questions. The trust and rapport built by the dietitian via verbal and nonverbal communication skills will help establish the strong relationship that is needed for continued work together for the patient to improve his health through nutrition.

RESEARCH UPDATE

An emerging dietary assessment method is the use of food pictures to increase the validity of dietary intakes. This opens up potential for telehealth in dietetics. Two studies have used this technology with different populations, both with positive results. A 2015 study by Ptomey and colleagues demonstrated three-day food records using mobile phones to take pictures of foods and beverages in adolescents with intellectual and developmental disabilities were more accurate than the traditional proxy-assisted food logs. Kato et al. were able to validate the use of photos taken with smartphones to estimations by dietitians. This method supports the use of technology for their type 2 diabetes self-management program.

Ptomey, L. T., Willis, E. A., Goetz, J. R., Lee, J., Sullivan, D. K., & Donnelly, J. E. (2015). Digital photography improves estimates of dietary intake in adolescents with intellectual and developmental disabilities. *Disabil Health J, 8*(1): 146–150. doi:10.1016/j.dhjo.2014.08.011

Kato, S., Waki, K., Nakamura, S., Osada, S., Kobayashi, H., Fujita, H., et al. (2016). Validating the use of phones to measure dietary intake: The method used by DialBetics, a smartphone-based self-management system for diabetes patients. *Diabetology International, 7*(3): 244–251.

To Sum It Up

- The dietitian's communication skills impact patient satisfaction.
- Communication is a complex system that risks breakdown if not attended to with care.

- Communication includes verbal, tone, and nonverbal components.
- Nonverbal communication accounts for the majority of communication.
- Reflective listening should be used to reduce confusion and bias.
- The dietitian directs the flow of the diet interview, starting with preparation.
- Diet interviews include information gathering about:
  o food/nutrition history
  o nutrition behaviors
  o dietary intake influencers
  o actual intake
- Dietary assessment techniques vary based on information needed for the patient and include:
  o 24-hour recall
  o Typical Daily Intake
  o Food Record
  o Food Frequency Questionnaire
  o Diet Screener
- Dietitians need to be aware of their verbal and nonverbal communication when interacting with patients.

Put It into Practice: Interviewing and Interpersonal Skills Evaluation

You can practice your verbal and nonverbal communication and interviewing skills with this exercise. Get a friend, family member, or classmate to act as your "patient" and another to act as the evaluator. Interview the patient to collect the suggested data below. Use the interviewing skills described in this chapter and as listed below in the evaluation form. Have the evaluator observe your interview and watch for the skills listed and evaluate your performance.

For this exercise, assume the patient has recently been diagnosed with type 2 diabetes, and you are conducting an initial interview to gather some data. Use the techniques described in this chapter to obtain some or all of the following information:

Data Gathering
Appetite; now and prior to admission
GI status (chewing/swallowing, nausea/vomiting, diarrhea/constipation)
Relevant social info (lifestyle related to living arrangements, food shopping and preparation, dining out, etc.)
Physical activity level/handicaps
Height
Weight; usual body weight, recent weight changes
Diet; usual diet at home; previous diets, total intake, food frequency, food intolerances, previous diet instruction
Interest in counseling/diet instruction:

Directions: Use an "X" to indicate satisfactory achievement;
Use an "O" to indicate an area needing improvement

Nonverbal Communication	Name:	Name:	Name:
Kinesics:			
Body positioning (faces speaker, attentive)			
Eye contact			
Continuing responses (appropriate head nods)			
Hand gestures, smiles			
Paralanguage:			
Vocal quality: rate, pitch, volume, tone			
Vocal characterizers: disrupting flow with yawning, whispering, laughing, etc.			
Vocal segregates: use of *um*, *uh*, *ah*, etc.			
Vocal qualifiers: intensity, pitch height			

Nonverbal Communication	Name:	Name:	Name:
Proxemics:			
Slight forward lean			
Physical distance (not too distant or too close to speaker)			
Verbal Communication			
Asking questions (open-ended)			
Probing (following speaker's communication)			
Continuing responses (reflecting, summarizing)			
Listening skills (versus talking, use of silent pauses)			
Does not interrupt patient			
Rapport			
Affective Demeanor (friendly, warm, encouraging)			
Introduction; ID patient, self, purpose			
Closing; follow-up, thank you			
Evaluation: Rate 1 to 5; 5 is highest			
Nonverbal Communication Good eye contact; body positioning Provided continuing responses (nods)			
Verbal Communication Majority of questions are open-ended Provided continuing responses			
Rapport Introduction/established rapport via speech; nonverbals; warmth, empathy			
Overall Interviewing Skills			

Self-Evaluation: Rate 1 to 5; 5 is highest	Rating	Areas to Strengthen
Nonverbal Communication		
Verbal Communication		
Rapport		
Overall Interviewing Skills		

Check for Understanding

1. The dietitian asks a patient how many cups of noodles he ate at lunch. The patient is confused, since they eat noodles in a bowl and not a plate. This is an example of:

   a. Feedback

   b. Proxemics

   c. Noise

   d. Diet history

2. If a patient has a doctorate degree, the dietitian should assume that she can use medical terminology during the interview.

   a. True

   b. False

3. Culture impacts which of the following:

   a. The sender

   b. Noise

   c. Nonverbal Cues

   d. All of the above

4. The gold standard for dietary intake assessments includes:

   a. Two consecutive 24-hour recalls

   b. Diet Screener

   c. Three-Day Food Record

   d. Modified Food Frequency Questionnaire

5. A dietitian is taking a diet recall with a hospitalized patient. They client says they usually eat one cup of mashed potatoes. The dietitian does not have any food models handy, so they could verify the portion by:

   a. Assuming they mean a coffee cup at the bedside

   b. No need to verify the portion as the client seems educated on portions

   c. Looking at a picture in a magazine

   d. Showing a woman's fist and asking how much more or less

Answers in Appendix B

References

1. Brammer, L. M. (1985). *The helping relationship: Process and skills.* Englewood Cliffs, NJ: Prentice-Hall.

2. De Negri, B., DiPrete Brown, L., Hernandez, O., Rosenbaum, J., & Roter, D. Improving Interpersonal Communication Between Health Care Providers and Clients. USAID, Quality Assurance Project. http://pdf.usaid.gov/pdf_docs/Pnace294.pdf. Accessed August 3, 2017.

3. Cant, R. P., & Aroni, R. A. (October 2008). Exploring dietitians' verbal and nonverbal communication skills for effective dietitian-patient communication. *J Hum Nutr Diet, 21*(5): 502–511. doi:10.1111/j.1365-277X.2008.00883.x

4. Hancock, R. E., Bonner, G, Hollingdale, R., & Madden, A. M. (June 2012). "If you listen to me properly, I feel good": A qualitative examination of patient experiences of dietetic consultations. *J Hum Nutr Diet, 25*(3): 275–284. doi:10.1111/j.1365-277X.2012.01244.x

5. Agarwal, O. P. (2009; 2010). *Effective communication-I.* Mumbai, India: Himalaya Publishing House.

6. Shannon, C. E., & Weaver, W. (1949). *The mathematical theory of communication.* Urbana: University of Illinois Press.

7. Berlo, D. K. (1960). *The process of communication: An introduction to theory and practice.* New York, NY: Holt, Rinehart and Winston.

8. Barnlund, D. (2008). A transactional model of communication. In C. D. Mortensen (Ed.), *Communication theory,* 2nd ed. Reference & Research Book News. Portland, OR: Ringgold, Inc.

9. DeFleur, M. L., Kearney, P., & Plax, T. G. (1993). *Mastering communication in contemporary America.* Mountain View, CA; Mayfield.

10. Mehrabian, A., & Ferris, S. R. (1967). Inference of attitudes from nonverbal communication in two channels. *J of Consulting Psychology, 31*: 248–252.

11. Birdwhistell, R. L. (1970; 1971). *Kinesics and context: Essays on body motion communication,* Vol. 2. Philadelphia: University of Pennsylvania Press.

12. Bavelas, J. B., & Chovil, N. (2002). Visible acts of meaning: An integrated message model of language in face-to-face dialogue. *J of Language and Social Psychology, 19*:163–194.

13. Safeer, R. S., & Keenan, J. (2005). Health literacy: The gap between physicians and patients. *Am Fam Physician, 72*(3): 463–468.

14. America's Health Literacy: Why We need Accessible Health Information. Office of Disease Prevention and Health Promotion. https://health.gov/communication/literacy/issuebrief/. Accessed on August 10, 2017.

15. Health Literate Care Model. Office of Disease Prevention and Health Promotion. https://health.gov/communication/interactiveHLCM/. Accessed August 10, 2017.

16. Best Practices for Creating Nutrition Education Materials. US Department of Agriculture. https://www.choosemyplate.gov/best-practices-creating-nutrition-education-materials. Accessed August 14, 2017.

17. Simple words and phrases. Improving Communication from the Federal Government to the Public. http://www.plainlanguage.gov/howto/wordsuggestions/simplewords.cfm. Accessed August 12, 2017.

18. Snetselaar, L. G. (2009). *Nutrition counseling skills for the nutrition care process*, 4th ed. Sudbury, MA: Jones and Bartlett.

19. Curry, K., & Jaffe, A., MS, RD, LD. (1998). *Nutrition counseling & communication skills*. Philadelphia, PA: W. B. Saunders.

20. Poyatos, F. (2002). *Nonverbal communication across disciplines, Vol. 2: Paralanguage, kinesics, silence, personal and environmental interaction*. Amsterdam, Netherlands: John Benjamins.

21. Wertheim, EG. The Importance of Effective Communication. Retrieved from https://www.helpguide.org/articles/relationships-communication/nonverbal-communication.htm#how on August 12, 2017.

22. Akechi, H., Senju, A., Uibo, H., Kikuchi, Y., Hasegawa, T., & Hietanen, J. K. (2013). Attention to eye contact in the West and East: Autonomic responses and evaluative ratings. *PLOS one, 8*: e59312.

23. Hadjikhani, N., Asberg Johnels, J., Zurcher, N. R., Lassalle, A., Guillon, Q., Hippolyte, L., et al. (2017). Look me in the eyes: Constraining gaze in the eye-region provokes abnormally high subcortical activation in autism. *Scientific Reports, 7*: 3163. doi:10.1038/s41598-017-03378-5

24. Hall, E. T. (1966). *The hidden dimension*, 1st ed. Garden City, NY: Doubleday.

25. Merriam-Webster Dictionary. https://www.merriam-webster.com/dictionary/empathy. Accessed September 3, 2017.

26. Berger, B. A. (2009). *Communication skills for pharmacists*, 3rd ed. Washington, DC: American Pharmacists Association.

27. Gable, J., & Herrmann, T. (2015; 2016). *Counselling skills for dietitians*, 3rd ed. UK: Wiley-Blackwell.

28. Egan, G. (2007). *The skilled helper: A problem-management and opportunity development approach to helping*, 8th ed. Pacific Grove, CA: Brookes Cole.

29. Lee, R. D., & Nieman, D. C. (2013). *Nutritional assessment*, 6th ed. New York, NY: McGraw-Hill.

30. Raper, N., Perloff, B., Ingwersen, L., Steinfeldt, L., & Anand, J. (2004). An overview of USDA's dietary intake system. *J Food Compos Anal, 17*(3–4): 545–555.

31. Boyle, M. A. (2017). *Community nutrition in action: An entrepreneurial approach.* Boston, MA: Cengage Learning.

32. Kris-Etherton, P., Eissenstat, B., Jaaz, S., Srinath, U., Scott, L., Rader, J., et al. (2001). Validation for MEDFICTS, a dietary assessment instrument for evaluation adherence to total and saturated fat recommendations of the National Cholesterol Education Program Step 1 and Step 2 diets. *J Am Diet Assoc, 101*(1): 81–86.

OUR CASE STUDY OF PATIENT SB: COMMUNICATION SKILLS

The importance of good communication skills in patient interviewing becomes evident in the accuracy and amount of information the RD is able to obtain from the patient. After collecting data from the medical record (chapter 2), the RD can prepare for interviewing the patient. In addition to the typical questions, information from the medical record will enable the RD to ask questions specific to the patient to be interviewed. Although most in-patient dietitians do not collect specific dietary information, when it is fairly clear that a diet instruction will be needed, it is important to obtain specific information on the patient's typical intake. In addition, it is important to become skilled in collecting dietary intake information, as it will be critical in other venues.

Dietitian Interview and Physical

Your patient speaks English and his wife is at bedside.

Appetite and intake: "My appetite is good, maybe too good! It was just as good before coming here, and I am eating all my meals. I could use more food! I've had diabetes for about 10 years, and I have cholesterol (I take pills for it), but I don't pay too much attention to what I eat; I never talked to anyone about diet. I eat everything my wife cooks."

Weight loss and UBW: "I don't weigh myself, but my clothes fit the same as a few years ago."

Food allergies: "Shellfish."

Cultural or religious food preference: "I am Muslim, but pork is the only food I don't eat."

Difficulty chewing or swallowing: "No."

Nausea, vomiting, constipation, or diarrhea: "No, but I get acid a lot, so I take two calcium tablets every day".

Preferences: "I eat all the traditional Lebanese foods, and I like meat and chicken; I have one or two pitas a day, and I like to put butter on it. We have rice every day. I also really like my potato chips, so I eat those every night! *Wife:* "I use olive oil to cook". every meal."

Musculoskeletal Depletion: None

Subcutaneous Fat Depletion: None

You talk to his nurse.

"Pt's wife has brought food every day, looks like lots of rice and pitas, and several desserts. They don't appear to be considering sugar or counting carbohydrates."

Problem Solving Matrix Assessment for SB Case Study

Typical Daily Intake/Food Frequency			
Food Category	**Specific Type/Preparation**	**Frequency**	**Amount**
Meat/Fish/Poultry	No pork, shellfish	Daily	Unsure
Dairy: Milk, Cheese, Yogurt	Only whole milk	Daily	1 cup
Eggs		Twice/week	2
Starch (bread, grain, cereal)	Pita, rice, wheat flakes cereal	Usually daily	1 lg pita; 2 cups cereal; 2 cups rice
Vegetables	Spinach, broccoli (sautéed in oil)	3 to 4/week	1 cup
Fruits	Only juice, usually orange	Daily	1 cup
Sugars, Sweets/ Desserts	Chocolate chip cookies, donut, baklava (one of these types/day)	Daily	2 cookies, 1 donut, 2 inch square baklava
Snack Foods (salted)	Potato chips	Daily	2 cups
Fats	Olive oil (for food prep), butter (on pita)		
Beverages: Coffee, Tea, Soda	Coffee (with cream)	Daily	3 cups
Alcohol	None		

Step: Collection of data from patient interview

1.0 Assessment

♦ Collect assessment data from: Review of the medical record & patient interview
♦ Analyze collected data: Use nutrition equations & standard lab parameters

Assessment Data Categories	Collect Data Fill-in the date collected from MR and interview	Analyze Data Calculate BMI, IBW, %UBW, %wt change, etc.; identify abnormal labs
Anthropometric	**Data collected**	**Analyze data (BMI, IBW, %UBW, %wt change, etc.)**
Weight/Height	Ht: 190.5cm (pt estimate); Wt: 106.5 kg (actual)	
Biochemical Data, Medical Test, Procedures	**Data collected**	**Analyze data (identify any abnormal lab values)**
VPS: albumin, RBP, transferrin, prealbumin, TLC (moderated by inflammation/stress)		
Lipids: TC, HDL, LDL, ratio, TG		
Dx/Disease-related (CVD, DM, GI, liver, renal)	Glu 208 (H); HbA1c-7.5% (H); Na 136; Cr 1.19; GFR-61	
Nutrition-Focused Physical Findings	**Data collected from NFPE and History & Physical (Review of Systems)**	**Analyze data (identify any physical findings that are outside the normal parameters)**
Physical appearance (muscle wasting, fat loss, edema, skin, hair, nails, etc.)		
Physical function (hand grip)		
Functional Problems (GI, etc.)	□N □V □D □C Oral motor: □ Intact □ Dysphagia □ Difficulty chewing □ Other: GERD	

History	Data collected
Food/ Nutrition: Food intake, appetite, wt history, physical activity, cultural, religious, food allergy & intolerances, medications, supplements, food availability	**Food intake**: Good appetite now at PTA on regular diet; Typical intake shows meat every day with rice and pita bread, desserts, potato chips, olive oil for food prep, butter on pita **Wt Hx**: No wt changes, but does not weigh self **Physical Activity**: Sedentary -owns a bookstore, no other activity **Culture/Religion**: Arabic (traditional foods); Muslim (no pork) **Food Allergy:** Shellfish **Meds/Supplements**: As noted in chart, no supplements **Food Availability**: Wife shops/cooks
Client History: Medical; nutritionally-relevant Dx	T2DM, HTN, GERD (uses OTC calcium CO_3) , peripheral neuropathy, foot ulcer x 1yr
Social History: Lives alone, support, occupation, income, education level, program participation	Positive for tobacco; Denies ETOH, drug use; Lives w/wife (wife cooks); owns bookstore
Determine/Estimate Nutrient Needs	**Estimated Nutrient Needs (Nutrition Prescription)**
Energy needs: use range equation, Mifflin, Harris-Benedict, etc (consider activity and stress or disease-specific factors)	
Protein needs: use facility intake standards (consider disease-specific needs)	
Fluid needs: use facility intake standards (consider disease-specific needs)	

CHAPTER 4

Nutrition Assessment

NUTRITION-FOCUSED PHYSICAL EXAMINATION

Nancy J. Park, MS, RDN-AP, CNSC

By the end of the chapter, the reader will be able to

- Identify the six characteristics for diagnosing malnutrition through nutrition-focused physical examination
- Describe the techniques and outline the steps used when conducting a physical examination
- Describe how to incorporate the nutrition-focused physical examination into the patient nutrition assessment
- Identify how the nutrition-focused physical examination can be used in conjunction with other patient data to determine nutrition risk

A n important component of nutrition assessment and the Nutrition Care Process (NCP) is the Nutrition-Focused Physical Examination (NFPE). Performing the NFPE is essential to understanding nutritional status in context of the patient's underlying disease state and condition. Every attempt to perform NFPE in all patients requiring an assessment should be made. The NFPE makes up *three* of the six categories utilized in describing and defining malnutrition.

MALNUTRITION AND THE ROLE OF THE DIETITIAN

The importance of the dietitian's role in determining nutrition risk, and malnutrition cannot be overemphasized. Malnutrition is linked to poor outcomes for patients, including increased length of stay, increased risk of falls, pressure ulcers, delayed wound healing, and increased need for alternate care post-discharge. Upwards of 50% of hospitalized patients are malnourished, and 69% continue to decline throughout their hospital stay (1). The Center for Medicare and Medicaid Services (CMS) recognizes malnutrition as a complicating/comorbid condition, and in 2007 changed reimbursement to reflect the impact of malnutrition on hospital costs. Malnutrition continues to be largely unrecognized by healthcare providers (2).

RESEARCH UPDATE

Corkins and colleagues reviewed 1,248,640 hospital discharges from the 2010 Healthcare Costs and Utilization Project (HCUP) and found the malnutrition diagnosis made it to the discharge summary in only 3.2% of patients.

Data from Corkins, M. R., Guenter, P., DiMaria-Ghalili, R. A., Jensen, G. L., et al., & the American Society for Parenteral and Enteral Nutrition. (2014). Malnutrition diagnoses in hospitalized patients: United States, 2010. *JPEN J Parenter Enteral Nutr, 38: 186–195.*

NUTRITION-FOCUSED PHYSICAL EXAMINATION

Nutrition-Focused Physical Examination in Relation to Malnutrition

Given the prevalence of malnutrition and the lack of understanding and recognition of this complex issue, the Academy for Nutrition and Dietetics (AND) and the American Society for Parenteral and Enteral Nutrition (A.S.P.E.N.) collaborated to standardize diagnosis of malnutrition. The 2012 Academy/A.S.P.E.N. consensus statement on malnutrition focuses on six specific characteristics/criteria in conjunction with an understanding of the etiology behind the condition (3). The etiology is based on the presence of inflammation and whether or not the inflammatory response is acute (< 3 months), or chronic

(> 3 months.) The six characteristics for diagnosing malnutrition can be found in Box 4.1. It is important to note malnutrition can exist in situations where inflammation is not present, such as anorexia nervosa. The malnutrition resulting from noninflammatory circumstances results from prolonged starvation.

BOX 4.1

Six Characteristics Defining Malnutrition

- Weight loss
- Inadequate energy intake
- Loss of muscle mass
- Loss of subcutaneous fat
- Fluid accumulation
- Hand grip strength

Data from reference 3: White, J. V., Guenter, P., Jensen, G., Malone, A., Schofield, M.; Academy Malnutrition Work Group; A.S.P.E.N. Malnutrition Task Force; A.S.P.E.N. Board of Directors. (May 2012). Consensus statement: Academy of Nutrition and Dietetics and American Society for Parenteral and Enteral Nutrition: Characteristics recommended for the identification and documentation of adult malnutrition (undernutrition). *JPEN J Parenter Enteral Nutr, 36*(3): 275–283.

The Inflammatory Process and Malnutrition

Inflammation is the normal biologic response to heal the body after a harmful or irritating insult. It is part of the body's immune response. Inflammation occurs so the body can localize and eliminate the cause of the injury, along with any damaged tissue or necrotic cells, and begin tissue repair. This healing process could last hours, days, weeks, months, and even years, depending on the degree and extent of injury. The differentiation between acute and chronic inflammation can sometimes be confounding. Diseases with a slower onset and persisting greater than three months are considered chronic, and diseases of sudden onset and persisting less than three months are considered acute. Examples of each type are listed in Table 4.1.

TABLE 4.1 Examples of Disease States Associated with Acute and Chronic Inflammation

Acute	Chronic
• Major infection	• Pancreatic Cancer
• Burns	• End-stage Organ Failure
• Trauma	• Rheumatoid Arthritis
• Closed head injury	• Sarcopenic Obesity
• Major abdominal surgery	• Inflammatory Bowel Disease

When injury is severe and/or prolonged, the ramping up of the inflammatory response can have deleterious effects. The release of cytokines increases production of acute phase reactants (such as C-reactive protein, tumor necrosis factor (TNF), interleukin VI) and metabolic demand, which accelerates muscle breakdown and fat loss. This process is illustrated in Box 4.2. Simultaneously, production of carrier proteins (such as albumin) is suppressed, which leads to fluid accumulation/edema. As the understanding of the immune response to illness has improved—as well as the relationship of the response to nutritional status and serum proteins—albumin, prealbumin, and transferrin are no longer considered as determining factors for malnutrition. These biochemical markers are negative-acute phase reactants and are affected by confounding factors, making them unreliable as indicators of malnutrition. Subsequently, protein markers were not included in the AND/A.S.P.E.N. consensus statement.

BOX 4.2

The Effect of Inflammation on Nutritional Status

Inflammatory Response → Release of Cytokines → Release of Acute-Phase Reactants →Increased Protein Catabolism and Decreased Carrier Protein Synthesis →Increased Energy Expenditure and Nitrogen Loss

Signs of inflammation can be visually seen on patient examination. The five cardinal signs of inflammation are pain, redness, immobility, swelling, and heat. Inflammation of internal organs is determined through diagnostic imaging and testing; for example, a chest X-ray to detect pneumonia. See Box 4.3 for conditions, procedures, and laboratory data that may indicate inflammation. Certain categories of acute illness, such as trauma or pancreatitis, create a milieu of inflammatory responses known as "SIRS": the *Systemic Inflammatory Response Syndrome*. The criteria for SIRS is noted in Box. 4.4. Other indicators of inflammation are not visible. Radiographic and CT imaging, as well as endoscopic or surgical procedures such as a diagnostic laparotomy, may reveal inflammation. Symptoms of inflammation often include elevation of white blood cells, an increase in body temperature, and an increase in heart or respiratory rate. Also, laboratory data holds keys to inflammation, typically evidenced by an elevated C-reactive protein and decreased albumin and/or prealbumin.

BOX 4.3

Evidence of Inflammation

Chart Location	Examples of Evidence
History and Physical Medical/Surgical History	*Chronic Inflammation:* Chronic pancreatitis, cancer, end-stage organ failure, AIDS, sarcopenic obesity, arthritis, asthma, diabetes *Acute Inflammation:* Trauma, severe burns, SIRS/sepsis, major abdominal surgery, closed head injury (CHI)
Laboratory Data	*Biochemistry:* Increased White Blood Cell count (WBC) Elevated blood sugar (hyperglycemia) Decreased Albumin, prealbumin Elevated C-Reactive Protein (CRP) *Microbiology:* Positive cultures from stool, urine, sputum, and/or blood Wound drainage

Diagnostic and Imaging Procedures	*Endoscopy/Colonoscopy:* Active Inflammatory Bowel Disease, colitis, radiation enteritis, strictures
	CT Scan/X-ray: Pulmonary infiltrates, pneumonia, bowel obstruction, pneumointestinalis
Vital Signs	Temperature > 38°C or < 36°C
	Heart Rate > 90 beats/min.
	Respiratory Rate > 20 breaths/min. or PaCO2 < 32 Torr

NIH US National Library of Medicine. Medline Plus: Vital Signs. https://medlineplus.gov/ency/article/002341.html. Accessed February 16, 2018.

BOX 4.4

SIRS Systemic Inflammatory Response Criteria

Two or more of these must be present to meet SIRS criteria.

- Temperature > 38°C or < 36°C
- Heart Rate > 90 beats/min.
- Respiratory Rate > 20 breaths/min. or $PaCO_2$ < 32 Torr
- WBC > 12,000 cells/mm^3, < 4000 cells/mm^3, or > 10% immature (band) forms

Source: Bone, R. C., Balk, R. A., Cerra, F. B., Dellinger, R. P., Fein, A. M., Knaus, W. A., Schein, R. M., & Sibbald, W. J. (June 1992). Definitions for sepsis and organ failure and guidelines for the use of innovative therapies in sepsis. The ACCP/SCCM Consensus Conference Committee. American College of Chest Physicians/Society of Critical Care Medicine. *Chest, 101*(6): 1644–1655.

Overview and History of the Components in NFPE

NFPE is a major component of the overall nutrition assessment of a patient. Muscle loss, subcutaneous fat loss, and presence of edema account for three of the six defining characteristics of malnutrition. The other components (as previously described in Chapters 2 and 3) rely on the practitioner's ability to obtain information through verbal communication and data review. While functional status, as measured by hand grip strength, is the last characteristic, this is not typically used in the hospital setting.

The loss of muscle and fat mass are closely linked to loss of functional status and malnutrition. The first concise and practical approach linking all these factors together was the *Subjective Global Assessment, SGA*. Detsky, McLaughlin, Baker and colleagues included assessment of muscle wasting and fat loss to determine if the patient was well nourished (A), moderately malnourished (B), or severely malnourished (C) (4). The loss of muscle mass is associated with decreased strength and mobility. For certain patients, such as the elderly, muscle loss can lead to impairment in the ability to perform activities of daily living, such as preparing meals and feeding oneself. Fat loss exposes bony prominences. Friction, shear, and pressure on bony prominences can lead to skin breakdown. Accurate assessment of findings on NPFE not only provides key and essential components of nutrition diagnosis, it helps to determine the overall plan of care for the patient and can determine placement needs post-discharge.

In order to assure consistency, reliability, and reproducibility, major body regions have been designated for inclusion. The assessment of muscle mass includes the temple region, clavicles, shoulders, scapula, hand, thighs, and calves. Regional areas for fat loss assessment include the orbital, triceps, and rib cage (5).

Getting Started with NFPE

The NFPE requires a "hands-on" approach. For many, this is a new skill set. As it is incorporated into the Nutrition Care Process, all dietitians must demonstrate competency with this skill. The easiest way to begin is to incorporate NFPE while obtaining the other components of nutrition assessment; weight history and intake history. Techniques associated with physical examination include inspection, palpation, percussion, and auscultation. Box 4.5 provides the definition of these techniques. Inspection and palpation are the two most commonly used in NFPE. As with any new skill, practice and experience increases comfort and competency. Reviewing the major muscle and fat regions, as well as locating areas of edema, should take place prior to assessing an actual patient.

BOX 4.5

Definitions Used in Physical Assessment

- **Inspection:** visual observation of color, shape, texture and size
- **Palpation:** use of touch to examine location, texture, size, temperature, tenderness, and mobility
- **Percussion:** tapping of fingers against body surfaces and listening for sounds that reflect solids, liquids, or gases
- **Auscultation:** used during exam of heart, lungs, and abdomen with a stethoscope

---

RESEARCH UPDATE

Updated standards of practice for registered dietitians include NFPE as part of professional competency. The ability to differentiate loss of muscle and fat, as well as assessing edema, is included.

Data from: The Academy Quality Management Committee and Scope of Practice Subcommittee of the Quality Management Committee. (2013). Academy of Nutrition and Dietetics: Revised 2012 standards of practice in nutrition care and standards of professional performance for registered dietitians. *J Acad Nutr Diet, 113:* S29–S45.

Put It into Practice

There are many workshops, including virtual, that offer tutorials on how to perform NFPE. Consider participating in a workshop to expand and hone NFPE skills. There are tutorials and workshops, and toolkits offered by the AND, as well as the Dietitians in Nutrition

Support (DNS) Practice Group, A.S.P.E.N., and even nutriceutical companies, such as Abbott and Nestlé. Seek out opportunities to learn more about NFPE.

How to Perform NFPE

In order to differentiate between normal, mild-moderate, and severe malnutrition, the dietitian visually inspects the overall appearance of the patient. Then, the designated areas are physically palpated to determine the amount of muscle mass in relation to fat. Certain areas may require lightly tapping, such as under the eye, and others may require grasping areas to gently roll the skin and separate muscle from fat. Tables 4.2 and 4.3 address the particular regions of the body assessed during NFPE. These tables also describe the typical findings on physical exam. It is divided into separate categories for patients who are well nourished, (normal), mild-moderate malnutrition, and severe malnutrition. Also, the last column in each of these tables provides the dietitian with tips for performing NFPE.

When looking at the major regions for muscle loss, the upper areas tend to deplete more quickly than lower areas. This is primarily due to the size of the muscle; quadriceps are large and take longer to deplete than the small temporal muscle. Obese and morbidly obese patients may have muscle loss even with significant fat stores. It is important to perform NFPE to discern between muscle and fat mass, and not to assume, based on weight or BMI, that a patient is adequately nourished.

TABLE 4.2 Body Regions to Assess for Muscle Loss

Region	Normal	Mild-Moderate	Severe	Hands-on Heads-up
Temples (Temporalis)	Well defined, easily seen	Slight depression	Hollow/ scooped appearance	Look face-on at patient; exam each side separately

(Continued)

TABLE 4.2 (*Continued*)

Region	Normal	Mild-Moderate	Severe	Hands-on Heads-up
Clavicle (Pectoralis, deltoid, trapezius)	Men: Clavicle not visible; Women: May be visible but not prominent	Men: visible Women: Protrusion of clavicle	Clavicle protruding and prominent	Have patient sit up straight if possible; look and feel for prominent bone
Clavicle and Acromion (Deltoid)	Well rounded curves at shoulder, arm, neck	Nonsquare; Acromion Process may protrude	"Squaring off" from shoulder to arm, prominent bones	Have patient drop arms to side for observation
Scapular (Trapezius, latissimus dorsi)	Bones not prominent	Bones may show slightly	Bones prominent, significant	Extend arms straight out, or if possible, have patient push against a wall
Hand (Interosseous)	Muscle protrudes	Slightly depressed	Depressed area between thumb and index finger	Observe muscle bulge by pressing thumb against index finger, or have patient touch index finger to tip of thumb.
Patellar (Quadriceps)	Well rounded, no depressions	Mild depression on inner thigh; kneecap somewhat prominent	Depression of muscle on thigh; bones prominent; minimal or no muscle definition	Grasp quadriceps to differentiate muscle from fat

Region	Normal	Mild-Moderate	Severe	Hands-on Heads-up
Calf (Gastrocnemius)	Well-developed bulb of muscle	Not well developed	Thin; minimal to no muscle definition	Grasp calf muscle to differentiate muscle from fat

Data adapted from White, J. V., Guenter, P., Jensen, G., Malone, A., Schofield, M.; Academy Malnutrition Work Group; A.S.P.E.N. Malnutrition Task Force; A.S.P.E.N. Board of Directors. (May 2012). Consensus statement: Academy of Nutrition and Dietetics and American Society for Parenteral and Enteral Nutrition: Characteristics recommended for the identification and documentation of adult malnutrition (undernutrition). *JPEN J Parenter Enteral Nutr, 36*(3): 275–283.

TABLE 4.3 Body Regions to Assess for Fat Loss

Region	Normal	Mild-Moderate	Severe	Hands-on Heads-Up
Orbital (around the eye)	Slightly bulged fat pads	Slightly darker circles; somewhat hollow look	Dark circles, hollow look; depression, loose skin	Look face-on at patient; gently touch above cheekbone
Upper Arm (Triceps)	Large space between fingers when pinching	Some depth pinch, but not ample. Fingers almost touch	Little space between fingers when pinching, fingers almost touch	Bend arm, and grasp skin; roll skin between fingers; try not to include muscle
Thoracic/Lumbar (ribs, lower back)	Ribs do not show	Ribs are apparent; however, gaps are not large	Ribs very apparent with depression between ribs	Assess patient from side if necessary to view

Data adapted from White, J. V., Guenter, P., Jensen, G., Malone, A., Schofield, M.; Academy Malnutrition Work Group; A.S.P.E.N. Malnutrition Task Force; A.S.P.E.N. Board of Directors. (May 2012). Consensus statement: Academy of Nutrition and Dietetics and American Society for Parenteral and Enteral Nutrition: characteristics recommended for the identification and documentation of adult malnutrition (undernutrition). *JPEN J Parenter Enteral Nutr, 36*(3): 275–283.

After assessing for muscle and fat loss (these two categories are often combined together), the dietitian then assesses for fluid accumulation. Edema is an accumulation of fluid in the body's tissues, cavities, and/or the space surrounding a body's cells (interstitial spaces). Interstitial spaces are those occurring outside of the organs or vessels, between the cells. Edema is most noticeable in dependent or lower parts of the body: feet, ankles, and genitalia, (scrotum and vulva). Fluid accumulation is assessed in the face, upper and lower extremities. In hospitalized patients, edema is usually related to the suppression of carrier protein synthesis due to inflammation. Edema is not typically seen in patients with starvation-related malnutrition.

To assess presence of edema, the dietitian presses the affected area with the index finger, and notes how long it takes the depression made in the skin to subside. The depth and duration of the indentation determine the severity of the edema. The hands-on assessment of edema and interpretation of findings are found in Box 4.6. It is important to take into consideration the many other conditions that may cause edema, and these are listed in Box 4.7.

BOX 4.6

How to Assess Edema

- Edema is the retention of fluid beneath the skin.
- Typical areas where edema is found are: from the feet to below the knee, hands, and face
- Skin that is *edematous* remains indented after pressing with the thumb or finger, and this is called *pitting edema*

Assessment of edema
- Use a graded scale from 1+ (mild) to 4+ (severe)
  - 1+ = 2 mm indentation
    - Space fills in rapidly (0–30 seconds)
  - 2+ = 4 mm indentation

- o   3+ = 6 mm indentation
- o   4+ = 8 mm indentation
  - ■   Space refills slowly (2–5 min.)
- With 4+ pitting edema, dependent parts of the body are grossly fluid filled and taut

---

BOX 4.7

Underlying Causes of Edema

- Excess fluids
- Heart, renal, or liver failure
- Immobilization
- Hypoalbuminemia
- Medications
- Heat
- Sodium intake
- Pregnancy/Menstruation
- Infection (cellulitis)

Put It into Practice

Practice NFPE with classmates, coworkers, family members, and friends prior to performing NFPE on a patient. Work with a partner or in a small group to check regional locations for inspection and palpation. Practice interview skills for introducing the procedure, as well as the hands-on portion, to gain skill and confidence in NFPE.

Incorporating NFPE into Patient Assessment

NFPE is best approached as part of the patient interview. As with all patient interaction, the dietitian should introduce him- or herself and explain the reason for the visit and for the hands-on examination. The patient should be properly identified. Hand washing takes place before donning gloves, and again when the exam is complete and the gloves are removed. When beginning NFPE, taking notes or checking boxes on a worksheet template may be helpful to remember findings. Some dietitians prefer to assess for muscle wasting first, then fat loss. Others prefer to assess the two categories together as the dietitian works from head to toe. As experience and confidence in the techniques associated with NFPE are gained, the dietitian will find the method that works best. After completing the NFPE, the dietitian combines this information with the findings from other data and works toward assessing the patient's nutritional status (6).

When Is NFPE Not appropriate?

Dietitians may be reluctant to start performing NFPE. It should always be considered part of the nutrition assessment. There are times when NFPE cannot be performed. If the patient is in extreme pain or discomfort, offer to come back at another time. The patient typically will not refuse NFPE if the appropriate introduction is made. Asking the nurse or another dietitian for assistance may be another way to accomplish the task if the situation is complicated or daunting. If the patient is in isolation, NFPE can and should still be performed. The hospital guidelines for isolation precautions should be followed. If the patient is considering hospice, or is at or near end of life, NFPE may be deferred. However, if unable to perform NFPE, the dietitian should document this in the assessment. Upon reassessment, the NFPE may be performed.

It is appropriate and possible to perform NFPE on critically ill patients. This situation may seem overwhelming due to the number of tubes, drains, and ongoing activities at the bedside. Taking a minute to assess the best way to gain access to the patient and working with the patient's nurse will usually enable the dietitian to perform NFPE. The actual hands-on approach to NFPE should only add a few minutes to the time spent with the patient. Time to perform NFPE should not be a deterrent to the dietitian.

NFPE in Context with Other Findings

The NFPE does not stand alone when determining nutrition risk. Perhaps the patient was always thin, or overweight? Typically, abnormal findings on NFPE are tied in with other concerning factors, such as weight loss, or the underlying disease state or condition, such as cancer. Obtaining this information is crucial to an accurate nutrition diagnosis and care plan. Performing NFPE in context with the patient's history helps pull the entire picture together. Chapters 5 explains how all the pieces fit together to determine nutrition status and risk, and come up with the correct nutrition diagnosis for the patient. This, is turn, sets the course for the nutrition care plan, interventions, and follow-up (chapters 6, 7, 8). In addition, while not part of the diagnostic criteria for determining malnutrition, the underlying disease and treatment for the disease or condition may predispose the patient to deficiencies of vitamins and minerals. Table 4.4 reviews major body systems and the signs of deficiency, along with the corresponding nutrient. When performing NFPE, careful observation for any signs or symptoms of nutrient deficiency should be noted.

TABLE 4.4 Clinical Signs of Nutrient Deficiency

Body System	Sign/Clinical Finding	Nutrient Deficiencies
Skin	Pressure ulcers, non-healing wounds	Vitamin C, zinc, protein
	Poor skin turgor	Water, protein
	Pallor	B12, folate, and/or iron
	Lesions and/or altered pigmentation dermatitis, flaky-paint dermatitis, pellagra	Essential fatty acid deficiency (EFAD), niacin and/or tryptophan
	Ecchymosis, petechiae	Vitamin C or K
	Dry, scaly skin	Vitamin A or EFAD

(*Continued*)

Body System	Sign/Clinical Finding	Nutrient Deficiencies
Nails	Spoon-shaped	Iron
	Dull	Protein
	Mottled, pale, non-blanchable	Vitamin A or C
Scalp/Hair	Dull, sparse, thin	Protein, iron, zinc, or EFAD
	Plucked with ease	Protein
Face	Moon-facies, temporal wasting	Protein and energy
Eyes	Sunken; hollow around eye sockets	Protein and energy
	Night blindness	Vitamin A
	Redness and cracking at edge of eyelids and eyebrows	Riboflavin or niacin
	Pale conjunctiva	Iron
	Foamy spots on cornea (Bitot's spots)	Vitamin A
	Dull, dry, rough appearance to inner eyelids	Vitamin A
	Milky or opaque cornea, or softening of corneas	Vitamin A
Nose	Greasy skin with yellow-gray material around the nares	Riboflavin or pyridoxine
Lips	Cracking and redness at corners of mouth (angular stomatitis)	Riboflavin, niacin, and/or pyridoxine
	Vertical cracking (cheilosis)	Riboflavin or niacin
Mouth (inspect dentition, as this influences ability to chew)	Pallor, inflammation	Iron, Vitamin C, B-complex vitamins

Body System	Sign/Clinical Finding	Nutrient Deficiencies
Tongue	Beefy-red color	Niacin, folate, riboflavin, iron
	Magenta color	Riboflavin
	Smooth, flattened papillae	Folate, niacin, iron, riboflavin, B12
	Altered taste; diminished or distorted	Zinc
Gums	Bleeding, spongy, receding	Vitamin C
	Pale	Iron
	Dry	Water
Neck	Enlarged thyroid (goiter)	Iodine
	Distended neck veins	Volume overload

To Sum It Up

- Dietitians are the health care professional with the skill set and knowledge to perform NFPE and pull together all other findings in the determination of nutrition risk and malnutrition diagnoses
- NFPE is now considered within the scope of practice for dietitians and is required for competency in clinical dietetics
- NFPE can be performed on most hospitalized patients at the bedside; reasons why NFPE cannot be done should be noted and documented, and attempted again at a future time and date
- NFPE is a major component of nutrition assessment comprising three of the six characteristics of malnutrition
- Understanding of NFPE findings in context with other patient information, such as intake history, weight history, past medical and surgical history, is essential in forming the nutrition diagnosis, nutrition care plan, and follow-up

Check for Understanding

1. The presence or lack of inflammation is now considered in the etiology of malnutrition.
    a. True
    b. False

2. Albumin and prealbumin, when used in conjunction with C-reactive protein, are useful biochemical markers in determining inflammation.
    a. True
    b. False

3. The two skills most commonly used when performing a Nutrition-Focused Physical Exam include:
    a. Inspection, auscultation
    b. Inspection, percussion
    c. Inspection, palpation
    d. Auscultation, percussion

4. When assessing muscle loss, the upper area of the body is more sensitive to change than the lower body.
    a. True
    b. False

5. Edema is a common finding in patients with starvation-related malnutrition.
    a. True
    b. False

Answers in Appendix B

REFERENCES

1. Somanchi, M., Tao, X., & Mullin, G. E. (March 2011). The facilitated early enteral and dietary management effectiveness trial in hospitalized patients with malnutrition. *JPEN J Parenter Enteral Nutr, 35*(2): 209–216.

2. Corkins, M. R., Guenter, P., DiMaria-Ghalili, R. A., Jensen, G. L., et al., & the American Society for Parenteral and Enteral Nutrition. (2014). Malnutrition diagnoses in hospitalized patients: United States, 2010. *JPEN J Parenter Enteral Nutr, 38: 186–195.*

3. White, J. V., Guenter, P., Jensen, G., Malone, A., Schofield, M.; Academy Malnutrition Work Group; A.S.P.E.N. Malnutrition Task Force; A.S.P.E.N. Board of Directors. (May 2012). Consensus statement: Academy of Nutrition and Dietetics and American Society for Parenteral and Enteral Nutrition: Characteristics recommended for the identification and documentation of adult malnutrition (undernutrition). *JPEN J Parenter Enteral Nutr, 36*(3): 275–283.

4. Detsky, A. S., McLaughlin, J.R., Baker, J. P., et al. (1987). What is subjective global assessment of nutrition status? *JPEN J Parenter Enteral Nutr, 11: 8–13.*

5. Malone, A., & Hamilton, C. (December 2013). The Academy of Nutrition and Dietetics/the American Society for Parenteral and Enteral Nutrition consensus malnutrition characteristics: Application in practice. *Nutrition in Clinical Practice, 28*(6): 639–650.

6 Litchford, M. (2013). Putting the nutrition focused physical assessment into practice in long-term care settings. *Annals of Long-Term Care: Clinical Care and Aging, 21*(11): 38–41.

OUR CASE STUDY OF PATIENT SB: NUTRITION ASSESSMENT: NUTRITION-FOCUSED PHYSICAL EXAM

Chapter 3 discussed the patient interview and how to appropriately obtain information through communication with the patient. The patient interview is the ideal time to conduct your nutrition-focused physical exam. This hands-on approach can initially feel like a daunting task, but as with any new skill, practice and experience will increase your comfort and competency.

The NFPE focuses on assessment of muscle loss, subcutaneous fat loss, and the presence of edema. Functional status can be measured using hand grip strength, but this step is currently not a typical part of the exam in the acute care setting.

Dietitian Interview and Physical

Your patient speaks English and his wife is at bedside.

Appetite and intake: "My appetite is good, maybe too good! It was just as good before coming here, and I am eating all my meals. I could use more food! I've had diabetes for about 10 years, and I have cholesterol (I take pills for it), but I don't pay too much attention to what I eat; I never talked to anyone about diet. I eat everything my wife cooks."

Weight loss and UBW: "I don't weigh myself, but my clothes fit the same as a few years ago."

Food allergies: "Shellfish."

Cultural or religious food preference: "I am Muslim, but pork is the only food I don't eat."

Difficulty chewing or swallowing: "No."

Nausea, vomiting, constipation, or diarrhea: "No, but I get acid a lot, so I take two calcium tablets every day."

Preferences: "I eat all the traditional Lebanese foods, and I like meat and chicken; I have one or two pitas a day, and I like to put butter on it. We have rice every day. I also really like my potato chips, so I eat those every night!

Wife: "I use olive oil to cook every meal."

Musculoskeletal Depletion: None

Subcutaneous Fat Depletion: None

You talk to his nurse.

"Pt's wife has brought food every day, looks like lots of rice and pitas, and several desserts. They don't appear to be considering sugar or counting carbohydrates."

Problem Solving Matrix Assessment for SB Case Study
Step: Collection of data from Nutrition-Focused Physical Examination

1.0 Assessment

+ *Collect assessment data from:* Review of the medical record & patient interview
+ *Analyze collected data:* Use nutrition equations & standard lab parameters

Assessment Data Categories	Collect Data Fill in the date collected from MR and interview	Analyze Data Calculate BMI, IBW, %UBW, %wt change, etc.; identify abnormal labs
Anthropometric	Data collected	Analyze data (BMI, IBW, %UBW, %wt change, etc.)

Weight/Height	Ht: 190.5cm (Pt estimate); Wt: 106.5 kg (actual)	
Biochemical Data, Medical Test, Procedures	**Data collected**	**Analyze data (identify any abnormal lab values)**
VPS: albumin, RBP, transferrin, prealbumin, TLC (moderated by inflammation/stress)		
Lipids: TC, HDL, LDL, ratio, TG		
Dx/Disease-related (CVD, DM, GI, liver, renal)	Glu 208 (H); HbA1c-7.5% (H); Na 136; Cr 1.19; GFR-61	
Nutrition-Focused Physical Findings	**Data collected from NFPE and History & Physical (Review of Systems)**	**Analyze data (identify any physical findings that are outside the normal parameters)**
Physical appearance (muscle wasting, fat loss, edema, skin, hair, nails, etc.)	Musculoskeletal depletion: None Subcutaneous fat depletion: None	
Physical function (hand grip)		
Functional Problems (GI, etc.)	☐N ☐V ☐D ☐C Oral motor: ☐ Intact ☐ Dysphagia ☐ Difficulty chewing ☐ Other: GERD	

History	Data collected
Food/ Nutrition: Food intake, appetite, wt history, physical activity, cultural, religious, food allergy & intolerances, medications, supplements, food availability	**Food intake:** Good appetite now as PTA on regular diet; typical intake shows meat every day with rice and pita bread, desserts, potato chips, olive oil for food prep, butter on pita **Wt Hx:** No wt changes, but does not weigh self **Physical Activity:** Sedentary—owns a bookstore, no other activity **Culture/Religion:** Arabic (traditional foods); Muslim (no pork) **Food Allergy:** Shellfish **Meds/Supplements:** As noted in chart, no supplements **Food Availability:** Wife shops/cooks
Client History: Medical; nutritionally relevant Dx	T2DM, HTN, GERD (uses OTC calcium CO3), peripheral neuropathy, foot ulcer x 1yr
Social History: Lives alone, support, occupation, income, education level, program participation	Positive for tobacco; denies ETOH, drug use; lives w/wife (wife cooks); owns bookstore
Determine/Estimate Nutrient Needs	**Estimated Nutrient Needs (Nutrition Prescription)**
Energy Needs: Use range equation, Mifflin, Harris-Benedict, etc. (consider activity and stress or disease-specific factors)	
Protein Needs: Use facility intake standards (consider disease-specific needs)	
Fluid needs: Use facility intake standards (consider disease-specific needs)	

CHAPTER 5

Nutrition Diagnosis

MAKING SENSE OF ASSESSMENT DATA

By the end of the chapter, the reader will be able to

- Identify the three components of the nutrition diagnostic statement: problem, etiology, and signs/symptoms
- Analyze and correlate assessment data collected and calculations derived from the data to identify the patient's nutrition concerns and needs
- Identify all possible nutrition diagnoses for the concerns and needs identified from the assessment using the Academy Standardized Terminology for the Nutrition Care Process
- Select the optimal nutrition diagnosis for each patient problem or need and the corresponding etiology and signs/symptoms for each nutrition diagnosis
- Write the nutrition diagnosis in "Problem-Etiology-Signs/Symptoms" (PES) format appropriate for documentation in the medical record
- Evaluate each nutrition diagnosis based on established criteria: assessment data support; within the RD's scope of practice; specificity, clarity, conciseness of statement; measurability of signs and symptoms

n many ways, the nutrition diagnosis step of the NCP is the most critical step in the entire process. In this phase, the RD analyzes all of the assessment data collected and calculations derived from the data to identify the patient's nutrition concerns and needs, and states this in the nutrition diagnosis written in the succinct "Problem-Etiology-Signs/Symptoms" (PES) format (Boxes 5.1 and 5.2) (1).

This is prerequisite for solving the patient's nutrition concerns and meeting their needs. It is different from a medical diagnosis of disease, given the RD's scope of practice versus that of the physician, and in that it focuses exclusively on nutritionally relevant concerns and needs that are within the RD's scope of practice to resolve. Critical thinking skills are essential in determining the patient's nutritional concerns and formulating the nutrition diagnosis in the PES format. After the nutrition assessment phase, the process of converting identified nutrition concerns into the nutrition diagnosis (ND), culminating in a statement expressed in PES format appropriate for documentation in the medical record, encompasses five steps.

The five steps of converting nutrition concerns into the ND consist of:

1. List All Nutrition Concerns from the Nutrition Assessment
2. Analyze and Correlate Nutrition Concerns
3. Select Optimal Nutrition Diagnostic Term
4. Identify Etiology, Signs and Symptoms
5. Write the Diagnosis in PES Format.

In order to make the most of this chapter's activities and the case studies in upcoming chapters, the reader is reminded to visit the Academy's NCP section and purchase either a subscription to the eNCPT or the print book (NCPT), https://ncpt.webauthor.com/. The following sections illustrate what the RD does in each step of the process to develop the nutrition diagnosis. At the end of each section is a table containing an exercise to apply the information for the corresponding step of the process. The answers to the exercise are at the end of the chapter (Tables 5.1–5.5).

BOX 5.1

Nutrition Diagnosis: Problem/Etiology/Signs

The problem (P) describes alterations in patient nutritional status concerns, or needs:

A diagnostic label (qualifier) is an adjective that describes the physiologic response, e.g., altered, impaired, risk of

The etiology (E) refers to cause(s) or contributor(s) to the problem:

It is linked to the problem by the words "related to" (RT)

The signs/symptoms (S) are clusters of subjective and objective factors that provide evidence that a problem exists:

- They also quantify the problem and describe severity
- They are linked to (E) by the words "as evidenced by" (AEB)
- They should be measurable

Adapted from reference 6: Abridged Nutrition Care Process Terminology (NCPT) Reference Manual: Standardized Terminology for the Nutrition Care Process. (2018). Academy of Nutrition and Dietetics.

BOX 5.2

Writing the Nutrition Diagnosis (ND) Statement in PES Format

Example for the ND statement format: (P)roblem/(E)tiology/(S)igns/symptoms

Excessive energy intake **(P)** related to frequent consumption of large portions of high-fat meals **(E)**, as evidenced by:

1. Daily caloric intake exceeding DRI by 500 kcal **(S)**
2. 12-lb weight gain during past 18 months **(S)**

LABELING NUTRITION PROBLEMS

Step 1: Identifying Potential Nutrition Concerns

After collecting patient data in the assessment step of the NCP—and much like a detective trying to solve a mystery—the RD must now sift through this data in order to determine the patient's concerns and needs. In reviewing assessment data, the RD makes note of all data that falls outside of the established standards, whether the specific abnormal datum is a laboratory value that is out of normal range or a patient's inability to swallow food properly, as seen in the Assessment section (1.0) of the Problem Solving Matrix (Table 5.1). This is essentially a list of potential concerns that are nutritionally relevant, in that they may adversely affect the patient's nutritional status, which in turn will impede recovery, or present a need, whether educational or related to specific nutrients.

An important aspect of the list of potential nutrition concerns is the word *potential*. This is perhaps one of the most difficult steps to work through: several parameters may be abnormal or out of range, but they may not represent actual problems. One common example is that of a patient reporting poor appetite. This could be highly significant, because most people with a poor appetite will consume less food, which generally produces unintended weight loss, one of the most important patient risk factors. However, if the patient has not reduced food intake and lost weight, the report of poor appetite may not be a problem.

TABLE 5.1 Step 1. List All Potential Nutrition Concerns

Problem Solving Matrix: 1.0 Assessment	
♦ *Collect assessment data from:* Review of the medical record & patient interview	
Assessment Data Categories	Collect Data Fill in the data collected from MR and interview
Anthropometric Weight/Height	Data collected
Biochemical Data, Medical Test, Procedures	Data collected

VPS: albumin, RBP, transferrin, prealbumin, TLC (moderated by inflammation/stress)	
Lipids: TC, HDL, LDL, ratio, TG	
Dx/Disease-related (CVD, DM, GI, liver, renal)	
Nutrition-Focused Physical Findings	Data collected from NFPE and History & Physical (Review of Systems)
Physical appearance (muscle wasting, fat loss, edema, skin, hair, nails, etc.)	
Physical function (hand grip)	
Functional Problems (GI, etc.)	□N □V □D □C Oral motor: □ Intact □ Dysphagia □ Difficulty chewing □ Other:
History	**Data collected**
Food/Nutrition: Food intake, appetite, wt history, physical activity, cultural, religious, food allergy & intolerances, medications, supplements, food availability	
Client History: Medical; nutritionally relevant Dx	
Social History: Lives alone, support, occupation, income, education level, program participation	
Determine/Estimate Nutrient Needs	Estimated Nutrient Needs (Nutrition Prescription)
Energy needs: Use range equation, Mifflin, Harris-Benedict, etc. (consider activity and stress or disease-specific factors)	
Protein needs: Use facility intake standards (consider disease-specific needs)	
Fluid needs: Use facility intake standards (consider disease-specific needs)	

Step 2: Analyze and Correlate Nutrition Concerns

The Diagnosis section (2.0) of the Problem Solving Matrix form (Table 5.2) provides the critical thinking steps to determining if nutrition concerns identified from the nutrition assessment are actual patient problems or needs. In this step, the RD analyzes all the potential concerns identified from the nutrition assessment. The concerns need to be considered both independently and especially as they relate to each other to determine if actual concerns exist that should be part of the nutrition diagnosis and requiring a nutrition intervention.

One example of whether an assessment parameter identified as falling outside the established standard might not be a nutrition concern is BMI in an elderly individual. In the elderly population, research has shown that a higher BMI is protective in most individuals when the higher BMI does not affect an existing condition, such as hypertension (2, 3, 4). In this case, because of the patient's age, and especially in certain venues such as long-term care, this would not be an actual concern for this particular patient. Another weight example would be a patient with a BMI below the normal range. If the patient has always been at this BMI, it is not an actual concern or problem for the RD.

In addition to considering abnormal assessment parameters independently, it's also important to look for correlations between parameters; for example, a patient may report diminished appetite. However, if there has been no change in oral intake or weight loss for the same time period, this may not be a concern that it is a problem requiring a nutrition intervention. Another related example of correlating parameters is that the RD notes that the patient reports diminished appetite and the patient's BMI is also below the normal range. If the patient's BMI has been stable for a significant period of time, and there has been no weight loss, this would not be an actual concern.

When the RD determines that abnormal assessment parameters are actual problems, it is vital that the RD also consider whether the problem falls within the dietetics scope of practice. This would indicate whether the RD can either resolve the problem or at least improve it with a nutrition intervention. An example of a problem that falls outside the RD's scope of practice but is an assessment parameter would be a symptom that represents a derangement in gastrointestinal function (5). While problems such as vomiting, diarrhea, and gastrointestinal pain clearly can severely affect appetite, oral intake, and nutrient absorption—all of which can ultimately adversely affect nutrition status—these problems are typically outside of the RD's scope of practice. If, however, they are the result of disease or condition that will respond to nutrition intervention, they would be part of the diagnostic statement as either the etiology along with the medical diagnosis, or the signs and symptoms.

TABLE 5.2 Step 2. Analyze and Correlate Nutrition Concerns

Analyze each nutrition concern by comparing it to all others listed and looking for correlations that verify only nutritionally relevant concerns; then determine if those can be resolved by the RD.

Problem Solving Matrix: 2.0 Diagnosis

♦ ***Compare analyzed data to standards:*** Use the data from 1.0 Assessment to identify all potential nutrition concerns; analyze each concern by comparing it to all others listed and looking for correlations that verify only nutritionally relevant concerns; then determine if those can be resolved by the RD and list nutrition diagnoses.

Data Categories	A. Identify & list all potential nutrition concerns (any abnormal parameters)	B. Analyze potential concerns as they relate to each other to determine if actual concerns exist; list only actual, nutritionally relevant current concerns
		(e.g.: Is low BMI d/t decreased appetite or does Hx show the patient's BMI has always been low?)
Anthropometric		

(Continued)

Biochemical, Test, Procedures		

NFPE Findings

History (Appetite/intake, knowledge & behavior, any other relevant history)

Current intake/Diet Rx status	Can patient meet EEN? Y/N	Is diet Rx tolerated? Y/N

Step 3: Select the Optimal Nutrition Diagnostic Term

After determining if all or any listed nutrition concerns and needs are actual problems, the RD reviews the Academy Nutrition Care Process Nutrition Diagnostic Terminology to find the optimal nutrition diagnosis or diagnoses to fit the patient's problems (6). The number of NDs will depend on the individual patient or client and their specific problems. Some RDs will focus on one diagnosis, and in many cases, this will suffice, but the number should not be limited in an effort to standardize one's documentation. In most cases, several ND terms can match the patient's problems from among the three domains (intake, clinical, behavioral-environmental) (Box 5.3).

For example, a major nutrition concern would be a patient who has lost 8% of body weight in the past two months. In the nutrition assessment, the RD finds that the patient has had diminished appetite and food intake. The first nutrition diagnostic term that would work is the weight loss, which is in the clinical domain and has its own category for several problems related to weight; in this case, "unintended weight loss." However, two other possible diagnostic terms in the intake domain would also work: inadequate oral intake and inadequate energy intake. In most cases, selecting a diagnostic term from the intake domain is the preferred choice because the RD is more likely able to have the most significant impact in problem resolution.

In some cases, the RD must distinguish between two seemingly similar diagnostic terms. One such example are the following terms in the intake domain:

1. Energy: Inadequate energy intake (1.2)
2. Oral or Nutrition Support: Inadequate oral intake (2.1)

The Academy provides background information on the terminology (6). The RD should use "inadequate oral intake" when food intake can be documented, as in the case of a calorie count being ordered with results reflecting this diagnostic term. In contrast, "inadequate energy intake" refers to the RD estimating a patient's energy intake and comparing this to the estimation of the patient's energy needs, as done with energy estimation equations in the nutrition assessment step of the NCP.

BOX 5.3

Nutrition Diagnostic Terminology Domains

Intake (NI)	Clinical (NC)	Behavioral-Environmental (NB)
Energy Balance	Functional	Knowledge and Beliefs
Oral or Nutrition Support Intake	Biochemical	Physical Activity and Function
Fluid Intake	Weight	Food Safety and Access
Bioactive Substances	Malnutrition Disorders	
Nutrient		

Adapted from reference 6: Abridged Nutrition Care Process Terminology (NCPT) Reference Manual: Standardized Terminology for the Nutrition Care Process. (2018). Academy of Nutrition and Dietetics.

TABLE 5.3 Step 3. Select the Optimal Nutrition Diagnostic Term

1) Determine all possible **Domains/Class/Subclass** and **Nutrition Diagnoses** for each of the common nutrition concerns. *Several may be possible, depending on the etiology, so list as many as are possible.*

2) Select the optimal nutrition diagnostic term for each common nutrition concern

Common Nutrition Concerns	Domain Class/ Subclass	All Possible Nutrition Diagnoses	Optimal Nutrition Diagnosis
Patient has lost weight			
Patient's appetite is poor			
Patient has a new nutritionally relevant Dx			
Patient does not have knowledge of Diet Rx			
Patient has difficulty swallowing			
Patient has high serum cholesterol			
Patient has gained weight			
Patient with diabetes has elevated BGL			
Patient with diabetes does not monitor BGL			
Patient has chronic constipation			

Step 4: Identify Etiology, Signs and Symptoms

In determining the nutrition diagnosis, the RD must also identify possible etiologies for each problem and finally select the most accurate etiology based on the nutrition assessment. The etiology is the cause of the nutrition problem, or when the exact cause is not known, a contributing factor to the problem. Several etiologies may be possible, so the RD must apply critical thinking skills to identify the most accurate etiology. This is an important step in the process of formulating the nutrition diagnosis because the nutrition intervention targets the etiology of the nutrition problem. Box 5.4 shows the ten etiology categories and a brief description of each. For each nutrition diagnostic term, the Academy eNCPT also provides possible etiologies (6).

The signs and symptoms included in the diagnostic statement should be specific and measurable. They serve a twofold purpose in the diagnostic statement: they provide the evidence for the diagnosis, and their measurement enables the RD to monitor patient progress and evaluate the nutrition interventions. In this latter function, specific and measurable signs and symptoms will help to identify whether the problem has been resolved or is beginning to improve. They become the basis for the fourth step of the nutrition care process: monitoring and evaluation.

BOX 5.4

Etiology Categories

Category	Causes/Contributing Risk Factors That *May Affect or Be Related to:*
Access	Dietary intake, availability of safe and healthy foods, water, supplies
Behavioral	Attainment of nutrition-related goals
Beliefs and Attitudes	Truth/facts of nutrition-related information; feelings regarding the truth/facts
Cultural	Values, social norms and customs, religion, political views
Knowledge	Understanding about food and nutrition, health, nutrition-related information
Physical Function	Physical ability to perform specific tasks; may also be cognitive function
Physiologic-Metabolic	Medical and health status that affects nutrition status
Psychological	Diagnosed or potential psychological problem
Social-Personal	Patient history
Treatment	Medical or surgical therapies and care that affect nutrition status

Adapted from reference 6: *Abridged Nutrition Care Process Terminology (NCPT) Reference Manual: Standardized Terminology for the Nutrition Care Process.* (2018). Academy of Nutrition and Dietetics.

TABLE 5.4 Step 4. Identify Etiology, Signs and Symptoms

— From the optimal nutrition diagnostic term selected, and using the eNCPT, list all possible etiologies

— Select the optimal etiology and a sign/symptom that correlates with the specific etiology

Common Nutrition Concerns	Nutrition Diagnosis	Possible Etiologies	Select one Etiology (optimal) "related to" (r/t)	Signs/ Symptoms "as evidenced by" (AEB)
Patient has lost weight				
Patient's appetite is poor				
Patient has a new nutritionally relevant Dx				
Patient does not have knowledge of Diet Rx				
Patient has difficulty swallowing				
Patient has high serum cholesterol				
Patient has gained weight				
Patient with diabetes has elevated BGL				
Patient with diabetes does not monitor BGL				
Patient has chronic constipation				

Step 5: Write the Diagnosis in PES Format

In formulating the optimal nutrition diagnosis in PES format, after identifying nutrition problems and needs, the components combine to become a succinct statement for documentation in the medical record (Box 5.2) (7). The RD should evaluate the ND in PES format by considering key evaluation points:

- All components are supported by the assessment data
- It is related to the patient concerns, now the problem
- It contains one etiology, with the etiology stated as the root cause
- The ND is within the RD's scope of practice, making the ND one that the RD can resolve or at least improve

Further, in constructing the PES statement, the goals include clarity and conciseness, specificity, measurability, and the ability to measure cited signs and symptoms, which will indicate whether the problem has been resolved or improved. Table 5.6 provides a checklist for evaluating the nutrition diagnosis in PES format.

TABLE 5.5 Step 5. Write the Diagnosis in PES Format

Write the Nutrition Diagnosis statement using the PES format and phrasing Create/add data, as would be needed for the statement (% weight loss, lab value, etc.)	
Common Nutrition Concerns	Nutrition Diagnosis in PES Format
Patient has lost weight	
Patient's appetite is poor	
Patient has a new nutritionally relevant Dx	
Patient does not have knowledge of Diet Rx	
Patient has difficulty swallowing	
Patient has high serum cholesterol	
Patient has gained weight	
Patient with diabetes has elevated BGL	
Patient with diabetes does not monitor BGL	
Patient has chronic constipation	

TABLE 5.6 Checklist for the Nutrition Diagnosis in PES Format

Evaluation Criteria	Yes	No
Does the assessment data fully support the ND and all PES components?		
Is the ND related to the patient problem?		
Is the ND related to one etiology listed as the root cause?		
Is the ND within the RD's scope of practice?		
Can the RD resolve or at least improve the ND?		
Is the PES statement clear?		
Is the PES statement concise (does not include extraneous words)?		
Is the PES statement specific?		
Are the signs and symptoms (those selected as indicators) measurable?		
Will measurement of signs/symptoms indicate problem resolution or improvement?		

To Sum It Up

1. In the nutrition diagnosis step of the nutrition care process, the RD analyzes all of the assessment data collected and calculations derived from the data to identify the patient's nutrition concerns and needs, and states this in the nutrition diagnosis written in the succinct "Problem-Etiology-Signs/Symptoms" (PES) format for documentation in the medical record.

2. The development of the nutrition diagnosis is a process of several steps requiring critical thinking: 1) List All Nutrition Concerns from the Nutrition Assessment; 2) Analyze and Correlate Nutrition Concerns; 3) Select Optimal Nutrition Diagnostic Term; 4) Identify Etiology, Signs and Symptoms; 5) Write the Diagnosis in PES Format.

3. In reviewing assessment data, the RD makes note of all data that falls outside of the established standards, which represents

a list of potential concerns that may adversely affect the patient's nutritional status. However, an important aspect of the list is the word *potential*, and the RD must determine if any of these are actual problems within the scope of practice to resolve or improve.

4. After identifying actual problems, the RD reviews the Academy Nutrition Diagnostic Terminology to find the optimal diagnostic term to fit the patient's problems because in many cases, several may be possible in all three domains (intake, clinical, behavioral-environmental). The Academy recommends that the RD select from the intake domain when possible.

5. Key evaluative criteria for the nutrition diagnosis in PES format include: assessment data support; within the RD's scope of practice; specificity, clarity, and conciseness of the PES statement; measurability of signs and symptoms.

Check for Understanding (Answers in Appendix B)

1. Which of the following accurately represents the development of the diagnostic statement
    a. RDs should limit the number of diagnostic statements to one
    b. The phrase "related to" is used with signs and symptoms
    c. The etiology is listed at the end of the diagnostic statement
    d. The intake domain is preferred over others whenever possible

2. The PES format of the nutrition diagnosis is an acronym for
    a. Problem, Etiology, Signs and Symptoms
    b. Problem, Evidence, Signs and Social History
    c. Potential Concern, Etiology, Symptoms and Signs
    d. Potential Problem, Evidence, Symptoms

3. The first of five steps in developing the nutrition diagnosis is
    a. Identifying the patient's actual nutrition problems
    b. Listing all abnormal assessment parameters

    c. Thinking critically to distinguish among etiologies

    d. Selecting an optimal diagnosis among many

4. The Academy distinguishes between inadequate energy intake and inadequate oral intake in that

    a. Energy intake refers to observation of a patient's actual intake in the hospital

    b. Energy intake refers to the estimation of the patient's projected energy needs

    c. Oral intake refers to beverages consumed by the patient upon admission

    d. Oral intake refers to foods consumed by the patient prior to admission

5. An important characteristic of the signs and symptoms is

    a. Measurability in order to monitor progress and evaluate interventions

    b. Specificity to the medical diagnosis so that interventions can be developed

    c. Ability to provide evidence for the medical diagnosis for the RD's documentation

    d. Correlational link to the nutrition intervention for medical record documentation

Answers in Appendix B

References

1. Writing Group of the Nutrition Care Process/Standardized Language Committee. (2008). Nutrition Care Process and Model Part I: The 2008 Update. *J Am Diet Assoc, 108*(7): 1113–1117.
2. Winter, J. E., MacInnis, R. J., Wattanapenpaiboon, N., et al. (2014). BMI and all-cause mortality in older adults: A meta-analysis. *Am J Clin Nutr, 99*: 875–890.
3. Flegal, K. M., Kit, B. K., Orpana, H., et al. (2013). Association of all-cause mortality with overweight and obesity using standard body mass index categories: A systematic review and meta-analysis. *JAMA, 309*(1): 71–82.
4. Batsis, J. A., Singh, S., & Lopez-Jimenez, F. (2014). Anthropometric measurements and survival in older Americans: Results from the third national health and nutrition examination survey. *J Nutr Health & Aging, 18*(2): 123–130.

5. Academy of Nutrition and Dietetics. Scope of Practice. Available at: http://www.eatrightpro.org/resources/practice/quality-management/scope-of-practice. Accessed June 21, 2017.

6. Abridged Nutrition Care Process Terminology (NCPT) Reference Manual: Standardized Terminology for the Nutrition Care Process. (2018). Academy of Nutrition and Dietetics.

7. Writing Group of the Nutrition Care Process/Standardized Language Committee. (2008). Nutrition Care Process and Model Part II: Using the International Dietetics and Nutrition Terminology to Document the Nutrition Care Process. *J Am Diet Assoc, 108*(8): 1287–1293.

OUR CASE STUDY OF PATIENT SB: NUTRITION DIAGNOSIS

Previous chapters covered the estimation of nutrient needs, assessment of the patient's ability to meet those needs, and assessment of potential nutrition risks. This chapter focuses on the next step of the nutrition care process: nutrition diagnosis. After collection and analysis of all the patient data from the nutrition assessment, the RD develops the nutrition diagnosis and expresses it in the PES format for documentation in the medical record.

Problem Solving Matrix Assessment for SB Case Study Step: Nutrition Diagnosis		
1.0 Assessment • *Collect assessment data from*: Review of the medical record & patient interview • *Analyze collected data:* Use nutrition equations & standard lab parameters		
Assessment Data Categories	*Collect Data* Fill-in the date collected from MR and interview	*Analyze Data* Calculate BMI, IBW, %UBW, %wt change, etc.; identify abnormal labs
Anthropometric	**Data collected**	**Analyze data (BMI, IBW, %UBW, %wt change, etc.)**
Weight/Height	Ht: 190.5cm (pt estimate); Wt: 106.5 kg (actual)	BMI: 29.3 (overweight); IBW: 89 kg/196# (119%IBW); 100% UBW
Biochemical Data, Medical Test, Procedures	**Data collected**	**Analyze data (identify any abnormal lab values)**
VPS: albumin, RBP, transferrin, prealbumin, TLC (moderated by inflammation/stress)		

Problem Solving Matrix Assessment for SB Case Study Step: Nutrition Diagnosis		
Lipids: TC, HDL, LDL, ratio, TG		Lipids not analyzed; pt on lipid-lowering and anti-HTN meds with PCP
Dx/Disease-related (CVD, DM, GI, liver, renal)	Glu 208 (H); HbA1c-7.5% (H); Na 136; Cr 1.19; GFR-61	BGL in poor control: no SMBG, no dietary changes or instruction on diet for DM
Nutrition-Focused Physical Findings	**Data collected from NFPE and History & Physical (Review of Systems)**	**Analyze data (identify any physical findings that are outside the normal parameters)**
Physical appearance (muscle wasting, fat loss, edema, skin, hair, nails, etc.)	Musculoskeletal depletion: None Subcutaneous fat depletion: None Excess abdominal girth	Swelling of RLE, foot ulcer x 1 yr (related to poor glycemic control)
Physical function (hand grip)		
Functional Problems (GI, etc.)	☐N ☐V ☐D ☐C Oral motor: ☐ Intact ☐ Dysphagia ☐ Difficulty chewing ☐ Other: GERD	GERD, uses OTC calcium tabs

History	Data collected
Food/Nutrition: Food intake, appetite, wt history, physical activity, cultural, religious, food allergy & intolerances, medications, supplements, food availability	**Food intake:** Good appetite now and PTA on regular diet; typical intake shows meat every day with rice and pita bread, desserts, potato chips, olive oil for food prep, butter on pita **Wt Hx:** No wt changes, but does not weigh self **Physical Activity:** Sedentary—owns a bookstore, no other activity **Culture/Religion:** Arabic (traditional foods); Muslim (no pork) **Food Allergy:** Shellfish **Meds/Supplements:** As noted in chart, no supplements **Food Availability:** Wife shops/cooks

Problem Solving Matrix Assessment for SB Case Study Step: Nutrition Diagnosis	
Client History: Medical; nutritionally relevant Dx	T2DM, HTN, GERD (uses OTC calcium CO3), peripheral neuropathy, foot ulcer x 1yr
Social History: Lives alone, support, occupation, income, education level, program participation	Positive for tobacco; denies ETOH, drug use; lives w/wife (wife cooks); owns bookstore
Determine/Estimate Nutrient Needs	**Estimated Nutrient Needs (Nutrition Prescription)**
Energy needs: Use range equation, Mifflin, Harris-Benedict, etc. (consider activity and stress or disease-specific factors)	2660–3200 cal (using 25cal–30/kg body wt): For T2DM and overweight status: 1800 cal
Protein needs: Use facility intake standards (consider disease-specific needs)	128 g (based on 1.2 g/kg actual body wt)
Fluid needs: Use facility intake standards (consider disease-specific needs)	2.6 L–3.2 L (based on 1 ml/cal)

Problem Solving Matrix Assessment for SB Case Study

Step: Nutrition Diagnosis

2.0 Diagnosis

• *Compare analyzed data to standards:* Use the data from 1.0 Assessment to identify all potential nutrition concerns; analyze each concern by comparing it to all others listed and looking for correlations that verify only nutritionally relevant concerns; then determine if those can be resolved by the RD and list nutrition diagnoses.

Data Categories	A. Identify & list all potential nutrition concerns (any abnormal parameters)	B. Analyze potential concerns as they relate to each other to determine if actual concerns exist; list only actual, nutritionally relevant current concerns (e.g., is low BMI d/t decreased appetite or does Hx show the patient's BMI has always been low?)	C. Determine if concerns listed in column B can be resolved by the RD, and then list all possible Nutrition Diagnoses for each domain (Intake, Clinical, Behavior-Environmental)		
			Intake	Clinical	B-E
Anthropometric	Overweight at BMI 29.3, 119% IBW	No recent weight change, but high BMI increases DM risks	1) Energy Balance: Excess energy intake	3) Weight: Overweight	1) Knowledge & Beliefs: Food and nutrition knowledge deficit 1.6) Limited adherence to nutrition-related recommendations 2) Physical Activity: Physical inactivity

Problem Solving Matrix Assessment for SB Case Study Step: Nutrition Diagnosis				
Biochemical, Test, Procedures	BGL in poor control, A1C 7.5%	Poor glycemic control increases risk for DM complications	5.8) Nutrient/ CHO: Excessive CHO intake; Intake of types of CHO inconsistent with needs	2) Altered nutrition-related labs (A1C, BGL)	1) Knowledge & Beliefs: Food and nutrition knowledge deficit 1.4) Self- monitoring deficit 1.6) Limited adherence to nutrition-related recommendations
NFPE Findings	Swelling of RLE, foot ulcer x 1 yr (related to poor glycemic control); Excess abdominal girth	Related to poor glycemic control			

(*Continued*)

Problem Solving Matrix Assessment for SB Case Study

Step: Nutrition Diagnosis

History (Appetite/intake, knowledge & behavior, any other relevant history)		Inadequate knowledge regarding DM risks and self-management (carbohydrate counting, excess weight, SMBG)		1) Knowledge & Beliefs: Food and nutrition knowledge deficit 2) Physical Activity: Physical inactivity 1.4) Self- monitoring deficit 1.6) Limited adherence to nutrition-related recommendations
No SMBG; no dietary changes for DM; no instruction on diet for DM; high salt intake; high CHO intake				
Current intake/ Diet Rx status	Can patient meet EEN? Y/N	Is diet Rx tolerated? Y/N		

Problem Solving Matrix Assessment for SB Case Study
Step: Nutrition Diagnosis

2.1 Diagnosis in PES format
♦ Describe all identified concerns from 2.0 C. as Nutrition Diagnoses in PES format

Nutrition diagnosis or problem (P)		Etiology (E)		Signs and/or Symptoms (S)
Self-monitoring deficit	*related to*	Knowledge deficit	*as evidenced by*	elevated BGL >300 mg/dL (10/13), 152, 147, 158, 297 (10/17) and diet Hx/pt report
Food and nutrition knowledge deficit	*related to*	Lack of previous instruction	*as evidenced by*	diet history

Determine Nutrition Status

From the Nutrition Diagnoses; identify the patient's Nutrition Status

1. **Normal**
2. **Mildly compromised**
3. **Moderately compromised**
4. **Severely compromised**

Normal. Although this patient is not nutritionally compromised, there are still nutrition knowledge deficits that need to be addressed.

(Continued)

CHAPTER 6

Nutrition Intervention

PLANNING DIETS AND COORDINATING CARE

By the end of the chapter, the reader will be able to

- Identify the nutrition interventions domains within the Nutrition Care Process
- Provide examples of interventions for all the domains
- Describe the use of the Evidence Analysis Library in evidence-based dietetic practice and particularly in determining nutrition interventions in the Nutrition Care Process
- Match common therapeutic diets with specific diseases and conditions
- After completing nutrition assessment and diagnosis for a patient case, select the most appropriate and evidenced-based nutrition intervention/s

n the nutrition intervention step of the nutrition care process, after collecting and assessing data to make the nutrition diagnosis, the RD determines the interventions to solve the nutrition problems identified in the nutrition diagnosis (1). This may consist of one or more of the following general steps in planning:

1. Gathering more data/requesting data
2. Coordinating the patient's care with other health care professionals or institutions

3. Modifying some aspect of the physical diet or how it is provided to the patient

4. Recommending or implementing education

The nutrition intervention step also includes development of the nutrition prescription, which refers to the patient's estimated nutrient needs based on reference standards and guidelines, and importantly, the nutrition diagnosis. The purpose of the nutrition prescription is to state in the patient's medical record the RD's recommendations based on the nutrition assessment and diagnosis. The estimation of energy needs, an important component of the nutrition prescription, is covered in Chapter 2.

NUTRITION INTERVENTION: SOLVING NUTRITION PROBLEMS AND MEETING NEEDS

The Nutrition Intervention Domains

Nutrition intervention encompasses the five domains of Food and/or Nutrient Delivery (ND), Nutrition Education (E), Nutrition Counseling (C), Coordination of Nutrition Care by a Nutrition Professional (RC), and Population-Based Nutrition Action (P) (Table 6.1) (1). Within each domain, there are classes and subclasses, so that the RD can be specific in selecting and documenting the intervention. Nutrition interventions generally should target the etiology of the nutrition diagnosis problem (problem/etiology/signs and symptoms). However, if the RD cannot affect the etiology of the problem, they may need to target the signs and symptoms in the diagnosis. Box 6.1 provides examples of how nutrition intervention targets the etiology of the problem of the nutrition diagnosis. This chapter focuses on the ND domain, as domains E and C are covered in Chapter 8. The RC domain will be covered briefly; however, the P domain occurs outside the clinical setting and will not be covered.

Medical nutrition therapy (MNT) is commonly used interchangeably with nutrition intervention to signify the use of a therapeutic diet or provision of nutrition education. For example, definitions on the Internet describe MNT as a "therapeutic approach to treating medical conditions and their associated symptoms via the use of a specifically tailored diet" (2). However, the Academy defines MNT more broadly to encompass the entire nutrition care process as the:

"Evidence-based application of the Nutrition Care Process. The provision of MNT (to a patient/client) may include one or more of the following: nutrition assessment/re-assessment, nutrition diagnosis, nutrition intervention and nutrition monitoring and evaluation that typically results in the prevention, delay or management of diseases and/or conditions" (3).

TABLE 6.1 Nutrition Intervention Domains

Domain	Domain Categories/Descriptions
Food and/or Nutrient Delivery	Meals and Snacks Enteral and Parenteral Nutrition Supplements Feeding Assistance Feeding Environment Nutrition-Related Medication Management
Nutrition Education	Brief diet instruction in hospital at bedside; outpatient instruction
Nutrition Counseling	In-depth collaboration between RD and client that may include advanced counseling techniques, such as the RD's use of cognitive-behavioral theory and motivational interviewing
Coordination of Nutrition Care by a Nutrition Professional	Collaboration and Referral of Nutrition Care Discharge and Transfer of Nutrition Care to New Setting or Provider
Population-Based Nutrition Action	Interventions for the improvement of nutritional health of a population

Reference: Academy of Nutrition and Dietetics. *Nutrition Terminology Reference Manual (eNCPT): Dietetics Language for Nutrition Care.* http://www.ncpro.org.

BOX 6.1

Nutrition Intervention Targets of the Nutrition Diagnosis

Nutrition Diagnosis	**Nutrition Intervention**
Inadequate oral intake (*problem*) related to **inability to self-feed** post-CVA (*etiology*) as evidenced by 60% PO and 5% weight loss x 1 month (*signs and symptoms*)	Targets the Etiology of the Problem Adaptive eating devices (plate and tableware) Domain: Food and/or Nutrient Delivery Class: Feeding Assistance
Swallowing difficulty (*problem*) related to paralysis from recent CVA (*etiology*) as evidenced by choking when eating and drinking (*signs and symptoms*)	Targets the Signs and Symptoms Pureed diet Domain: Food and/or Nutrient Delivery Class: Meals and Snacks Subclass: Texture modified diet

Evidenced-Based Practice

It is clear from the Academy definition that nutrition interventions must be grounded in evidence-based dietetic practice, which the Academy defines as "the process of asking questions, systematically finding research evidence, and assessing its validity, applicability and importance to food and nutrition practice decisions; and includes applying relevant evidence in the context of the practice situation and the values of clients, customers and communities to achieve positive outcomes" (3).

For dietitians, the best resource for ensuring that nutrition interventions are the most current evidence-based interventions is the Academy's Evidence Analysis Library (EAL). Academy members have access to the online EAL at no cost. In addition to providing citations for research and other articles included in the review, the EAL also includes patient education resources that are available for purchase. At the EAL site, topics can be accessed at the "Projects" tab or in an alphabetized "Index" (Box 6.2) (4). Topics include nutritionally relevant diseases, such as hypertension; nutrients, foods, and dietary compounds, such as dietary fatty acids and fruit juice; nutrition needs and concerns in specific age groups, such as older adults; and nutrition issues, such as nutrition screening and telenutrition.

BOX 6.2

Evidence Analysis Library FAQs

What is it?
— An online tool that incorporates nutrition research and in key areas of dietetic practice; it includes systematic reviews with conclusive statements on key nutrition topics, as well as: bibliographies, grades for conclusive statements, and recommendations

How often are guidelines updated?
— Every five years

Who can use it?
— Free to Academy members

How do I learn how to use it?
— The EAL includes an orientation tutorial: https://www.andeal.org/tutorials

Why is the EAL important to dietitians?
— The EAL contributes to and ensures evidence-based practice for high-quality patient care and outcomes

Reference: Academy of Nutrition and Dietetics Evidence Analysis Library. Available at: https://www.andeal.org/

As part of the nutrition prescription, the dietitian can only recommend diet changes outlined in the facility's diet manual. A diet manual includes all therapeutic diets that the facility provides. The diet manual can be one that the facility or its contract company, if the facility uses a contract company, has developed, or a commercially produced manual such as the Academy's Nutrition Care Manual (5). A thorough knowledge of the facility's manual is essential, as it provides the dietitian with all therapeutic diets available, as well as a description of the circumstances in which the diet is used and its recommended duration, which is important for some diets. Some therapeutic diets are intended only as a transitionary regimen, also known as transition diets. These diets usually consist of liquids or soft solid foods that most people easily tolerate, often used after surgery. Transition diets typically do not provide adequate essential nutrients; for example, as with a clear liquid diet.

FOOD AND/OR NUTRIENT DELIVERY

Within the first classification of the food and nutrient delivery domain, the dietitian will find the most commonly used interventions, modification of the physical diet or how it is delivered to the patient. This first classification, "Meals and Snacks: General, Modify, Specific Foods," includes the various modifications to the physical diet and how it is provided to the patient (1).

The diet and how it is provided may be modified as to any of the following aspects:

- Essential nutrients
- Dietary/food constituent
- Texture, consistency
- Route of administration
- Energy level
- Feeding environment

Diet modifications may be temporary, such as not feeding a patient (NPO status, or *nil per os*) or with a transition diet, or long term. A patient on NPO status may be undergoing diagnostic procedures or awaiting surgery. A key point regarding diet modification is that even a seemingly minor change can adversely affect appetite and food intake; therefore, the RD needs to monitor oral (PO) intake after a modification, as well as nutritional status and needs if intake declines. For this reason, after a modification is made, it is important to try to progress back to a regular diet, if and when possible. An example is a texture or consistency modification, such as providing only ground meat. A patient may find this unappetizing and reduce his intake of the typical protein source in the diet, so the dietitian should make all possible effort at diet progression.

Another common example of the impact of diet modification is sodium reduction, which for a patient accustomed to a high intake, may result in a reduction in appetite and intake. In an elderly patient, who may already have lost weight, this could present a significant risk to nutritional status. In this example, the modification is likely to be long term or permanent, as it may be related to a chronic disease. Therefore, while a modification may be necessary and likely permanent, it's important for the dietitian to assess appetite, intake, and any potential effect on nutritional status.

Essential Nutrients

Any of the essential nutrients, the micronutrients of vitamins and minerals, and the macronutrients (energy-yielding nutrients) of protein, fat, and carbohydrate, may be modified for therapeutic purposes (Table 6.2). The diet may be modified, or essential nutrients may be given in supplemental form. In addition, it may also be necessary to modify water (fluid) intake in patients with specific diseases and in certain conditions. In general, essential nutrients are more typically increased in the diet rather than reduced. For example, in a patient who has lost weight and is nutritionally compromised, it is usually important to recommend higher protein and energy intake. However, in the case of protein, a patient with chronic kidney disease (depending on the stage) will need to monitor protein intake to not exceed the DRI, which the typical American diet exceeds by up to 75% (6, 7). Energy (caloric) level, not relative to a specific macronutrient, can also be modified for the purposes of weight gain or weight loss. In the assessment phase of the NCP, the RD estimates the patient's energy needs by using various techniques, usually with equations (see Chapter 2).

TABLE 6.2 Essential Nutrient Modifications

Nutrient	Modification	Disease / Condition*
Nutrient: Protein		
Total amount	Higher	Compromised nutrition status, kidney disease, kidney dialysis
	Lower	Kidney disease
Specific amino acids	Higher	Amino acids shown to enhance GI function (glutamine, arginine, cysteine)
	Lower	Congenital metabolic diseases, such as PKU and Krabbe disease
Nutrient: Fat / Fatty Acids		
Total amount	Higher	
	Lower	Fat malabsorption
Specific type	Unsaturated	Cardiovascular diseases
	n-3 fatty acids	Cardiovascular diseases, inflammatory diseases
	Saturated	Cardiovascular diseases
	Long-Chain	Congenital metabolic diseases
	Medium-Chain Triglyceride	Fat malabsorption
Nutrient: Minerals		
Sodium	Lower	Hypertension and other cardiovascular diseases, edema, ascites, liver disease, kidney disease, dialysis
Potassium	Lower	Kidney disease
Calcium	Adequate intake	Kidney stones
Phosphorus	Lower	Kidney disease, dialysis

Nutrient	Modification	Disease / Condition*
Nutrient: Carbohydrate		
Total amount	Higher	When protein is either restricted or when higher, for protein-sparing effect
	Consistent/ Controlled	Diabetes, using carbohydrate counting
Specific type	Fiber—Lower	Reduce GI peristalsis/ stimulation in diarrhea, or exacerbation of GI diseases (diverticular disease, inflammatory bowel disease)
Nutrient: Fluid (Water)	Higher	Kidney stones, kidney disease (Fanconi's syndrome)
	Lower	Kidney disease, heart failure, overhydration

* Not intended as a comprehensive list

References: Academy of Nutrition and Dietetics. *Nutrition Care Manual.* Available for subscription at: https://www.nutritioncaremanual.org/

Protein and Amino Acids

The most common protein modification is providing additional protein to a patient who is nutritionally compromised. In addition to this modification in a patient with general malnutrition, patients undergoing dialysis may require higher protein intake, depending on the specific type of dialysis and their nutrition status. When an increase in protein is indicated, it is also important to provide additional energy (calories) from other macronutrients in order to spare the protein for protein synthesis (8).

Protein may also be modified as to specific amino acids, by either an increase or reduction. The most common example is the addition of glutamine, arginine, and cysteine, amino acids that some studies show can enhance gut function (9). However, specific amino acids must be restricted in various congenital metabolic diseases in which the body cannot metabolize a particular amino acid. For example, in phenylketonuria, the patient lacks the phenylalanine hydroxylase, the enzyme that metabolizes phenylalanine. If intake of this amino acid is not restricted, phenylalanine can reach toxic levels (10).

The trio of branched chain amino acids (BCAA)—leucine, isoleucine, and valine—can also be increased in various liver diseases in which the organ is not functioning adequately, since the liver does not metabolize these amino acids. However, in the case of Krabbe disease (maple-syrup urine disease), another congenital metabolic disease, patients lack branched chain-alpha-keto acid dehydrogenase, the enzyme that metabolizes the BCAA, and these amino acids must be restricted (11).

The amino acid tyramine, which can be synthesized from tyrosine, must be restricted when a patient is taking a medication known as a monoamine oxidase inhibitor (MAOI) (Box 6.3). The MAO enzyme normally counters the blood pressure–raising effect of tyramine, but this action is inhibited by these drugs. If the patient has a high level of dietary tyramine, this can cause a hypertensive crisis leading to a stroke.

Specific proteins can also damage the intestinal mucosa in genetically susceptible individuals, as in the case of people with celiac disease, an autoimmune disease. The damaging compound is gliadin, the storage protein fraction of grain endosperms, and a fraction of the gluten protein (5). Foods that contain these proteins are wheat, barley, rye, and ingredients made from these grains, which all must be avoided by those with celiac disease to prevent damage to the small intestine, by being on a gluten-free diet.

BOX 6.3

Monoamine Oxidase Inhibitor (MAOIs) Drugs and Foods to Avoid

MAOIs

Isocarboxazid

Phenelzine

Selegiline

Tranylcypromine

Tyramine-Containing Foods to Avoid

Aged Cheese

Alcohol

Dried and Overripe Fruits

Fermented/Pickled Foods

Legumes: Fava Beans, Snow Peas

Meat Tenderizer

Processed/Smoked Meats

Soybeans/Soy-Containing Foods and Sauces

Yeast-Containing Foods

Reference: Mayo Clinic. Diseases and Conditions. https://www.mayoclinic.org/
diseases-conditions/depression/in-depth/maois/art-20043992

Dietary Fat: Total Fat and Specific Fatty Acids

The most typical fat modifications are related to the prevention and treatment of cardiovascular disease via the effects of fatty acids on blood lipids. These modifications follow the American Heart Association and the American College of Cardiology guidelines with reduction in saturated fatty acids and a shift toward unsaturated fatty acids (12) (Table 6.3). In addition, although not a triglyceride, dietary cholesterol is also reduced in accordance with the guidelines. Dietitians help patients who have had a cardiovascular event, usually a myocardial infarction, in hospitals and cardiac rehabilitation programs, as well as in outpatient settings to reduce the risk for an event in patients with various dyslipidemias.

Many diseases or conditions can cause fat malabsorption (Box 6.4), which can cause several nutrition-related problems (Box 6.5). One of the most important of these is weight loss because of the loss of energy from fat, the most calorically dense of the macronutrients. Medium-chain triglycerides (MCTs), in which the fatty acids are six to 12 carbons in length, are sometimes used to replace the loss of energy from fat malabsorption because they require no emulsification and minimal digestion to be absorbed (13). They are commercially hydrolyzed from longer-chain fatty acid sources, usually palm kernel and coconut oil. The MCTs provide 8.3 kcal/gram, close to typical dietary triglycerides of 9 kcal/gram, although they do not contain the essential fatty acids of linoleic and linolenic acids. The MCTs can be provided as ingredients in formulas or as stand-alone products for patient use.

Another fat modification is the use of short-chain fatty acids (SCFAs), which are two to six carbons in length, specifically propionate, butyrate, and acetate. These fatty acids are produced by gut microbes, for which soluble fiber serves as a substrate (14). Because SCFAs reduce the pH of the large intestine, they may have a laxative effect, which may be problematic for some patients. However, they also positively affect the intestine by limiting uptake of ammonia, reducing dehydroxylation of bile acids, which renders these compounds potential carcinogens (15). The SCFAs are an important energy source for gut cells, particularly butyrate, which provides 70% of the energy for these cells, enhancing gut function and repairing damage from intestinal diseases and surgery (14).

TABLE 6.3 AHA/ACC Lifestyle Modifications to Reduce Cardiovascular Risk

Diet	1) Emphasize: Vegetables, fruits, and whole grains; low-fat dairy, poultry, fish, legumes, nontropical oils and nuts
	2) Limit intake of sweets, sugar-sweetened beverages, red meats
	3) Follow plans such as DASH, AHA Diet, USDA Food Pattern
	4) Lower sodium intake to 2300mg daily,1500mg more desirable
	5) SFA: Aim for a dietary pattern of 5% to 6% of calories from SFA
	6) TFA: Reduce percent of calories from trans fat
Physical Activity	40 minutes of moderate to vigorous intensity 3 to 4 days weekly

Reference: Eckel, R. H., Jakicic, J. M., Ard, J. D, et al. (2014). 2013 AHA/ACC Guideline on lifestyle management to reduce cardiovascular risk: A Report of the American College of Cardiology/American Heart Association Task Force on Practice Guidelines. *Circulation, 129.* S76–S99

BOX 6.4

Fat Malabsorption

Significant nutritional concern
– Loss of energy, fat-soluble nutrients, loss of calcium and magnesium with steatorrhea

General causes

– Interference with bile action; liver, gallbladder; biliary tract obstruction

– Gut stasis/bacterial overgrowth (many causes)

– Interference with lipases, pancreas, or pancreatic duct

– Ileal dysfunction

Specific causes

Blind Loop; Celiac Disease; Medications; Endocrine Disorders; Fistulas; Gastrectomy; Inflammatory Bowel Disease; Liver Disease; Pancreatic Disease; Short Bowel Syndrome (Removal/Resection); Intestinal Bypass Surgery

References: Medscape. Malabsorption Clinical Presentation. History. Available at: https://emedicine.medscape.com/article/180785-clinical. Causes.

https://emedicine.medscape.com/article/180785-clinical#b5

BOX 6.5

Consequences of Fat Malabsorption

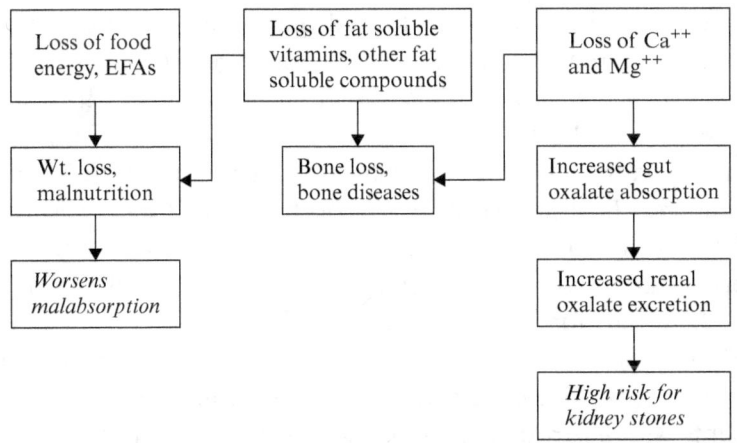

Carbohydrate: Total Amount and Type

Dietary carbohydrate is most often controlled in the management of diabetes. However, several diseases necessitate the restriction of one of the other macronutrients, and carbohydrate is increased to replace the energy from the restricted macronutrient. Although carbohydrate had historically been restricted in diabetes, the current approach is to control the total amount for a more consistent daily intake and focus on foods containing complex carbohydrate and dietary fiber over simple carbohydrates and sugar, as stated in the 2018 Guidelines: "an emphasis on foods higher in fiber and lower in glycemic load is preferred over other sources, especially those containing added sugars" (16). The patient teaching approach involves the use of carbohydrate choices (Box 6.6), in which the dietitian determines the optimal carbohydrate level (in grams) for individual patients to balance with either endogenous insulin, exogenous insulin, or medications, and physical activity. This is divided by 15 for a specific number of daily carbohydrate choices for the patient to consume a consistent amount and type of carbohydrate to manage their diabetes for optimal glycemic control.

Specific types of carbohydrates must sometimes be restricted, usually a disaccharide, in response to inadequate synthesis of the enzyme needed for hydrolysis, or disease-induced damage to the intestinal cells that produce the enzyme. This is referred to as carbohydrate intolerance and malabsorption, or disaccharidase deficiency, although a monosaccharide may also be malabsorbed, such as fructose. The most common of the disaccharide malabsorptions are of lactose, sucrose, and maltose (17, 18). The prevalence of lactose malabsorption is 65% internationally, with some groups as high as 90%, leading some to consider it the more normal state.

Dietary fiber encompasses an array of carbohydrate compounds that the human digestive tract does not have enzymes to degrade. Patients with gastrointestinal diseases may require modification of dietary fiber, either an increase or a reduction. These diseases and conditions include irritable bowel syndrome, inflammatory bowel disease, diverticular disease, surgical intestinal resections, diarrhea, and constipation. The recommended daily levels of dietary fiber for healthy men and women under the age of 50 are 38 grams and

25 grams, respectively (19). At ages 51 and above, the recommended levels are 30 grams for men and 21 grams for women. However, the estimated average intake is 16 grams daily, well below the recommended levels (20). As with many nutrient modifications relative to actual patient intake and recommended levels, both restrictions and increases must consider patient intake.

BOX 6.6

The Carbohydrate Choices Approach for Diabetes

1. Determine the level of carbohydrate (in grams) for the patient to maintain optimal glycemic control, based on:
   - Exogenous insulin (Type 1 or Type 2 Diabetes)
   - Endogenous insulin (Type 2 Diabetes)
   - Medications (Blood glucose–lowering agents)
   - Physical activity

   Example, based on above, patient needs:
   - 2000 calories, 50% as carbohydrate; 1000 carbohydrate calories
   - Divide carbohydrate calories (1000) by 4 calories per gram to yield carbohydrate in grams; 250 grams of carbohydrate

2. Divide the carbohydrate (in grams) by 15 grams to yield daily carbohydrate choices

   Example:
   - 250 grams carbohydrate/15 grams
   - 16.7 carbohydrate choices, round to 17

3. Teach patient to match carbohydrate choices with insulin, or medications, and physical activity

Micronutrients: Vitamins and Minerals

In general, vitamins would not be restricted or controlled, but one exception is vitamin K. Anticoagulant and antiplatelet medications interfere with clot formation, which is crucial to prevent cardiovascular events, such as stroke or heart attack, in high-risk patients. The vitamin is a cofactor for a carboxylase that activates seven protein components of the blood-clotting cascade (21). Patients on these medications must consume a consistent level of vitamin K to avoid interfering with the medication. High dietary intake or supplements reduce the effectiveness of the drugs.

Several minerals must often be modified for various diseases and conditions. The most commonly restricted mineral is sodium. Although the recommendation for the healthy public is less than 2300 mg/day (12), the average daily intake in the United States is well above this level at 3400 mg/day (22). Because the average intake exceeds the recommendation, some hospitals still consider sodium restrictions at levels that also exceed the recommended level, varying from 1500 mg to 4000 mg (23). Sodium restriction is used for volume-dependent conditions that cause edema and ascites, including cardiovascular diseases such as heart failure and hypertension, liver diseases, kidney diseases, and balance disorders such as Meniere's disease. In addition, specific medications may necessitate a sodium-restricted diet, as is the case with prednisone, an anti-inflammatory drug that causes fluid retention (24).

One of the most important mineral restrictions is that of potassium in kidney disease because it can be life threatening. When the kidney loses the ability to adequately filter potassium, serum levels rise and can cause cardiac arrest. Another mineral that may require restriction in kidney disease is phosphorus. In addition to dietary restriction, patients may be prescribed drugs that bind these minerals: phosphate binders and potassium binders (25). However, common medications such as potassium-wasting diuretics deplete the body of potassium, and a dietary increase in foods high in potassium or supplement is sometimes necessary (26). Another common medication that may necessitate an increase in potassium intake is digoxin, prescribed for heart failure or arrhythmias (27).

Dietary/Food Constituent

Several compounds in foods or types of foods must be restricted for specific diseases and conditions (Table 6.4). One example is a patient with esophagitis, in whom the esophagus is inflamed and irritated from any number of possible causes. Foods high in acid, such as fruits, will aggravate the inflamed tissue, causing pain, so these should be avoided. Patients with gastritis or peptic ulcers, in contrast, do not need to restrict high acid foods since the pH of the stomach is lower than any food. However, it's important to reduce gastric secretions, primarily gastric acid, so these patients need to restrict food ingredients and beverages that stimulate sections or irritate gastric mucosa, such as alcohol, black pepper, chili pepper/powder, cocoa, caffeine, coffee, and tea, including these latter two beverages in decaffeinated form.

Another example of a dietary constituent that is restricted is oxalate (oxalic acid), an organic acid contained in some plant foods that binds to essential minerals like calcium and iron, rendering them unabsorbable. The compound is also endogenously produced as a metabolite of amino acids and ascorbic acid (28). As calcium oxalate, it is the most common type of kidney stone, found in up to 80% of kidney stones. For patients with this type of stone, or patients who are high risk for kidney stones, such as those with fat malabsorption, avoiding foods high in oxalate is important (Box 6.7).

Oxalate can't be metabolized, so it is degraded by colonic bacteria, excreted in urine and stool as calcium oxalate (29). Since dietary calcium is not fully absorbed, some will bind to the oxalate, and the amount of calcium available is important in the normal excretion of oxalate. High urinary oxalate (hyperoxaluria), either from high dietary intake, a metabolic problem, or the lack of adequate unbound calcium to bind oxalate, promotes the formation of kidney stones. One of the consequences of fat malabsorption arising from a disease or as the result of bariatric surgery is that calcium and magnesium form soaps from the unabsorbed fatty acids, which pass into the stool, producing steatorrhea (Box 6.5) (30). Because calcium, which would normally bind to oxalate, instead is bound to unabsorbed fatty acids, urinary oxalate is high, which increases the risk for stone formation.

TABLE 6.4 Dietary Constituent Modifications

	Modification	Disease / Condition
Acidity	Avoid citrus fruits and juices, pineapple, tomato, coffee and tea (regular and decaffeinated), beverages containing caffeine	Irritated or inflamed esophagus, as in GERD, hiatal hernia, esophageal varices
Gastric Stimulants/ Irritants	Alcohol, black pepper, chili pepper/powder, cocoa, caffeine-containing beverages/foods, coffee, and tea, including these decaffeinated	Gastritis, peptic ulcer disease
Gluten	Products containing wheat, barley, rye, triticale (limit oats, based on individual response), beer, malt, soy sauce	Celiac disease, gluten intolerance
Oxalate	See Box 6.7	Kidney stones, fat malabsorption, as can occur in diseases of the liver, biliary tract, pancreas; short bowel syndrome; bariatric surgeries involving intestinal bypass

References: Jackson Siegelbaum Gastroenterology. Gastroesophageal reflux disease. Available at: https://www.gicare.com/diets/gerd/; HealthHype.com. Gastritis diet. Available at: https://www.healthhype.com/gastritis-diet-peptic-ulcer-diet-foods-to-avoid-and-lifestyle.html; Celiac Disease Foundation. What Is Gluten? Available at: https://celiac.org/live-gluten-free/glutenfreediet/what-is-gluten/

BOX 6.7

Foods High in Oxalate

Grains: Wheat bran

Legumes and Nuts: Nuts, soybeans

Vegetables: Beets, chards, okra, potatoes, rhubarb, spinach, sweet potatoes

Other: Black pepper, chocolate, coffee, tea

References: Mayo Clinic. Available at: https://www.mayoclinic.org/diseases-conditions/kidney-stones/diagnosis-treatment/drc-20355759

Stewart, C. S., Duncan, S. H., & Cave, D. R. (2004). *Oxalobacter formigenes* and its role in oxalate metabolism in the human gut. *FEMS Microbiol Lett, 230* (1): 1–7.

Texture and Consistency

Modifying the texture and consistency is important in several conditions and in many situations serves as a transition to a regular diet. The reasons for modifying the diet are varied, as are the diets, which include clear liquid, full liquid, blenderized, and mechanically altered (5) (Table 6.5). In a mechanically altered diet, sometimes called a mechanical soft diet, specific foods will be modified in texture to varying extents, such as ground meats up to all pureed foods for patients with difficulty chewing. Facilities use a variety of names for these diets; for example, some facilities use a gastrointestinal (GI) soft diet, or a soft diet, which is typically low in fiber, soft in texture, and readily digestible for most patients. The purpose of the GI soft, which is a transitional diet, is to reduce gastrointestinal discomfort in patients with GI diseases or those who have had abdominal surgery (31). Patients with swallowing difficulty (dysphagia) for various reasons will require a staged approach to consistency for foods and liquids (32).

TABLE 6.5 Texture and Consistency Modified Diets

	Modification/s	Disease / Condition
Blenderized	Any regular foods are blenderized to pureed consistency; can be thinned to desired consistency by adding water	Problems causing chewing difficulties or having difficulty eating solid foods; jaw surgery
Clear Liquid	Clear liquids only: examples include water, broth, gelatin, coffee and tea (no cream), soda, popsicles	Preparation for diagnostic or medical procedures; digestive problems such as diarrhea
Dysphagia	Staged approach with different levels of consistency of foods and thickness of liquids	Stroke, head and neck injuries/cancer
Full Liquid	Any liquids, typically milk-based, strained cream-based soups; includes all liquids from clear liquid list	Preparation for diagnostic or medical procedures; post-surgery for gastric or intestinal disorders; problems with chewing or swallowing; can be progression from clear liquid
Gastrointestinal Soft (Bland Diet)	Foods typically soft in texture, low fiber; avoid foods that are raw (fruits and vegetables) spicy, fried; avoid alcohol and caffeine	Reduce peristalsis GI stimulation/irritation; peptic ulcer disease, chronic gastritis, GERD (and hiatal hernia), excessive flatulence
Mechanical Soft (Dental Soft)	Foods are modified in texture to the specific needs of the patient; foods may be ground, mashed, minced, or even pureed	Chewing and swallowing problems

References: Academy of Nutrition and Dietetics. *Nutrition Care Manual.* Available for subscription at: https://www.nutritioncaremanual.org/; Today's Dietitian. Blenderized Diet. Available at: http://www.todaysdietitian.com/newarchives/011315p30.shtml; Mayo Clinic. Clear Liquid Diet. Available at: https://www.mayoclinic.org/healthy-lifestyle/nutrition.../clear-liquid-diet/art-20048505; International Dysphagia Diet Standardisation Initiative. Complete IDDSIF Framework-Detailed definitions. Available at: http://iddsi.org/Documents/IDDSIFrame-work-CompleteFramework.pdf; NIH U.S. National Library of Medicine. MedlinePlus. Liquid diet—full. Available at: https://medlineplus.gov/ency/patientinstructions/000206.htm

Route of Administration

The route of administration refers to providing nutrients in the normal manner (oral, or by mouth), enteral, and parenteral. Providing enteral nutrition consists of using the GI tract by means of insertion of a feeding tube and the infusion of a formula. The tube can be inserted at various points, and it can deliver the formula to specific parts of the GI tract. In parenteral feeding, the GI tract is bypassed, and a solution of nutrients is infused directly into the bloodstream. Both forms are invasive, which means that they present potential risks to the patient, and they are costlier than oral feeding, with parenteral nutrition presenting more risk and cost. The main reason for using parenteral nutrition is a situation in which the GI is either not functional or can't be used. Parenteral nutrition can also be used when a patient's energy needs exceed their ability to consume this level, such as in a patient with severe burns. At times, it may be beneficial to use a combination of administration routes, such as small amounts of enteral feeding in addition to parenteral nutrition supplying most of the patient's needs.

Whether a patient will be fed enterally or parenterally, the dietitian plays a major role in nutrition intervention for the patient. This begins with the nutrition assessment phase of the nutrition care process, in which the RD determines the patient's energy needs. Since this type of patient is typically relying solely on the nutrition provided and not consuming food on his own, it is even more crucial that the energy, nutrients, and fluid provided are sufficient to meet the needs.

In addition, in the case of an enteral formula, the RD makes recommendations as to any special modifications to the nutrients contained in the formula that would benefit the patient. For example, a patient who has lost significant weight may require a formula high in energy and protein (based on formula density) compared to a standard formula that usually provides 1 kcal/ml and 0.38 grams of protein/ml (33). Disease-specific formulas are designed to meet the needs of patients with certain conditions or diseases with various modifications of nutrients, additional therapeutic ingredients, and concentration of the constituents for volume-sensitive conditions (34).

Energy Level

The energy or calorie level may be modified to promote weight gain, as discussed relative to the high-calorie, high-protein diet, or to promote weight loss. In overweight and obese patients, even modest weight loss can improve several conditions, such as type 2 diabetes, hypertension, and other cardiovascular diseases. To plan a weight loss regimen, dietitians often use the Exchange Lists System (ELS), developed in 1950 by the American Diabetes Association and the American Dietetic Association (now the Academy of Nutrition and Dietetics), and the U.S. Public Health Service (35). The ELS was originally used exclusively for people with diabetes, both type 1 and type 2. However, with the focus in diabetes now on controlling carbohydrate with the use of Carbohydrate Counting, the ELS is now best used in planning a nutrition regimen, especially for promoting weight loss.

The ELS consists of groups of foods with similar macronutrient (energy-yielding nutrient) profiles (36) (Table 6.6). Within each list, the foods that may be selected or exchanged for each other vary as to the amount or serving size of each individual food that provides the macronutrients and calories for the entire group, which is considered one exchange for that group. In diet planning, the RD begins with an estimate of the patient's current caloric intake, which would maintain the patient's current weight (Box 6.8). The next step is to subtract from that estimate the calories sufficient to produce safe and effective weight loss of one to two pounds weekly (37).

Although the estimate of 3,500 calories for one pound of weight loss (38) has been discredited, it is still widely used since it is divisible by seven (for a daily level) and since an exact caloric value is not possible (39). This yields a figure of 500 to 1000 calories daily to subtract from the current caloric intake in order to produce weight loss. To reduce the level of calories that must be subtracted, RDs can recommend the addition of daily exercise. Once the diet plan energy level has been determined, the RD decides on the macronutrient distribution; i.e., the percentages of carbohydrate, fat, and protein.

Specific reasons may direct the decision on the macronutrient distribution, such as client preference or use of a Mediterranean pattern moderately higher in fat, or a typical distribution may be used consisting of 50% carbohydrate, 30% fat, and 20% protein. The percentages are converted into calories for each macronutrient and then converted to totals in grams; for example, a 1500-calorie diet plan using the typical macronutrient distribution would yield 750 calories from carbohydrate, which converts to 188 grams. From this point, the RD calculates the number of exchanges from each of the groups, from which the client can plan meals and vary the food choices using the exchanges in each group.

TABLE 6.6 Exchange Lists

Group	Carbohydrate (grams)	Protein (grams)	Fat (grams)	kcals
Milk, fat free or 1%	12	8	0	90
Veg	5	2	0	25
Fruit	15	0	0	60
Starch	15	3	1	80
Very Lean Protein	0	6 to 7	1	35
Lean Protein	0	7	2 to 3	55
Medium Lean Protein	0	7 to 8	5	75
Fat	0	0	5	45

Reference: National Heart, Lung, and Blood Institute. Available at: https://www.nhlbi.nih.gov/health/educational/lose_wt/eat/fd_exch.htm

---

BOX 6.8

Steps in Diet Planning

1. Using either equations or from analysis of actual client dietary intake, estimate the current average daily energy intake
2. From the current energy intake, subtract 500 to 1000 calories daily
3. Add back to energy intake calories for regular planned physical activity

4. Determine the macronutrient distribution for the diet plan; consider client preferences or special dietary needs. If no special considerations, use 50% carbohydrate, 30% fat, 20% protein

5. Determine calories from each macronutrient, then convert the calories to grams for each macronutrient

6. Start with minimum servings from specific groups based on current recommendations; in adults, for example: 3 milk/dairy, 5 to 8 fruits and vegetables, etc.

7. From the number of exchanges for each group from #6, calculate the grams for each macronutrient

8. Use up all carbohydrate sources except for starch

9. Total the carbohydrate, use remaining as starch

10. Total the protein; use client preference for proteins to add (lean, medium, etc.)

11. Total the fat; use fat exchanges to arrive at the goal grams of fat for the plan

Evaluation of the plan
- Actual calories should be within 25 of the diet plan
- Plan should follow all dietary guidelines and recommendations
- Plan should be tailored to the client's preferences

Feeding Environment

Patients may need assistance of various types with eating. This may involve a caregiver feeding a patient, as in the case of a patient recovering from neck surgery or stroke or a patient with dementia. Some patients may require an accommodation to facilitate their ability to feed themselves, such as adaptive eating equipment, which includes plates with rims and ridged sections and flatware with grips. And still other patients may only require help with meal set-up, such as a caregiver to open food packages, insert straws into beverages, or precut food. It may also be beneficial in a long-term care setting to bring a nonambulatory resident into the dining room for the experience of eating with others, which can improve their food intake.

COORDINATION OF NUTRITION CARE (RC)

The Academy defines the Coordination of Nutrition Care domain as "facilitating service or interventions with other professionals, institutions, or agencies on behalf of the patient/client prior to discharge from nutrition care" (1). In general, this consists of collaboration with others, both within or outside of one's facility. An example in long-term care is the periodic resident care conferences in which health professionals from various disciplines discuss each resident's status and goals. In hospitals and within one's facility, the dietitian may also confer with social work to discuss a patient's discharge to a long-term or rehabilitation facility, as to specific nutrition interventions that need to continue.

Other types of interventions within the RC domain are referrals to other health care professionals within one's facility or to agencies that offer services and programs that may be of benefit to the patient after discharge. Within one's facility, the dietitian may request a speech pathology consult for a patient who is experiencing swallowing difficulty, dysphagia. The speech pathologist, in turn, will conduct procedures called swallowing evaluations, one of which may be done at the bedside, while another is more extensive involving video fluoroscopy, a video fluoroscopic swallowing exam (VFSE). The VFSE is a radiologic examination that assesses the patient's ability to swallow foods and beverages of varying consistencies.

Outside of the facility, the dietitian can make referrals for important services that may be beneficial to the patient. For example, patients being discharged may not be able to purchase groceries or prepare their meals. Community programs that provide home-delivered meals, including therapeutic diets, on a temporary basis can facilitate the transition for the patient to full recovery. Another example of referral to community agencies is making patients of limited income aware of government programs that provide supplemental foods for which they may be eligible.

SELECTING NUTRITION INTERVENTION/S AND DOCUMENTING IN THE MEDICAL RECORD

The nutrition intervention/s, also called the nutrition care plan, should flow logically from the nutrition assessment and diagnosis.

As discussed, the intervention typically is aimed at the etiology of the problem of the nutrition diagnosis, the cause of the problem. However, sometimes the intervention may target the signs and symptoms in the diagnosis (Box 6.1). Since the goal is to solve nutrition problems and address the patient's nutritional needs, it is useful to consider what the desired goal or outcome is for each problem. A model representing this can help to determine the optimal intervention: the components of **P**roblem, **G**oal, **I**ntervention, **E**vidence-based rationale (PGIE) (Table 6.7).

The PGIE model begins with the nutrition diagnoses (P), which describes the nutrition problem in terms of etiology and the evidence that the problem exists. In the next step, a consideration of the goal (G) represents what the problem will look like after its resolution, so it represents the ideal situation for the patient. The example in Table 6.7 presents the nutrition diagnosis for a patient who has had inadequate energy intake, resulting in weight loss. The goal or ideal outcome would be that the patient would regain the weight lost.

In the third step, the RD identifies an appropriate intervention that would bring about the goal, the ideal outcome, of regaining lost weight; an appropriate intervention would be to provide additional energy and protein to support weight regain. In this example, the RD determines after the nutrition assessment that the most effective way to implement this is to provide an oral supplement. And in the final step, the RD must always incorporate evidence-based practice (E) into planned interventions, which in this case is straightforward: provision of an additional 500 calories daily should produce weight gain of approximately one to two pounds per week.

The other problem (P) in the same example relates to the patient's lack of knowledge about diet, which the dietitian determines after conducting a food/nutrition-related history in nutrition assessment (Table 6.7). The ideal outcome, or goal (G), would be that the patient would understand the diet prescription, which will facilitate adherence to the plan. The intervention (I) that is most likely to lead to the goal is for the dietitian to instruct the patient about the diet prescription, an intervention from the Nutrition Education domain. As for the final step, the evidence-based rationale (E) for the intervention, based on education theory and research, if a learner is able to meet learning objectives for the diet instruction, this indicates learning and higher potential for behavior change.

TABLE 6.7 Nutrition Intervention Planning Model (PGIE)

1) Problem / Etiology *(Nutrition Diagnosis)*	2) Goal	3) Plan/Intervention	4) Evidence-Based Rationale
1) Inadequate Energy intake (Intake domain; Energy Balance)	Pt will regain lost visceral protein and body weight	Provide extra kcals/ protein Provide nutrition supplement BID (Food/Nutrient Delivery domain; Medical Food Supplement Therapy)	Supplement will provide additional 500 kcals/ day, resulting in ~ 1–2 lb gain/week
2) Food and nutrition-related knowledge deficit (Behavioral-Environmental domain; Knowledge and Beliefs)	Pt will understand Diet Rx and follow plan	Provide diet instruction (Nutrition Education domain)	Pt meets learning objectives to adhere to Diet Rx

Nutrition Diagnoses: Problems identified from the Nutrition Assessment

Goal: Represents what the problem will "look like" when it is resolved (the ideal)

Plan/Intervention: What to do to reach the goal

Rationale: The "why" of the plan, which must be "evidence-based"

Put It into Practice: Nutrition Interventions

1. Determine all possible and appropriate Nutrition Intervention/s (NI) for each patient case, listing the corresponding NI Domains and Categories.

2. Go to the Academy eNCPT and Evidence Analysis Library (EAL) sites and log in.
3. At the EAL, go to the Index tab and find the relevant topic area. In the EAL column, list key points and any recommendations.

Patient	**Possible NI Domain/Category**	**EAL**
Elderly patient in a long-term care facility who has lost 8% body weight in past 3 months		
A 48-year-old man in the hospital with a new diagnosis of type 2 diabetes; BMI of 32, sedentary lifestyle		
A 20-year-old woman with a new diagnosis of celiac disease in outpatient clinic		

To Sum It Up

1. The intervention phase of the nutrition care process represents the dietitian's strategies and plans for resolving nutrition problems and needs identified in the nutrition assessment phase and stated in the nutrition diagnosis. The intervention domains are 1) Food/Nutrient Delivery; 2) Nutrition Education; 3) Nutrition Counseling; 4) Coordination of Nutrition Care; and 5) Population-Based Nutrition Action. From within each domain, the dietitian selects the most appropriate intervention to solve the individual patient's problems and meet their needs.
2. The intervention targets the etiology of the problem, as stated in the nutrition diagnosis. Several interventions may be necessary, based on the number of nutrition diagnoses for a patient, and this is sometimes called the nutrition care plan. Interventions must be evidence based, and the Academy's Evidence Analysis Library is a useful online tool for ensuring that interventions meet this critical standard.

3. In the clinical setting, dietitians will most often use interventions in the Food/Nutrient Delivery domain. Within this domain, the RD may need to modify several aspects of the physical diet or its delivery, including food and beverage texture and consistency, essential nutrients, bioactive substances, enteral and parenteral nutrition, medical food supplements, and accommodations to patient feeding.

4. The Coordination of Nutrition Care domain contains interventions that focus on the dietitian's collaboration with and referral to other health care professionals, both within the RD's facility and outside the facility to include other types of facilities and community agencies. The purpose is to enhance the patient's recovery and meet ongoing needs after discharge from the RD's facility.

5. Nutrition interventions should flow logically from the nutrition assessment and diagnosis. The PGIE model can be useful in representing linkages between the steps to ensure that interventions are appropriate; the model components are problem, goal, intervention, evidence-based rationale.

Check for Understanding

1. In most cases, what should the nutrition intervention target?
   a. signs and symptoms of the assessment
   b. etiology of the problem of the diagnosis
   c. patient-estimated energy and protein needs
   d. possible collaboration with other professionals
2. Dietitians in hospitals most often use which of the following intervention domains?
   a. population-based nutrition action
   b. nutrition counseling
   c. coordination of nutrition care
   d. food/nutrient delivery

3. Which of the following is the most accurate definition of medical nutrition therapy?

   a. evidence-based application of the nutrition care process

   b. specialized enteral formulas to treat specific diseases

   c. nutrition assessment and diagnosis of hospitalized patients

   d. modifications to both the physical diet and delivery of the diet

4. One way to ensure that the RD's nutrition interventions are evidence based is to use

   a. the hospital diet manual, policies and procedures manual

   b. the Academy's online Evidence Analysis Library

   c. the Standards for Professional Performance for RDs

   d. National Heart, Lung, and Blood Institute MedIndex

5. Which domain contains interventions for the modification of the texture and consistency of foods and beverages?

   a. Feeding Assistance

   b. Bioactive Substance Management

   c. Food/Nutrient Delivery

   d. Coordination of Nutrition Care

Answers in Appendix B

References

1. Academy of Nutrition and Dietetics. *Nutrition Terminology Reference Manual (eNCPT): Dietetics Language for Nutrition Care.* http://www.ncpro.org. Accessed January 16, 2018.

2. Wikipedia, the Free Encyclopedia. Medical Nutrition Therapy. Available at: https://en.wikipedia.org/wiki/Medical_nutrition_therapy. Accessed January 29, 2018.

3. Academy of Nutrition and Dietetics. Scope of Practice. Academy Definition of Terms. Available at: http://www.eatrightpro.org/~/media/eatrightpro%20files/practice/scope%20standards%20of%20practice/academydefinitionoftermslist.ashx. Accessed January 29, 2018.

4. Evidence Analysis Library. Available at: http://www.eatrightpro.org/resources/research/applied-practice/evidence-analysis-library. Accessed December 7, 2017.

5. Academy of Nutrition and Dietetics. *Nutrition Care Manual*. Available for subscription at:https://www.nutritioncaremanual.org/. Accessed January 27, 2018.

6. National Kidney Foundation KDOQI Guidelines. Available at: http://kidney-foundation.cachefly.net/professionals/KDOQI/guidelines_nutrition/nut_a24.html. Accessed March 15, 2018.

7. Evidence Analysis Library. CKD Protein Requirements. Available at: https://www.andeal.org/topic.cfm?conclusion_statement_id=251472&cat=4484. Accessed March 15, 2018.

8. Kocher, R. A. (1916). The mechanism of the sparing action of carbohydrates on protein metabolism. *J Biol Chem, 25*: 571–576.

9. Ruth, M. R., & Field, C. J. (2013). The immune modifying effects of amino acids on gut-associated lymphoid tissue. *J Anim Sci Biotechnol, 4*(1): 27.

10. National Institutes of Health. National Center for Advancing Translational Diseases. Genetic and Rare Diseases Information Center. Phenylketonuria. Available at: https://rarediseases.info.nih.gov/diseases/7383/phenylketonuria. Accessed April 6, 2018.

11. National Institutes of Health. National Center for Advancing Translational Diseases. Genetic and Rare Diseases Information Center. Krabbe disease. Available at: https://rarediseases.info.nih.gov/diseases/6844/krabbe-disease. Accessed April6, 2018.

12. Eckel, R. H., Jakicic, J. M., Ard, J. D., et al. (2014). 2013 AHA/ACC Guideline on lifestyle management to reduce cardiovascular risk: A Report of the American College of Cardiology/American Heart Association Task Force on Practice Guidelines. *Circulation, 129*: S76–S99.

13. Shah, N. D., & Limketkai, B. N. (February 2017). The use of medium-chain triglycerides in gastrointestinal disorders. *Prac Gastroenterol,* 20–28. Available at: file:///C:/Users/Admiral/Dropbox/TR%20WSU%20files/5250/1%20Lecture%20Materials/8%20LGI/2019/MCT%20in%20GID.pdf. Accessed April 6, 2018.

14. LeBlanc, J.-G., Chain, F., Martín, R., et al. (2017). Beneficial effects on host energy metabolism of short-chain fatty acids and vitamins produced by commensal and probiotic bacteria. *Microb Cell Fact, 16*: 79.

15. Wang, X., Fu, X., Van Ness, C., et al. (2013). Bile acid receptors and liver cancer. *Curr Pathobiol Rep, 1*(1): 29–35.

16. American Diabetes Association. (2018). Lifestyle management: Standards of medical care in diabetes. *Diabetes Care, 41*(Suppl): S38–S50.

17. National Institutes of Health. U.S. National Library of Medicine. Genetics Home Reference. Congenital sucrase-isomaltase deficiency. Available at: https://ghr.nlm.nih.gov/condition/congenital-sucrase-isomaltase-deficiency#statistics. Accessed April 6, 2018.

18. National Institutes of Health. U.S. National Library of Medicine. Genetics Home Reference. Lactose intolerance. Available at: https://ghr.nlm.nih.gov/condition/lactose-intolerance#statistics. Accessed April 6, 2018.

19. The National Academies. Health and Medicine. Dietary Reference Intakes Tables and Application. Table: Macronutrients Summary. Available at: http://nationalacademies.org/hmd/~/media/Files/Activity%20Files/Nutrition/DRI-Tables/8_Macronutrient%20Summary.pdf?la=en. Accessed April 6, 2018.

20. U.S. Department of Agriculture. Agricultural Research Service. Fiber intake of the U.S. population: What We Eat in America, NHANES 2009–2010. Available at: https://www.ars.usda.gov/ARSUserFiles/80400530/pdf/DBrief/12_fiber_intake_0910.pdf. Accessed April 6, 2018.

21. Dowd, P., Ham, S. W., Naganathan, S., et al. (1995). The mechanism of action of vitamin K. *Annu Rev Nutr, 15*: 419–440.

22. Centers for Disease Control and Prevention. Get the Facts: Sodium and the Dietary Guidelines. Available at: file:///C:/Users/Admiral/Dropbox/1%20CPD%20Stuff/2017%20Book%202/Chp%207%20Interventions/Articles%20Cited/sodium_dietary_guidelines.pdf. Accessed April 5, 2018.

23. Children's Hospital of Wisconsin. Sodium and fluid restriction. Available at: https://www.chw.org/medical-care/dialysis-and-renal/tests-and-treatments/sodium-and-fluid-restriction. Accessed April 5, 2018.

24. University of California–San Francisco. *ILD Nutrition Manual*: Prednisone and Weight Gain. Available at: https://www.ucsfhealth.org/education/ild_nutrition_manual/prednisone_and_weight_gain/. Accessed April 6, 2018.

25. Chaitman, M., Dixit, D., Barna Bridgeman, M., et al. (2016). Potassium-binding agents for the clinical management of hyperkalemia. *PT, 41*(1): 43–50.

26. Mayo Clinic. Diuretics: A cause of low potassium? Available at: https://www.mayoclinic.org/diseases-conditions/high-blood-pressure/expert-answers/blood-pressure/FAQ-20058432?p=1. Accessed April 6, 2018.

27. U.S. National Library of Medicine. Medline Plus. Digoxin. Available at: https://medlineplus.gov/druginfo/meds/a682301.html#special-dietary. Accessed April 6, 2018.

28. Nazzal, L., Puri, S., & Goldfarb, D. S. (2016). Enteric hyperoxaluria: An important cause of end-stage kidney disease. *Nephrol Dial Transplant, 31*(3): 375–382.

29. Stewart, C. S., Duncan, S. H., & Cave, D. R. (2004). *Oxalobacter formigenes* and its role in oxalate metabolism in the human gut. *FEMS Microbiol Lett, 230*(1): 1–7.

30. Kumar, R., Lieski, J. C., Collazo-Clavell, M. L., et al. (2011). Fat malabsorption and increased intestinal oxalate absorption are common after Rouxen-Y gastric bypass surgery. *Surgery, 149*(5): 654–661.

31. Cleveland Clinic. Gastrointestinal soft diet overview. Available at: https://my.clevelandclinic.org/health/articles/15637-gastrointestinal-soft-diet-overview. Accessed April 8, 2018.

32. International Dysphagia Diet Standardisation Initiative. Complete IDDSIF Framework: Detailed definitions. Available at: http://iddsi.org/Documents/IDDSIFramework-CompleteFramework.pdf. Accessed April 11, 2018.

33. Collins, N. (2011). Selecting the right tube-feeding formula. *Ostomy Wound Management, 57*(2).

34. Abbott. Adult. Available at: https://abbottnutrition.com/adult. Accessed April 10, 2018.

35. Caso, E. K. (1950). Calculation of diabetic diets. *J Am Diet Assoc, 26*: 575–583.

36. National Heart, Lung, and Blood Institute. Food Exchange Lists. Available at: https://www.nhlbi.nih.gov/health/educational/lose_wt/eat/fd_exch.htm. Accessed April 11, 2018.

37. Centers for Disease Control and Prevention. Healthy Weight. Losing Weight. Available at: https://www.cdc.gov/healthyweight/losing_weight/index.html. Accessed April 11, 2018.

38. Wishnofsky, M. (1958). Caloric equivalents of gained or lost weight. *Am J Clin Nutr, 6*(5): 542–546.

39. Thomas, D. M., Gonzalez, M. C., Pereira, A. Z., et al. (2014). Time to correctly predict the amount of weight loss with dieting. *J Acad Nutr Diet, 114*(6): 857–861.

OUR CASE STUDY OF PATIENT SB: NUTRITION INTERVENTION

Chapter 5 covered the nutrition diagnosis step of the NCP, and this chapter focuses on the next step of nutrition intervention. After determining the nutrition diagnosis, which represents the patient's nutrition problems and needs, the RD determines the nutrition intervention/s to resolve the problems and meet the patient's needs. The interventions should flow from the assessment and diagnosis steps, and each intervention targets the etiology or problem of each nutrition diagnosis.

3.0 Nutrition Prescription / Interventions			
♦PGIE Model For Planning (Problem/Goal/Intervention/Evidence)			
Nutrition Prescription: 1800 ADA, Na 2g (high protein)	**Current Diet Order:** 1800 ADA, Na 2g (high protein)	**Estimated Needs for Energy:** 2660–3200 cal	**Estimated Needs for Protein:** 128 g
Nutrition Diagnosis	**Goal/Expected Outcome**	**Intervention/s**	**Evidence-Based Rationale**
Nutrition Diagnoses are those problems identified from the assessment section and written in PES format	Goal represents what the problem will look like when it is resolved (the ideal)	The Prescription is the estimated nutrient needs, and Intervention is what to do to reach the goal (these are the plan components); Interventions usually target ND problem etiology	Rationale is the "why" of the plan; it must be **"Evidence Based"** Use ADA Evidence Analysis Library (EAL)

3.0 Nutrition Prescription / Interventions			
◆PGIE Model For Planning (Problem/Goal/Intervention/Evidence)			
Self-monitoring deficit r/t knowledge deficit AEB elevated BGL >300 mg/dL (10/13), 152, 147, 158, 297 (10/17) and diet Hx/ pt report	Patient will do SMBG as directed to facilitate glycemic control	NE: Instruction on the use of SMBG in conjunction with tracking diet (Carb Counting) and physical activity	EAL Topic/s: –DM Major Recommendations; Nutrition Intervention: Education on Glucose Monitoring
Food and nutrition knowledge deficit r/t lack of previous instruction AEB diet Hx	Patient will meet learning objectives regarding the nutrition prescription to facilitate behavior change for improved glycemic control and modest weight loss	NE: Instruction on 1800 ADA, using Carb Counting, 2 gram sodium (higher protein for wound healing)	EAL Topic/s: –DM Major Recommendations; Nutrition Intervention: Carbohydrate Mgt Strategies –HTN: Sodium –DM: Energy Intake –Wound Care: Protein

CHAPTER 7

Nutrition Intervention

NUTRITION EDUCATION AND CULTURAL COMPETENCY

Tilakavati Karupaiah, PhD, APD, AN

LEARNING OBJECTIVES

By the end of the chapter, the reader will be able to

- Describe the implications of demographic projections relative to the diversity of the population and prevalence of nutritionally relevant chronic diseases and health disparities
- Identify how cultural competence relates to all steps of the nutrition care process
- Identify the process by which the RD can become culturally competent and the resources to assist in the process
- Outline basic teaching and learning principles relating to the development of all steps of the teaching plan
- Develop a teaching plan based on client assessment data

The United States is home to diverse minority groups, who currently make up 36% of the current population, a figure expected to rise to 40% by 2030 (1). Minority groups are mainly of Alaska Native, Native American, African American, Latino/ Hispanic, Asian and Pacific Islander descent, with 21 million non-English speakers (2). Some minority groups are in the highest risk group for chronic diseases with nutrition links, such as diabetes and cardiovascular diseases (3–5) (Box 7.1). A landmark study by the Institute of Medicine (IOM) highlighted racial and ethnic disparities in the US health care system at the local, state and national levels (6). The IOM study suggests "bias, stereotyping, prejudice, and clinical uncertainty on the part of health care providers may be major contributing factors to health disparities."

The probability is very high that the RD will have clients from a special minority group. Effective dietetic service calls for culturally appropriate practices to enable clients to achieve goals of medical nutrition therapy. The Academy of Nutrition and Dietetics has stated that "the goal of credentialed dietetics practitioners is to provide safe, culturally competent and quality care" (7). While important in all steps of the nutrition care process (NCP), the RD needs to be culturally competent in designing outcome-focused education appropriate to the client when incorporating nutrition education as part of the intervention strategy. Capabilities of dietitians will therefore be driven by the nature of the client, which is multidimensional and contextual.

BOX 7.1

Vulnerable Ethnic Groups

Compared with White Americans with the same BMI, South Asians have more risk factors for heart disease, including type 2 diabetes, low HDL ("good") cholesterol and more abdominal obesity (4). "Many Canadians of South Asian descent—as well as those of Aboriginal, African and Chinese descent—are experiencing historic levels of risk for heart disease and stroke" (5).

THE CULTURALLY COMPETENT DIETETIC PROFESSIONAL

What Is Cultural Competency?

The term *cultural competence* is fluid and appears to be defined according to different stakeholders, as is the definition of *culture* (Box 7.2). The Academy suggests that skills such as "recognizing and forming one's attitudes, beliefs, skills, values, and levels of awareness to provide culturally-appropriate, respectful, and relevant health care services" would constitute cultural competencies required in an RD (8). The position statement on cultural competency by the American Evaluation Association (9) describes "learning, unlearning and relearning" as the foundational core to developing these skills.

BOX 7.2

What Is Culture?

- Culture is the shared experiences of people, including their languages, values, customs, beliefs, and mores. These are shaped into philosophies and knowledge, which are transferred through generations. Significant factors shaping culture are race/ethnicity, religion, social class, language, disability, sexual orientation, age, and gender. Geographic region and socioeconomic circumstances also shape culture.

- Cultural groupings refer to individuals not related by lineage, such as organizational culture, gay culture, or disability community culture.

- Culture is dynamic, fluid, and reciprocal.

- Elements of culture are passed on from generation to generation, but culture also changes from one generation to the next.

- Culture not only influences members of groups, it also delineates boundaries and influences patterns of interaction among them.

Adapted from reference 10: Chapter 27. Cultural Competence in a Multicultural World | Section 7. Building Culturally Competent Organizations. http://ctb.ku.edu/en/table-of-contents/culture/cultural-competence/culturally-competent-organizations/main. Accessed September 23, 2017.

---

1. Cultural competence is a process involving awareness of self, reflection on one's own cultural position, and awareness of others' positions (10). The process incorporates *learning* new knowledge about clients relating to lifestyle, language, foods, their country and religion; *unlearning* prejudices and biases about the clients; and *relearning* how to adapt and apply techniques of communication and counseling in the engagement process with clients of a specific community.

Interpretation and Application: A predominantly Middle-Eastern community has distinct food habits compared to a South Asian community. Middle-Eastern communities are predominantly Muslim, while South Asians may be Hindus, Buddhists, Muslims, or Sikhs. A white American RD of a Christian denomination and who may or may not be an agnostic will be challenged during the client engagement process of learning, unlearning, and relearning. Biases and prejudices may be within, which need to be acknowledged and shed during this process. This is at the macro level.

At the micro level, consider differences in food practices if a dietitian is challenged by a pregnant client who is a vegetarian and her issue is iron-deficiency anemia. The RD should be able to inform on iron-rich plant foods familiar to the client, as well as discuss why compliance to prescription iron supplements is critical.

2. The client engagement process of *learning, unlearning, and relearning* will take time and occurs along a continuum, but the process can be facilitated by networking with health worker colleagues with experience, as well as referencing guidelines from experts in the field.

3. The American Evaluation Association states that, "Cultural competence is defined in relation to a specific context or location, such as geography, nationality, and history. Competence in one context is no assurance of competence in another." (9)

Interpretation and Application: When working with a specific group of people or practicing in a particular community, the RD must familiarize herself with local history and the culturally determined values and beliefs of the people with whom she is working.

An RD who becomes culturally competent in dealing with a Hispanic community's health issues will not be able to translate these skills into handling Vietnamese clients. The RD will need to unlearn previous skills, set to learn about the new community, and this relearning process will develop new knowledge and skills specific to the new community. This will include language, lifestyle, food habits, religion, and the country from which the community is drawn from.

4. Cultural competence means to be respectful and responsive to the health beliefs and practices—and cultural and linguistic needs—of diverse population groups. This is the basis of effective health communication to ensure the needs of all community members are addressed.

    Interpretation and Application: The RD should be able to interact genuinely and respectfully with others of different cultures.

5. Modification of client behavior based on theories of change should be adapted to fit the cultural context.

    Interpretation and Application: The culturally competent RD draws upon suitable nutrition assessment methods and engages in nutrition education approaches that are culturally sensitive and appropriate to the client's background.

Factors Affecting Cultural Competency

Researchers have applied a type of logic model known as structural equation modeling (SEM) to study cultural competence in the nursing profession (11). An SEM incorporates a varying set of models, such as mathematical, statistical, and computer algorithms, to apply to data. Using SEM, they identified factors associated with the successful building of cultural competence in nurses working with patients from other cultures. Other researchers have developed process models for cultural competency that include situational, modifying, and transitional factors, showing how these contribute to shaping intrinsic personal development required before cultural competency outcomes can be demonstrated (12).

Exposure to multicultural experience determines confidence levels in attitudes toward ethnic diversity. Organizational support to learn culturally responsive behaviors from peers can positively moderate the experiential *learning process* of cultural competencies. Personal response through biases and prejudices toward intercultural experiences can be modified again through an *unlearning process*, which will moderate professional coping behaviors with clients from a diverse culture. This *relearning process* will allow the development of cultural competence, which embodies awareness, knowledge, sensitivity, and skills. Building on these conceptual models, RDs can apply nine cultural competency techniques to the NCP model steps to reduce racial and ethnic health disparities (Figure 7.1).

Much of the cultural competency research focuses on the goal of reducing racial and ethnic disparities in health and disease and within the health care system, one of the four goals of Health People 2020, a program of the US Department of Health and Human Services (USDHHS) that establishes target objectives to improve the nation's health. Investigators at the Agency for Healthcare Research and Quality (AHRQ), an agency within USDHHS, conducted a comprehensive literature review to identify the techniques for achieving the goal of reducing disparities (12). In order to accomplish this goal, they determined that health care systems and providers should employ nine key techniques:

1. Provision of Interpreter Services: For clients and patients who can only communicate in their native language, the employment of interpreters is crucial in the provision of care. These interpreters may be full time, part time, or contractual, depending on the need and the resources of the institution.

2. Minority Recruitment and Retention Policies: Having a diverse staff can make the environment more conducive to serving the needs of minority culture groups. In addition, minority staff can serve as a source of information for health care providers in meeting the needs of clients and patients. For these reasons, it is vital for institutions to have strong recruitment and retention programs.

3. Staff Training in Cultural Competence: Perhaps one of the most important techniques is that of developing and implementing high-quality training programs for staff. Training covers many aspects of cultural competence, including best practices for interacting with specific groups; task oriented, such as how to work with interpreters.

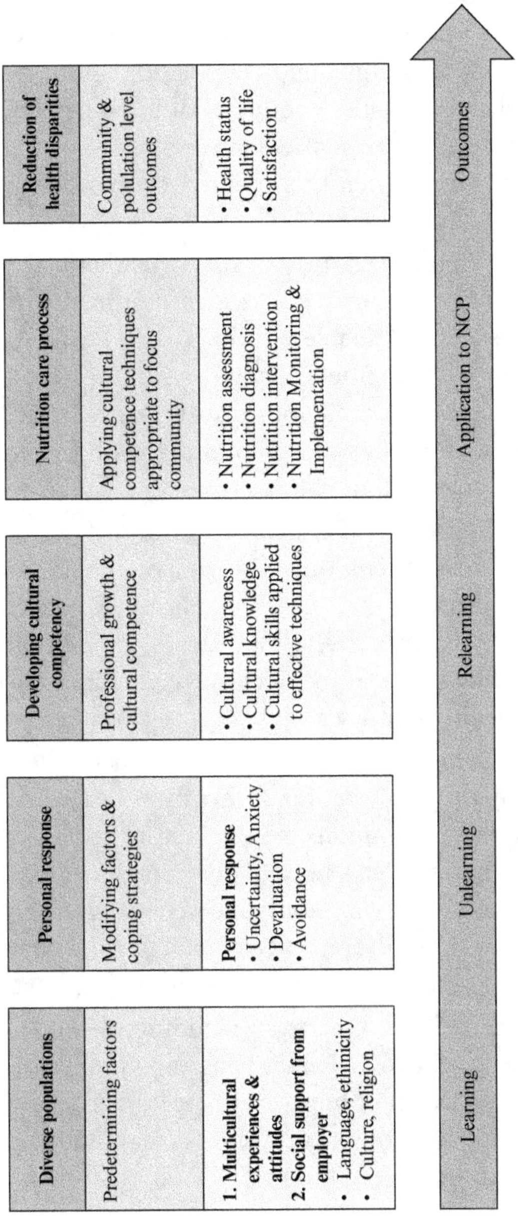

Diverse populations	Personal response	Developing cultural competency	Nutrition care process	Reduction of health disparities
Predetermining factors	Modifying factors & coping strategies	Professional growth & cultural competence	Applying cultural competence techniques appropriate to focus community	Community & polulation level outcomes
1. Multicultural experiences & attitudes **2. Social support from employer** • Language, ethinicity • Culture, religion	**Personal response** • Uncertainty, Anxiety • Devaluation • Avoidance	• Cultural awareness • Cultural knowledge • Cultural skills applied to effective techniques	• Nutrition assessment • Nutrition diagnosis • Nutrition intervention • Nutrition Monitoring & Implementation	• Health status • Quality of life • Satisfaction
Learning	Unlearning	Relearning	Application to NCP	Outcomes

FIGURE 7.1 Cultural Competence and the Nutrition Care Process

4. Coordination with Traditional Healers: Traditional healers are no longer on the fringes of many societies, now enjoying wide use in many countries. For some minority groups, this may be even more significant, depending on the specific culture. It's important for dietitians and other health care providers to be aware of and informed about traditional healers, as well as coordinating with them when possible, to avoid potential complications when therapeutic regimens may involve adverse interactions.

5. Use of Community Health Workers: Members of the community that are themselves of the race or ethnicity of specific client groups can be valuable additions to the health care team. These community members may be on staff at local agencies, community centers, or religious institutions. Identifying and networking with these key community members can greatly enhance the provision of care.

6. Culturally Competent Health Promotion: Dietitians and all members of the team must be vigilant when developing materials and promoting their programs and services to the community to project cultural competence. In addition to print and video materials, this includes messaging in news releases as well as media interviews.

7. Inclusion of Family and Community Members: By including either family or key community members in a client's treatment, both in decision making and actual implementation, the health care team can potentially improve outcomes. For example, a family or community member can participate in a diet instruction with the patient to facilitate understanding, if needed, and if privacy issues have been cleared with the patient.

8. Immersion into Other Cultures: In addition to educating the dietitian on specific foods, ingredients, and practices, cultural immersion can lessen or remove ethnocentrism, the tendency to inaccurately base one's perceptions of another culture on one's own culture.

9. Administrative Accommodations to the Local Cultures: While most dietitians are not able to make administrative decisions

regarding hours of operation and locations, they can provide valuable input to administration regarding how these variables can better serve minority group clients and patients. And dietitians at the managerial level can and should consider these operational decisions that may improve services for specific cultural groups.

In summary, dietitians who provide direct client and patient service can use many of these techniques for themselves, such as ensuring that their health promotion efforts are culturally competent and immersing themselves in local cultures. An example of this latter technique would be going to an ethnic grocery store and restaurant to directly learn about a specific group's traditional foods and ingredients. Dietitians at the managerial level within their institution can recommend the development and use of other techniques, such as the provision of interpreter services and staff training in cultural competence. In either case of the dietitian's role in direct service or management, openness and enthusiasm to learn about other cultures and become culturally competent are essential in providing high-quality and evidence-based care to clients and patients.

Another useful model for dietitians in developing cultural competency is to use a problem-based approach relating to specific cultural groups and nutritional issues. An understanding of the culture's worldview and cultural norms can provide a wealth of information that can greatly improve the provision of quality client and patient care. The following case scenarios from the literature demonstrate this approach:

Case Scenario 1: East Asian Population and Type 2 Diabetes

Background: Australian dietitians work with significantly diverse racial and ethnic groups, and one such group is Chinese immigrants to that country. Researchers studied the cultural variables and how best to provide diabetes education to this group in three different settings, China, Singapore, and Australia (13).

Problem: Although the prevalence of type 2 diabetes (T2DM) is rising in many countries, East Asian populations represent a major high-risk group. In addition, because of the size of the population, this is a particular problem in China and among Chinese people immigrating to other countries. Educational guidelines for this group are primarily based on Western culture, and as such have not been as effective as needed.

Situational Analysis: Researchers studied delivery of diabetes education and the learning behaviors and preferences of this group in the three countries. Using the case study model for their research by conducting interviews and observing education sessions, they identified important client attitudes and beliefs rooted in culture that affected the educational process and client behavior, referring to these as "themes." Based on this, the researchers pointed to the importance of incorporating these themes into the development of culture-specific education programs and strategies to enhance learning and promote behavior change.

Findings: Confucianism, which encompasses a philosophical and religious system originating in ancient China, is crucial in an individual's formation of moral values and social behavior that underpin Chinese society. In order to promote social stability, this system teaches that each individual must conform to their respective roles in the social structure. The researchers described the importance of Confucianism and its application in the nutrition education as follows:

- A heavy reliance on educating oneself predominates in the group, and only when this fails do they consider the use of a health care professional.
- They prefer a hierarchical approach in receiving information in which the dietitian provides specific instructions instead of flexibility and more individual choices.
- While the Western approach to client-focused care emphasizes active participation in planning nutrition intervention and specific goals, Chinese clients prefer to be directed by the dietitian. In addition, they were unlikely to voice concerns regarding their educational plan or progress.
- The importance of the individual's concept of their willpower was a predominant feature among Chinese clients. This emphasis on willpower led to an "all-or-nothing" way of thinking, which is often unproductive in efforts at dietary behavior change.

Cultural Competency Relevance: For Chinese clients, the client-focused Western approach to nutrition education is not effective. Rather, the educational program should be highly structured and hierarchical with the dietitian leading the sessions (13). This can be a difficult targeted approach for dietitians, but is essential to enhancing the learning process for Chinese clients to promote behavior change.

Case scenario 2: African American Population and Micronutrient Deficiency in Pregnancy (14)

Background: Dietitians working with pregnant women in various settings know the importance of adequate micronutrient intake to support a healthy pregnancy and promote a positive pregnancy outcome. For this reason, the recommendation for the use of prenatal vitamin and mineral supplementation is routine. However, adherence to supplement use is poor among African American women, as is micronutrient dietary intake (14). Researchers studied the problem to determine how to improve dietary micronutrient intake in this population and promote positive pregnancy outcomes.

 Problem: Micronutrient intake is crucial for fetal development and positive pregnancy outcomes, particularly to prevent anemia and gestational hypertension (preeclampsia). A high-risk group for inadequate micronutrient intake, anemia, and gestational hypertension is African American women of low socioeconomic status (SES).

 Situational Analysis: Researchers studied 93 African American women who were less than 20 weeks of gestation. They determined dietary micronutrient status and identified the major food groups from which this population typically obtained the nutrients, in order to inform dietitians how to more effectively counsel pregnant African American women.

 Findings: As expected, most of the women failed to meet the Estimated Average Requirement (EAR) or Adequate Intake (AI) for several key micronutrients from dietary sources: 66% for folate, 100% for vitamin D, 89% for iron, and 100% for choline. In addition, higher weight gain, and presumably overconsumption of energy, did not improve micronutrient intake. In this population, the major sources of the inadequate micronutrients included reduced-fat milk, eggs, mixed egg dishes, pasta dishes, and ready-to-eat cereal.

Cultural Competency Relevance: For African American women of low SES, who are at high risk for adverse pregnancy conditions, such as anemia and gestational hypertension in which micronutrient status is crucial, micronutrient intake is likely to be inadequate. It is important for the dietitian to carefully evaluate the adequacy of micronutrient intake in this population and base nutrition counseling on culturally appropriate food sources of these micronutrients in order to more effectively assist women in improving dietary intake.

Case scenario 3: Osteoporosis Risk in Chinese Americans

Background: Osteoporosis is a major health risk to the aging population in the United States, with Whites and Asians having the highest risk. Calcium intake is essential to prevent this disease, but the Chinese American population's intake of calcium is well below the daily recommendation (15). Researchers studied the dairy intake of Chinese American families to learn ways to increase their acceptance of dairy products.

Problem: Chinese Americans are at a high risk of osteoporosis due to suboptimal calcium intake from limited use of dairy products. To date, little has been done to reduce this risk in first-generation Chinese Americans.

Situational Analysis: Researchers conducting a qualitative study in Pennsylvania recruited and interviewed 20 first-generation Chinese American couples with children on their perceptions toward dairy products. Participants were asked a series of questions regarding "how they view dairy products, how they use them in the family food system, and how these influence their dietary behavior or intake" (15).

Findings: The responses from the couples indicated that although most of the parents knew the importance of providing calcium to their children, they did not realize that adults had an equally important need for this nutrient. Among the reasons that dairy was not often served was the concern with food additives, such as growth hormones, the perception that American yogurts were too sweet compared to Chinese yogurt, and the custom to have warm foods for breakfast versus cold cereal with milk or yogurt. Typically, there was more flexibility in dairy use at breakfast and lunch for the children. However, as the traditional head of the household, the father's views on dairy use and his preference for Chinese-based dinners dictated the limited use of dairy at dinner.

Cultural Competency Relevance: As a nutrition educator, the RD should encourage introduction of dairy products into the traditional meal patterns of Chinese Americans. Activities such as tasting opportunities for unfamiliar dairy products and demonstrating the use of dairy products in cooking and food preparation should target both parents. The RD should also provide evidence-based resources on the importance of calcium to bone health for both adults and children, and the proper amounts required for each group (15).

RD Approaches to Cultural Competency

The RD needs to know the demographics of his/her practice venue. If there is a specific cultural group among the clientele, the focus should be on that specific group. In addition, the RD should be aware of the country of origin versus the broad category of a patient; for example Mexico, Puerto Rico, El Salvador, or Peru versus Latino/ Hispanic. However, RDs should also be aware of general approaches to understanding culture (Table 7.1). And as the demographics of a society are continually changing, the RD must stay informed of new information on cultural competence by seeking additional resources in this vital area (Box 7.3).

TABLE 7.1 General Approaches to Understanding Culture

HISTORY	• Historical and social perspective
	– Influences of geography/climate
	o Food availability, accessibility
	– Interactions with neighboring countries/cultures
	o Political, religious factors
	• Effect the above has on food habits
RELIGION	• Inclusion or exclusion of specific foods or food groups
	– Consider subgroups in a diverse population; e.g., vegetarianism among Indians: Buddhism, Jainism, Hinduism
	• Special practices surrounding religious holy days
	– Fasting or abstention from certain foods/ beverages

(Continued)

SPECIFIC FOOD HABITS Focus on related nutrients/dietary constituents that may need to be modified in therapeutic diets for disease states	• Staple items—Wheat, rice, etc. • Protein foods—Plant based or animal • Predominant fat used in cooking and flavoring—Olive oil, lard, coconut oil, peanut oil • Spices and herbs—Gastric stimulants • Cooking methods • Frying, roasting

EVALUATION OF DIETARY INTAKE	• Potential dietary shortcomings
	  – E.g., low in calcium
	  – E.g., high in trans fat

HEALTH BELIEFS & FOOD HABITS	• Some cultures practice specific food habits related to beliefs about health and illness
	• Based on both religion and nonreligious beliefs
	  – Seventh Day Adventists
	    o Illness is a result of overindulgence, not following health rules
	  – Ayurvedic Medicine (India)
	    o Traditional medicine system, the science of longevity uses combination of herbs as disease prevention and therapy; encompasses rest, relaxation, exercise, and diet

BOX 7.3

Additional Resources for Cultural Competence

Georgetown University, National Center for Cultural Competence https://nccc.georgetown.edu/resources/title.php

US Dept. of Health & Human Services, National Partnership for Action to End Health Disparities https://minorityhealth.hhs.gov/npa/

University of Kansas, Center for Culturally and Linguistically Appropriate Services http://www.ctb.dept.ku.edu/en/table-of-contents/culture/cultural-competence/multicultural-collaboration/main

NUTRITION INTERVENTIONS: PATIENT EDUCATION

The Dietitian and Nutrition Education

A significant number of dietitians are continually involved with the educational process in teaching others, whether with individuals or groups, and in a variety of venues. This teaching usually involves nutrition education to bring about behavior change, although it may also include teaching other health care professionals and employees about nutrition or management issues in food service operations or in community programs. In the NCP, various forms of nutrition education are included in the nutrition intervention step and represent two of the four nutrition intervention domains as nutrition education and nutrition counseling (Box 7.4) (16).

BOX 7.4

Nutrition Intervention Domains

13 Interventions

- 4 Domains
  - Food and Nutrient Delivery (ND) – 8
  - Nutrition Education (E) – 2
  - Nutrition Counseling (C) – 1
  - Coordination of Nutrition Care (RC) – 2

Adapted from reference 16: Academy of Nutrition and Dietetics. Nutrition Terminology Reference Manual (eNCPT): Dietetics Language for Nutrition Care. Available by subscription at: http://www.ncpro.org. Accessed March 12, 2018.

The Commission on Dietetic Registration (CDR) Entry-Level Dietetics Practice Audit identifies education as one of the core activities of entry-level RDs (17). CDR defines a core activity as one in which at least 40% of all entry-level dietitians are involved for a minimum of five days every month in their positions. They further describe education as applying the principles of education. These principles typically include all aspects of the educational process; the assessment of learning needs, development of teaching plans, implementation of instruction, and evaluation of learning outcomes in both the knowledge and performance of the learner.

Depending on the area of dietetics—inpatient versus outpatient, acute care versus long-term care, or community—an RD will be using educational principles with varying frequency and levels of depth. An informal nonscientific survey of local large hospitals in urban areas suggests that clinical inpatient dietitians may do only two to four diet instructions per week. In addition, they will use only a minimum number of steps of the educational process. In contrast, an outpatient RD is mainly involved with educating clients and will use all aspects of the educational process. A diet instruction at the bedside of a hospitalized patient is considerably different than a nutrition counseling session, which RDs can conduct in hospital outpatient clinics, rehabilitation facilities, physicians' offices, and community programs (Box 7.5). Dietitians are also involved in group nutrition education, primarily in community settings, and the same educational principles will apply.

BOX 7.5

The Difference Between a Diet Instruction and Nutrition Counseling

- **Diet Instruction**: Provision of information on a prescribed diet (*inpatient, bedside*)
    - Generally of a cursory nature to enable patient to follow diet Rx after discharge ("survival skills")
    - Venues: inpatient settings; hospitals and nursing homes
    - Short in duration, averaging 10 minutes; possibly longer if topic is more complex
- **Nutrition Counseling**: Process of providing client (*outpatient*) with ability to self-manage their own nutritional care
    - Involves interview, assessment, counseling, follow-up consulting
    - Counseling involves development of rapport, empathy, and trust; *and*
    - Implementation of specific ***behavior change strategies*** aimed at client problem

- Venues: physician's office, hospital outpatient clinic, private counseling
- Longer in duration; typically 45 minutes for first session

EDUCATIONAL PRINCIPLES AND BEHAVIOR CHANGE

True Learning Means Behavior Change

In the 1970s John Travis, a preventive medicine physician, developed a model to describe the varying approaches to health and wellness, the Illness-Wellness Continuum (18). It described the traditional approach to illness at one extreme of the continuum (leading to early death), in which physicians responded to discernible signs and symptoms of disease and focused only on treating illness (Figure 7.2). At the opposite end of the continuum was the state of optimal health, or "high-level wellness." To achieve optimal health, he proposed that one should progress from the stages of awareness, education, and finally growth. The recognition of the importance of the role of nutrition in lowering the risk for disease and achieving wellness has increased dramatically over the past several decades. And Travis's model incorporates the concept that the goal of education and true learning results in behavior change, and ultimately, wellness. This involves the acquisition of knowledge, skills, and a change in attitude, or how an individual feels about a health issue, which bring about behavior change.

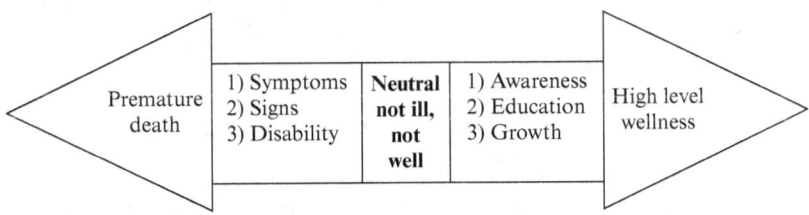

FIGURE 7.2 John Travis's Illness-Wellness Continuum

Adapted from reference 18: Wilcox, D. A., & Travis, J. W. (2015). How Culture Interacts with the Concept of Wellness: The Role Wellness Plays in a Global Environment. *Am J Health Promot, 29*(5): TAHP 6–8.

Theories abound on why and how people make behavioral changes, and two theories have particular importance for nutrition and health. The first of these theories, the Health Belief Model (HBM), originated in the 1950s, although the exact time and location is impossible to identify (19). The HBM developed from within the US Public Health Service from a range of independent research problems that many investigators were working to solve. The HBM suggests that the individual may make behavior changes under specific conditions: perception of a threat or risk ("it might hurt me, I might die" if no change), expectation of a beneficial outcome with change, the sense of self-efficacy, which is the belief that one has the capability to make the behavior change. One of the key implications of the HBM for dietitians is that a health crisis, at least for some people, may serve as an impetus or enhance the motivation to make dietary changes. Another implication is that a person needs to believe that they can make the changes necessary, so the dietitian's ability to adequately explain and provide strategies for change is important.

The second theory is perhaps one of the most important innovations in health promotion of the past few decades, the Transtheoretical Model (TTM), also known as the Stages of Change Model (20). This theory developed from research of smoking cessation programs and represents an integrated temporal framework for understanding and influencing health behavior. The TTM views behavior change as a process, not a dichotomous outcome, and posits that individuals are in various change stages relative to making behavioral changes toward some improved health parameter, cycling through the stages (Figure 7.3). These six stages of behavioral change, and the estimated percentage of individuals at the stages leading to the action stage are as follows:

- Precontemplation (40%): At this preliminary stage, the person is not considering a change and in some cases is not aware of the need for change.
- Contemplation (40%): The person is considering making a change but has not yet decided to do so.
- Determination/preparation (20%): At this stage within the TTM cycle, the person has decided to make the change and is preparing.

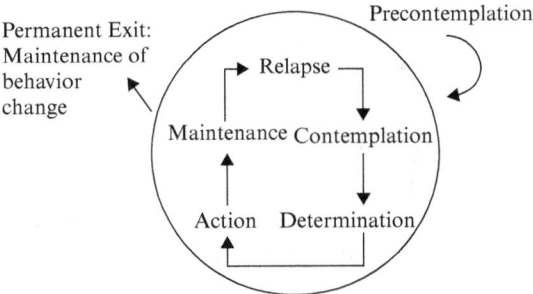

FIGURE 7.3 Transtheoretical Model

- Action: The person has made the behavioral change.
- Maintenance: The person must now maintain the change and will either continue with the new behavior and permanently exit the cycle or will relapse.
- Relapse: The person has failed to maintain the behavioral change.

Important implications from TTM for the dietitian include that a person needs to be ready to change, known as "readiness to change," and if the stage can be identified, stage-targeted education can improve the odds of success, known as stage-matched intervention. An important implication for both the dietitian and the patient is the recognition that relapse is the more common outcome for most people, but it can and does still lead to permanent success, so discouragement is unwarranted and can counter the sense of self-efficacy.

Educational Principles

Various theories of learning that guide the educational process have been proposed over decades, although much of the early research focused on children, i.e., pedagogy (21). The most basic theories suggest that learning requires, and is enhanced by, repetition, association, motivation, and involvement of the senses. In addition, various aspects of learning are organized into domains and taxonomies that can assist in the understanding and application of the learning process to develop education or teaching plans. Genuine learning, which results in behavior change, takes place within three domains; teaching plans should involve all domains when possible: 1) cognitive (knowing, thinking); psychomotor (neural activity + motion); affective (attitudes, feelings).

Bloom's Taxonomy, developed in 1956 and later revised in 2001, refers to a framework for classifying educational goals. The original six categories consist of knowledge, comprehension, application, analysis, synthesis, and evaluation, with the term *create* replacing synthesis and placed above evaluation in a later revision (22, 23). The taxonomy reflects a progression from the lowest level of learning (knowledge) to the highest (synthesis and evaluation) (Figure 7.4). For the highest form of learning to occur, an educational plan should move the learner through this progression. The taxonomy is useful in enabling the targeting of verbiage to the learning level, which is used to develop measurable objectives or learning outcomes. The following are definitions for each category:

1. **Knowledge:** the learner acquires knowledge of a topic and is able to recall the information.

2. **Comprehension:** the learner understands the information acquired and can use the information, although not necessarily associating it with other content or even understanding the information's total implications.

3. **Application:** the learner is able to transfer the information (apply the knowledge) to other situations.

4. **Analysis:** the learner can break down the information into its basic components with an understanding of the relative order of the components.

5. **Synthesis:** the learner can combine all the components to form an entire concept, which involves the creation of a new product. (*2001 Revision places above level 6, termed "Create."*)

6. **Evaluation:** the learner can judge the value of materials and methods for specific purposes.

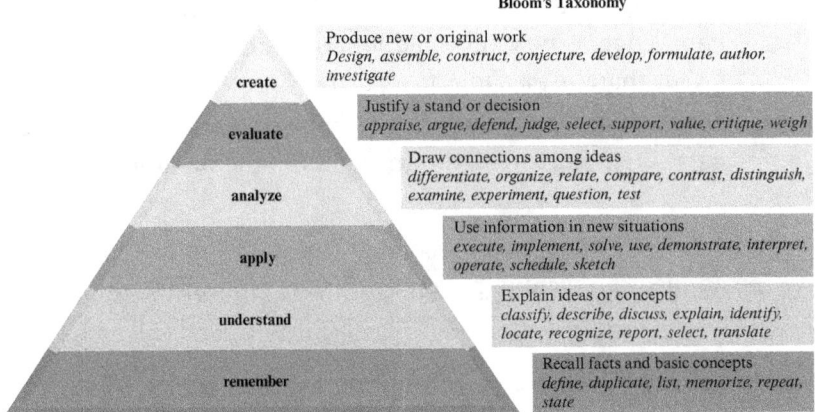

FIGURE 7.4 Bloom's Taxonomy

From Vanderbilt University Center for Teaching: https://cft.vanderbilt.edu/
guides-sub-pages/blooms-taxonomy/

Since most dietitians work with adults, the work of Malcolm Knowles is especially useful, as he proposed that adult learners are significantly different from children (24). He used the term *andragogy* to reflect the principles of teaching adults and described six important characteristics of adult learners that differentiated them from children:

1. **Relevance and Need:** Adults need to know why they need to learn something new.

2. **Self-Concept:** In adulthood, a person's self-concept in the learning process changes from that of being a dependent learner to being a self-directed learner, in which the adult takes responsibility for learning and has autonomy in the process; they need to be recognized as being autonomous.

3. **Life Experiences:** Adults' learning is enhanced when their life experiences are shared and used in teaching.

4. **Readiness to Learn:** Adults are prepared to learn when and what becomes relevant to their needs.

5. **Learning Orientation:** Adults need immediate application of knowledge, so new information should be focused on problems rather than just a subject.

6. **Motivation:** While adults can be somewhat responsive to external motivating forces, they need internal motivation to learn.

Boxes 7.6–7.8 illustrate how some of these educational principles can be applied in teaching patients and clients in different practice settings.

BOX 7.6

Learning Domains: Application in Outpatient Nutrition Education

Cognitive:
Present content on importance of matching/balancing blood glucose level, carbohydrate intake, and insulin dose

Psychomotor:
Teach blood glucose testing; recording on chart: CHO intake, BGL, insulin dose; fill out meal plan for typical meal, with possible substitutions

Affective:
Convey concepts of "self-management," wherein the patient takes control of their nutrition regimen to help prevent future health complications

---

BOX 7.7

Bloom's Taxonomy: Application in Community Nutrition Education

The learning plan should reflect progression from lower to higher levels of learning:

Stage 1: WIC participants in group education will watch a video on breastfeeding

Knowledge; Comprehension

Stage 2: WIC participants will discuss specific problems with breastfeeding and apply strategies from the video and each other to their personal approach

Application; Analysis

Stage 3: WIC participants return to group after implementing strategies discussed previous class; now discuss what worked, what didn't, and problem solve

Synthesis; Evaluation

BOX 7.8

Knowles's Adult Learner: Application in Community Nutrition Education

Use learners' life experiences in teaching
– Class discussion in which learners give personal strategies for coping with specific eating problems discussed in class by the instructor

Apply new knowledge immediately
– Use of activities with new concepts: learners will develop a daily meal plan based on the content presented about carbohydrate counting

Adult learner's self-concept and sense of autonomy
– Avoid "correct/incorrect" approach typically used in testing
– Use a game show–style approach with teams

Consider internal motivation, individually
– Try to assess each learner (issues, needs)
– Develop goals and objectives that drive the individual's motivation to learn

Nutrition Intervention: Developing the Teaching Plan

The basic steps to developing a teaching plan in any practice setting: 1) assess learning needs; 2) develop the plan; 3) implement the instruction; and 4) evaluate (21, 25). Depending on the practice setting, these steps may be of a more cursory nature, as in the inpatient setting, or more comprehensive, such as in an outpatient or community venue. However, all of these steps are important for effective education and learning outcomes. In any practice setting, the nutrition diagnosis is critical in guiding the dietitian to developing an optimal teaching plan, since it describes the nutrition problems (therapeutic diet and educational needs).

Assessment of Learning Needs

From the nutrition diagnosis, the RD knows the general learning needs and the first step in the education process is to assess the specific learning needs of the patient (16). Depending on the practice setting, in the nutrition assessment phase of the NCP, the RD may have collected some of the information for the assessment of learning needs, although an inpatient RD, who determines that the patient requires diet instruction after the initial nutrition assessment, will need specific details about dietary intake, food procurement, and preparation. Many aspects of the client and food and nutrition history are critical in assessing learning needs and planning instruction (Table 7.2).

TABLE 7.2 History Information for Teaching Plan

History Category	Specific Information
Personal History	Age, sex
Educational and cognition	Cognitive function
	Ability to perform daily functions
	Education level attained
Cultural/ethnic identity	Language, communication barriers
Occupation/economic status/family	Use of or eligibility for government programs

History Category	Specific Information
	Income
	Person responsible for grocery shopping, meal preparation
	Access to transportation
	Recent loss of spouse

Food and Nutrition History

Food intake	Food intolerances or allergies
	Typical daily intake (types and amounts of foods and beverages consumed)
Appetite, weight, habits and patterns	Appetite (current and prior to admission)
	Weight history (recent weight loss in particular)
	Physical handicaps affecting food preparation or intake
	Meal pattern
	Religious dietary restrictions
	Ethnic dietary habits
Lifestyle patterns	Alcohol consumption
	Frequency of dining out; types
	Exercise, physical activity (type and frequency)
Knowledge and attitudes	Attitude regarding nutrition and health
	Previous diet instruction (location, year, topic)
	Knowledge about nutrition
	Knowledge about the current therapeutic diet
	Interest in diet instruction or outpatient counseling
	Stage of change/readiness to learn

The gap between the RD's identification of the ideal level of nutrition knowledge needed (from the nutrition diagnosis and therapeutic diet) and the patient's current level of knowledge represents the actual learning needs of the patient. For example, an outpatient RD has the following diagnosis:

Excessive caloric intake (P) related to frequent consumption of large portions of high-fat meals, as evidenced by 1) Daily caloric intake exceeding DRI by 500 kcal; and 2) 12-lb weight gain during past 18 months.

The nutrition prescription consists of a 1500 kcal plan to produce safe and effective weight loss. It would be helpful for such a patient to be aware of the relative energy density of the energy-yielding nutrients in order to eat a more balanced diet and help in following the nutrition prescription. From the assessment of the patient's knowledge of this concept, the RD determines that a gap exists between what the patient needs to know and the patient actually knows—a learning need. Addressing learning needs helps to motivate the adult learner when the learner recognizes the gap between what they know and what they need and want to know (24). The learning needs form the foundation for the teaching plan and lead to the next step of developing goals and objectives.

Develop the Teaching Plan: Goals and Objectives

The learning needs give rise to the statement of goals for the learning process and in the teaching plan. Goals are not usually measurable but rather represent broad statements of expected learning outcomes. In contrast, objectives are specific statements of observable behaviors that can be measured, and when attained, contribute to realizing the goals. An example would be in diabetes education:

Uncontrolled diabetes leads to a higher risk of all serious long-term and short-term disease complications, and patient self-management is critical in controlling the diabetes.

Given the above, one of the goals for teaching a patient about diabetes would be:

The patient will value the role of taking responsibility for managing his diabetes.

It is clear that the patient needs to form an attitude of recognizing the key role he or she plays in preventing complications. However, while this goal is important in developing measurable objectives and providing a framework for learning, it is not itself measurable. From the goals, the RD needs to develop the learning objectives. Many different terms exist for the various types of objectives that can help distinguish among the types; however, use of more specific terms does not always occur. Indeed, the term *outcomes* is often used to label an objective. Yet knowing the different types of objectives can help the RD in developing the teaching plan.

Objectives have been described as being process objectives, behavioral objectives, performance objectives, and knowledge-based objectives. The most important distinction for the RD is the difference between knowledge—the prerequisite step to learning is the lowest level in Bloom's Taxonomy—and behavior. More simply put: what the client *knows* versus what the client *does*. From a nutritional standpoint, it's clear that having knowledge about a healthy diet does not necessarily translate into eating a healthy diet. However, in a hospital, the RD does not have the opportunity to see behavior change, in contrast to an outpatient or community RD, so knowledge is at least a starting point for the patient.

A measurable objective begins with expressing one of the key teaching points, based on the content needed to achieve the learning goals, and it specifies the task the learner will do, how well it will be done, how it will be done, and depending on the concept and task, sometimes a time frame for doing it. In developing an optimal objective, the RD should:

1. Focus on the patient's behavior by isolating the concept the patient will learn and how they will perform or demonstrate understanding of the concept.

2. Identify the level of learning the patient is expected to perform using Bloom's Taxonomy.

3. Use an action verb that is measurable and observable to describe the patient's behavior.

4. Identify the condition under which the action will be observed in order to be measured.

From the earlier example of diabetes education and an important goal for the learner, the following is a measurable objective that relates to the goal:

- Goal 1: The patient will value the role of taking responsibility for managing his diabetes.

- Objective 1: Given a hospital menu, the patient will identify six carbohydrate choices high in fiber suitable for the carbohydrate choices in her nutrition prescription.

  Since effective learning progresses from lower levels to higher, an objective that builds on the basic knowledge-based Objective 1, a learning objective that reflects the patient's ability to move beyond simple knowledge to Bloom's level five or six is as follows:

- Objective 2: The patient will plan one dinner meal pattern using the carbohydrate choices in her nutrition prescription.

  Another example of writing learning objectives that move from lower to higher learning levels and based on a learning goal is as follows:

- Goal 1: WIC participants in individual counseling will understand the role of iron in the growth and development on toddlers and its importance in preventing learning difficulties.

- Objective 1: The client can list five foods that are high in iron, which her toddler will eat on a regular basis, based on the completed food frequency questionnaire.

- Objective 2: The client will plan three lunch meals for her toddler that reflects foods high in iron to provide at least 30% of the DRI.

The number of goals and objectives the RD should develop depends on the practice setting and the client, with outpatient and community settings more conducive to a higher number compared to what the inpatient RD can hope to achieve. In the hospital, and depending on the patient, one goal and three learning objectives may be all that can be expected. Several useful mnemonics and acronyms can help to ensure that an objective has all the key components that are possible and practical for the specific practice setting, such as the SMART Objective and the ABCD Method (Table 7.3) (26). The use of Bloom's Taxonomy in conjunction with specific verbs helps to ensure that the objectives progress from lower levels to higher levels (Table 7.4). In addition, the teaching plan should include objectives for all three learning domains (cognitive, psychomotor, affective) when possible. In the brief inpatient diet instruction, this is not typically possible.

TABLE 7.3 Writing Objectives

Write SMART Objectives		
S	Specific	Significant, Simple
M	Measurable	Manageable, Meaningful, Motivational
A	Attainable	Appropriate, Achievable, Agreed, Actionable, Ambitious
R	Relevant	Realistic, Resourced, Resonant
T	Time-bound	Time-oriented, Timely, Time-Specific
Write Objectives Using the ABCD Method		
A	Audience	Identify the learner
B	Behavior	Describe the action the learner will do using an action verb based on Bloom's Taxonomy
C	Condition	Define the requirements for the task; what the learner will need in order to perform the task
D	Degree	Identify the extent to which the task must be performed (degree of accuracy, number of times, etc.)

Adapted from reference 26: Doran, G. T. (1981). There's a S.M.A.R.T. way to write management's goals and objectives. *Management Review, 70*(11): 35–36.

TABLE 7.4 Bloom's Levels of Learning and Action Verbs

Learning Level	Verbs
Level 1 – Knowledge	Define, identify, list, select, state
Level 2 – Comprehension	Compare, contrast, describe, differentiate, discuss, explain
Level 3 – Application	Apply, calculate, demonstrate, illustrate, modify, use
Level 4 – Analysis	Analyze, appraise, categorize, prioritize, review
Level 5 – Synthesis	Create, compose, design, develop, formulate, plan
Level 6 – Evaluation	Evaluate, assess, critique, decide, grade judge, recommend

Reference 22: Bloom, B. S., Engelhart, M. D., Furst, E. J., et al. (1956). Taxonomy of educational objectives: The classification of educational goals. Handbook I: Cognitive domain. New York, NY: David McKay Company.

Reference 23: Anderson, L. W., Krathwohl, D. R., Airasian, P. W., et al. (2001). *A taxonomy for learning, teaching, and assessing: A revision of Bloom's Taxonomy of Educational Objectives (Complete Edition)*. New York, NY: Longman.

DEVELOP THE TEACHING PLAN: LEARNING SESSION CONTENT, METHODS, MATERIALS, AND ACTIVITIES

Learning Session Content

The next step in developing the teaching or learning plan is to map the learning session content and select the instructional method, materials for the patient, and activities in which to engage the patient. The goals and objectives describe the learning session content. For example, an inpatient RD would begin with basic points regarding the therapeutic diet. The teaching plan content for a patient who has had a myocardial infarction might include the 1) amount and quality of dietary fats; 2) soluble and insoluble dietary fiber; 3) foods that either promote or reduce inflammation; 4) refined or low fiber carbohydrate; and 5) salt and hypertension. Depending on the assessed learning needs, the RD can expand on or limit the specific topics. For each basic point, the RD may have one or more learning objectives. In outpatient or community settings where a more extensive teaching plan and more than one learning session is possible, each key point may have several objectives.

Methods, Materials, Activities

The method of instruction refers to different ways to present the information to the learner. These methods can include lecture, discussion, demonstration, and simulations. For both individual and group instruction, but particularly for individual instruction (which is what most RDs do), the method is a hybrid of primarily lecture and discussion is most typical. However, demonstration is also useful in this presentation method, as in reading food labels with the patient or doing a food demonstration in teaching a community group.

Another method that is conducive to individual and group learning sessions is learning from worked examples, known also as example-based learning (27). This method involves first presenting the learner with the information needed to ultimately solve problems on their own. The next step consists of showing a worked example and each of the steps performed to solve the problem. The final step is to have the learner solve the problem on their own. For example, the RD may use this method to guide a patient through the steps of learning how to incorporate carbohydrate-to-insulin ratio into their regimen.

Various teaching aids or materials, such as printed information, audio-visual materials, and models can enhance learning (21). The extent to which these materials can be incorporated into the teaching plan depends on the practice setting and time constraints. For inpatient instruction, this will be typically limited to printed materials. However, it may be crucial to provide printed materials, given that the majority of patients may not remember up to 80% of what their physicians tells them (28). Perhaps even more alarming is that almost 50% of the information they claim to remember is incorrect. Effective printed materials can bridge these gaps, so that the patient has the accurate information they need after discharge.

The RD must carefully review printed materials before deciding on their use. The general evaluation criteria are 1) content; 2) literacy;

3) graphics; 4) layout and typography; 5) motivating principles; 6) cultural relevance; and 7) feasibility (29). Table 7.5 shows the criteria and their specific components. Dietitians who use a wide variety and high number of printed materials in the course of their practice can use more detailed evaluation tools: the Bernier Instructional Design Scale (BIDS), the DISCERN tool, the Suitability Assessment of Materials (SAM) instrument, and the Tool to Evaluate Materials Used in Patient Education (TEMPtEd) (29).

TABLE 7.5 Evaluating Educational Materials

Criteria	Components
Content	Accurate, current (3–5 yrs.), evidence based, relevant to patient's diagnosis
Literacy	Patient-appropriate: reading grade level, writing style, avoidance of esoteric terms and passive voice
Graphics	Visual presentation: charts, lists, graphs, images
Layout & Typography	Organization of print, white space, font, print size, color
Motivating Principles	Question and answer, quizzes
Cultural Relevance	Primary factors: race, religion, ethnicity, language; Secondary factors: age, gender, income level
Feasibility	Cost, availability, translations, and Braille available

Reference 29: Clayton, L. H. (2010). Strategies for selecting effective patient nutrition education materials. *Nutr Clin Pract, 25*: 436–442.

Implementation and Evaluation

Once the teaching plan has been developed, the last two steps of the process are to implement the instruction and evaluate the results. An important aspect of implementing the instruction is to follow the plan but allow for deviations in all settings, and particularly with an individual patient. With a patient in the hospital, the dietitian should be prepared to be flexible and realize that the patient's situation and needs are fluid and be ready to work the patient as effectively as possible at that moment. It may sometimes be necessary to reschedule the instruction due to changing circumstances, although the RD must be cognizant of the discharge day and time. During the instruction, the RD should strive to make the environment conducive to a relaxed exchange with the patient, which is more difficult in the inpatient instruction. And in all practice settings, even with being flexible, the RD should attempt to conform to the previously stated duration of the learning session, which reflects respect for the learner's time.

After the learning session is completed comes perhaps the most important step: evaluating the results. The most important outcomes to evaluate are achievement of the learning objectives, which provides evidence for effectiveness of the plan. For the inpatient and outpatient settings, documentation is important and should indicate that the patient demonstrated understanding based on the specific objectives, as well as an assessment of the patient's level of interest and engagement, which should promote motivation and potential adherence to the therapeutic diet. In addition, the evaluation also includes an instructor self-evaluation, and when appropriate, participant evaluation of the instructor and the learning session.

In summary, a complete teaching plan includes all the steps of the educational process, assessment of learning needs, development of the plan, implementation, and evaluation. The comprehensiveness and detail of the plan is highly dependent on the dietetic practice setting, but even in the inpatient setting, all of the components should be included. Box 7.9 shows a form for developing a teaching plan, which can be expanded or limited in applying it to various venues. The importance of cultural competence is evident throughout the NCP, particularly with the integration of the nutrition intervention of patient education in the prevention and treatment of disease to bring about positive health outcomes for patients and clients (Figure 7.5).

BOX 7.9: THE TEACHING PLAN

Teaching Plan: Instructional Planning for the Nutrition Education

Diet Prescription:

I. General Components of the Therapeutic Diet

A. List Dietary Components/Nutrient Controlled and other Dietary Changes

1.	3.	5.
2.	4.	6.

B. Key Instructional Points for Implementing Above Changes

1.

2.

3.

4.

II. Nutrition Assessment (Data Collection)

A. Food and Nutrition History

1. Food/Eating Patterns

a) Typical intake pattern around which to tailor Diet Rx:

b) Aspects of typical intake (food or behavior) which impede realization of Diet Rx:

---

2. Knowledge and Behavior Re: Diet Rx

a) Previous instruction and level of knowledge on current Diet Rx:

b) Cognitive abilities related to instruction (patient or significant other/s):

c) Knowledge patient needs to know; knowledge patient wants to know:

d) Readiness to change/learn (Staging: Precontemplation, contemplation, preparation, action, maintenance); Interest/motivation to follow Diet Rx:

III. Nutrition Intervention: Teaching Plan

A. Learning Goal/s:

B. Key Content Points	Learner Objectives for Content	Method/Materials/ Activities/
1.	1.	1.
2.	2.	2.
3.	3.	3.

IV. Evaluation

A) Patient demonstrated understanding based on specific objectives:

B) Assessment of patient interest/motivation and potential adherence:

C) Instructor self-evaluation (of plan/implementation):

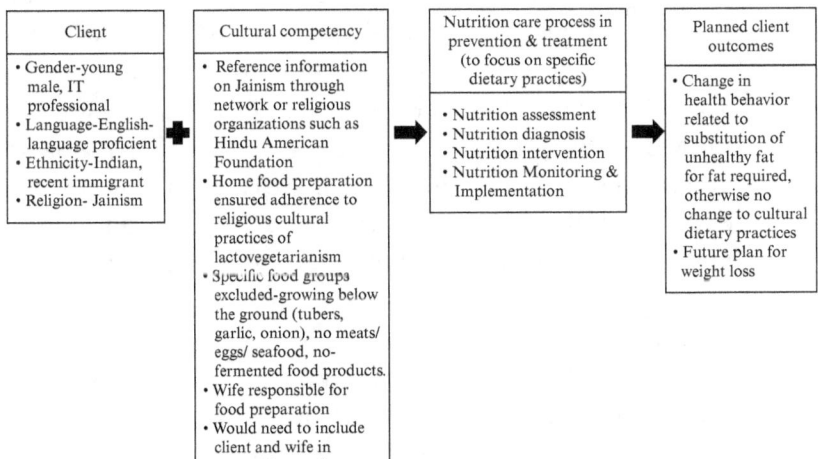

FIGURE 7.5 The Nutrition Care Process and Patient Education

Put It into Practice: Learn About Your Community

1. Research the demographics of your local community (city or county) by accessing the state health department statistics.
2. Select the minority group that is most prevalent in your community.
3. Research the major health issues facing this minority group, and select the issue that accounts for the highest mortality and morbidity and is nutritionally relevant.
4. Visit both a grocery store and restaurant in your community that serves the minority group and collect information on common food products (nutrition labels) and menu items.
5. Plan a diet instruction for a patient using the information you have collected and following the steps of developing an educational plan.

To Sum It Up

1. The US population is diverse, with minority groups consisting of 36% of the current population, which will rise to 40% by 2030. Some minority groups are in the highest risk group for nutritionally relevant chronic diseases. In addition, racial and ethnic disparities exist in the US health care system at all levels.
2. The RD must be culturally competent in conducting all steps of the NCP in order to improve outcomes for individual patients and clients and also reduce health disparities that currently exist. This is particularly important when planning and implementing nutrition intervention that involves patient nutrition education.
3. Cultural competence begins with knowledge of the demographics of the practice venue, and when there is a specific cultural group among the clientele, the focus should be on that specific group. However, RDs should also be aware of general approaches to understanding culture and stay informed of new information on cultural competence by seeking additional

resources in this vital area, as societal demographics continue to change.

4. Teaching individuals and groups; i.e., the educational process, with the ultimate goal of bringing about behavior change, is an important function of many dietitians. CDR has reported that education is a core activity of entry-level dietitians, with 40% performing this activity at least five times monthly.

5. In the NCP, two of the four nutrition intervention domains are nutrition education and nutrition counseling. Within the nutrition education domain, the two levels are initial/brief nutrition education and comprehensive nutrition education. The nutrition counseling domain consists of applying advanced counseling strategies and implies a more long-term client relationship.

6. The steps of the educational process include assessment of learning needs, development of the teaching plan, implementation of instruction, and evaluation of outcomes (learner's attainment of objectives and instructor self-evaluation).

Check for Understanding

1. In implementing the NCP and working with a diverse population, the Academy of Nutrition and Dietetics has stated that the goal of credentialed dietetics practitioners is to
   a. learn the languages of minority patients and clients
   b. provide safe, culturally competent, and quality care
   c. remove barriers to health care access in practice venues
   d. use an SEM to ensure interactions are culturally sensitive

2. What are the three aspects of the foundational core to developing cultural competency skills, as stated in the position statement by the American Evaluation Association?
   a. plan development, data assessment, implementation of plan
   b. knowledge of demography, sensitivity, understanding

      c.   predetermining factors, modifying factors, professionalism

      d.   a continuum of learning, unlearning, relearning

3.   In Step 1 in the process of Cultural Formulation, the RD needs to determine whether ethnic identity matters for the patient

      a.   ask the patient how well they've adapted to their new culture

      b.   assess the degree to which the patient has assumed new habits

      c.   inform the patient of any preconceptions the RD has about the culture

4.   One of the important ways an adult learner is different from a child is that an adult

      a.   does not need to see a reason to learn new content

      b.   views his life experiences as an impediment to learning

      c.   needs immediate application of new information

      d.   responds more strongly to external motivation

5.   A measurable learning objective is one that

      a.   is a broad statement of the desired learning outcome

      b.   identifies the task to be performed by the learner

      c.   specifies the duration of the learning session

      d.   reinterpretation of original medical orders

Answers in Appendix B

References

1. U.S. Department of Commerce, Economics and Statistics Administration U.S. Census Bureau. Humes, K. R., Jones, N. A., & Ramirez, R. R. (March 2011). Overview of race and Hispanic origin: 2010. C2010BR-02. Available at: https://www.census.gov/prod/cen2010/briefs/c2010br-02.pdf. Accessed August 30, 2017.

2. American Community Survey 2015. Characteristics of people by language spoken at home, 2011–2015 American Community Survey 5-year estimates. Available at: https://factfinder.census.gov/faces/nav/jsf/pages/community_facts.xhtml. Accessed August 31, 2017.

3. National Center for Health Statistics. Mortality Multiple Cause Micro-data Files. Public-use data file and documentation. NHLBI tabulations. Available at: http://www.cdc.gov/nchs/products/nvsr.htm. Accessed August 31, 2017.

4. Jiali, Y., Rust, G., Baltrus, P., et al. (2009). Cardiovascular Risk Factors among Asian Americans: Results from a National Health Survey. *Ann Epidemiol, 19*(10): 718–723.

5. Creatore, M. I., Moineddin, R., Booth, G., et al. (2010). Age- and sex-related prevalence of diabetes mellitus among immigrants to Ontario, Canada. *CMAJ, 182*(8): 781–789.

6. Nelson, A. (2002). Unequal treatment: Confronting racial and ethnic disparities in health care. *J Natl Med Assoc, 94*(8): 666–668.

7. Writing Group of Academy of Nutrition and Dietetics. (2013). Academy Quality Management Committee and Scope of Practice Subcommittee of Quality Management Committee. *J Acad Nutr Diet, 113*(6 Suppl).

8. Johnson-Askew, W. L., Gordon, L., & Sockalingam, S. (2011). See comment in PubMed Commons belowPractice paper of the American Dietetic Association: Addressing racial and ethnic health disparities. *J Am Diet Assoc, 111*(3): 446–456.

9. American Evaluation Association. Public Statement on Cultural Competence in Evaluation. Available at: www.eval.org. Accessed on September 1, 2017.

10. Center for Community Health and Development at the University of Kansas. Cultural Competence in a Multicultural World. Building Culturally Competent Organizations. Available at: http://ctb.ku.edu/en/table-of-contents/culture/cultural-competence/culturally-competent-organizations/main. Accessed September 1, 2017.

11. Ahn, J.-W. / Structural Equation Modeling of Cultural Competence of Nurses Caring for Foreign Patients. (2017). *Asian Nursing Research, 11*: 65–73.

12. Brach, C., & Fraserirector, I. (2000). Can Cultural Competency Reduce Racial and Ethnic Health Disparities? A Review and Conceptual Model. *Med Care Res Rev, 57*(Suppl 1): 181–217.

13. Choi, T. S. T., Walker, K. Z., Lombard, C. B., et al. (2017). Optimising the effectiveness of diabetes education in an East Asian population. *Nutrition & Dietetics 74*: 253–260.

14. Groth, S. W., Stewart, P. A., Ossip, D. J., et al. (2017). Micronutrient Intake Is Inadequate for a Sample of Pregnant African-American Women. *J Acad Nutr Diet, 117*(4): 589–598.

15. Ly, N., & Brown, J. L. (2011). Impact of a nutrition education program to increase intake of calcium-rich foods by Chinese-American women. *J Am Diet Assoc, 111*(1): 143–149.

16. *Abridged Nutrition Care Process Terminology (NCPT) Reference Manual: Standardized Terminology for the Nutrition Care Process.* (2018). Academy of Nutrition and Dietetics.

17. Griswold, K., Rogers, D., Sauer, K. L., et al. (2016). Entry-Level Dietetics Practice Today: Results from the 2015 Commission on Dietetic Registration Entry-Level Dietetics Practice Audit. *J Acad Nutr Diet, 116*(10): 1632–1684.

18. Wilcox, D. A., & Travis, J. W. (2015). How Culture Interacts with the Concept of Wellness: The Role Wellness Plays in a Global Environment. *Am J Health Promot, 29*(5): TAHP6–8.

19. Rosenstock, I. M. (1974). Historical origins of the health belief model. *Health Education & Behavior, 2*(4): 328–335.

20. Prochaska, J. O., & DiClemente, C. C. (1983). Stages and processes of self-change of smoking: Toward an integrative model of change. *J Consult Clin Psychol, 51*(3): 390–395.

21. Rankin, S. H., Stallings, K. D., & London, F. (2005). *Patient education in health and illness* 5th ed. Philadelphia, PA: Lippincott Williams & Wilkins.

22. Bloom, B. S., Engelhart, M. D., Furst, E. J., et al. (1956). Taxonomy of educational objectives: The classification of educational goals. Handbook I: Cognitive domain. New York, NY: David McKay Company.

23. Anderson, L. W., Krathwohl, D. R., Airasian, P. W., et al. (2001). *A taxonomy for learning, teaching, and assessing: A revision of Bloom's Taxonomy of Educational Objectives (Complete Edition)*. New York, NY: Longman.

24. Knowles, M., Holton, E. F., & Swanson, R. A. (2005). *The adult learner: The definitive classic in adult education and human resource development*, 10th ed. Houston, TX: Gulf Publishing.

25. Holli, B. B., & Beto, J. A. (2014). *Nutrition counseling and education skills for dietetics professionals*, 6th ed. Baltimore, MD: Lippincott Williams & Wilkins.

26. Doran, G. T. (1981). There's a S.M.A.R.T. way to write management's goals and objectives. *Management Review, 70*(11): 35–36.

27. Wittwer, J., & Renkl, A. (2010. How effective are instructional explanations in example-based learning? A meta-analytic review. *Educ Psychol Rev, 22*: 393–409.

28. Kessels, R. P. C. (2003). Patients' memory for medical information. *J R Soc Med, 96*: 219–222.

29. Clayton, L. H. (2010). Strategies for selecting effective patient nutrition education materials. *Nutr Clin Pract, 25*: 436–442.

OUR CASE STUDY OF PATIENT SB: CULTURAL COMPETENCY AND PATIENT EDUCATION

In this chapter, the Problems Solving Matrix is not included because there are no additions with the education step. However, the teaching plan is shown based on the data collected from the patient interview. The RD must be culturally competent in conducting all steps of the NCP in order to improve outcomes for individual patients and clients, and it is particularly important when planning and implementing nutrition intervention that involves patient education. Cultural competence begins with knowledge of the demographics of the practice venue, and when there is a specific cultural group among the clientele, the focus should be on that specific group. The ultimate goal of patient education is to bring about behavior change, although when conducting inpatient diet instruction, most objectives focus on patient knowledge and skills. Incorporating assessment data on the patient's culture, education, and ethnicity is critical in developing an effective plan for the patient.

Dietitian Interview and Physical

Your patient speaks English and his wife is at bedside.

Appetite and intake: "My appetite is good, maybe too good! It was just as good before coming here, and I am eating all my meals. I could use more food! I've had diabetes for about 10 years, and I have cholesterol (I take pills for it), but I don't pay too much attention to what I eat; I never talked to anyone about diet. I eat everything my wife cooks."

Weight loss and UBW: "I don't weigh myself, but my clothes fit the same as a few years ago."

Food allergies: "Shellfish."

Cultural or religious food preference: "I am Muslim, but pork is the only food I don't eat."

Difficulty chewing or swallowing: "No."

Nausea, vomiting, constipation, or diarrhea: "No, but I get acid a lot, so I take two calcium tablets every day."

Preferences: "I eat all the traditional Lebanese foods, and I like meat and chicken; I have one or two pitas a day, and I like to put butter on it. We have rice every day. I also really like my potato chips, so I eat those every night! *Wife:* "I use olive oil to cook every meal."

Musculoskeletal Depletion: None

Subcutaneous Fat Depletion: None

You talk to his nurse.

"Pt's wife has brought food every day, looks like lots of rice and pitas, and several desserts. They don't appear to be considering sugar or counting carbohydrates."

Typical Daily Intake / Food Frequency

Food Category	Specific Type/Preparation	Frequency	Amount
Meat / Fish / Poultry	No pork, shellfish	Daily	Unsure
Dairy: Milk, Cheese, Yogurt	Only whole milk	Daily	1 cup
Eggs		Twice/ wk	2
Starch (bread, grain, cereal)	Pita, rice, wheat flakes cereal	Usually daily	1 lge pita; 2 cups cereal; 2 cups rice
Vegetables	Spinach, broccoli (sautéed in oil)	3 to 4/wk	1 cup

Fruits	Only juice, usually orange	Daily	1 cup
Sugars, Sweets/ Desserts	Chocolate chip cookies, donut, baklava (one of these types/day)	Daily	2 cookies, 1 donut, 2 in. -square baklava
Snack Foods (salted)	Potato chips	Daily	2 cups
Fats	Olive oil (for food prep), butter (on pita)		
Beverages: Coffee, Tea, Soda	Coffee (with cream)	Daily	3 cups
Alcohol	None		

Teaching Plan for SB Case Study

Teaching Plan: Instructional Planning for Nutrition Education
Diet Rx: 1800 ADA, Na 2g

I. General Components of the Therapeutic Diet
A. Dietary Components/Nutrients Controlled and Other Dietary Changes
1) Energy restriction: 1800; 2) Carbohydrate Counting/coordinate w/meds & physical activity
3) Sodium restriction: 2 gm

B. Key Instructional Points for Implementing Above Changes
1) Relative difference in calories for energy nutrients; sources of carbohydrate
2) Carbohydrate counting using ADA Booklet and meal plan; coordinate with total regimen
3) Sources of sodium and salt in patient's diet

II. Nutrition Assessment (Data Collection)
A. Food and Nutrition History
1. Food/Eating Patterns
a) Typical intake pattern around which to tailor Diet Rx: Middle Eastern cuisine; no pork, no shellfish
b) Aspects of typical intake which impede realization of Diet Rx: Salty snacks; daily desserts

2. Knowledge and Behavior Re: Diet Rx

a) Previous instruction and level of knowledge on current Diet Rx: Inadequate

b) Cognitive abilities related to instruction (patient or significant other/s): No obstacles

c) Knowledge patient needs to know; knowledge patient wants to know: No conflicts

d) Readiness to change/learn (Staging: Precontemplation, contemplation, preparation, action, maintenance); Interest/motivation to follow Diet Rx: Moderate level of interest – Contemplation Stage

III. Nutrition Intervention: Teaching Plan

A. Learning Goal/s: Patient and spouse will understand the importance of carbohydrate counting, SMBG, coordination of these with physical activity to manage BG and prevent complications of DM

B. Key Content Points

Specific Objectives (possible discussion topics)	Learner Objectives for Content — Method	Activities	Method/Materials/ Activities/ Tools
– Energy nutrients (fat vs. CHO); CHO counting – Higher fiber CHO choices vs. high sugar – Substitutions for high-fat snack foods	Pt and spouse will plan 3 meals reflecting plan of 15 CHO choices (in coordination w/meds + activity) and reduction in high fat/ sugar foods by 50% of current level		ADA CHO Counting Booklet
– Importance of SMBG and coordinating w/ CHO intake and meds	Pt will verbalize recommended SMBG schedule and demonstrate correction for BG excursions based on CHO plan and meds		
– Sources of Na in Pt's diet; packaged foods, salty snacks; – Spouse's use of salt in food preparation	Pt and spouse will identify 5 typical high-salt/Na foods in Pt's diet and 5 appropriate substitutions		Actual food labels; FDA Food Label hand-out

IV. Evaluation

A) Patient demonstrated understanding based on specific objectives: Pt and spouse achieved all objectives

B) Assessment of patient interest/motivation and potential adherence: Moderate; Expect good compliance

C) Instructor self-evaluation (of plan/implementation): All objectives covered; Time exceeded

CHAPTER 8

Monitoring and Evaluation

ASSESSING THE NUTRITION INTERVENTIONS AND DOCUMENTING IN THE MEDICAL RECORD

Elise Kowalski, RDN

O nce the nutrition assessment, diagnosis, and intervention are complete, the next step in the nutrition care process (NCP) is monitoring and evaluation. Monitoring and evaluation reflect the intervention's impact on nutrition problems. The NCP steps often overlap with documentation, which is the written evidence of the NCP and a tool to measure nutrition intervention efficacy. NCP documentation follows the assessment, diagnosis, intervention, monitoring, and evaluation in the ADIME format, although other formats may be used.

MONITORING AND EVALUATION

Setting Goals and Monitoring Parameters

After planning the intervention, nutrition goals and monitoring parameters must be established to determine its efficacy. A common goal and objective setting model used in business and education, called the SMART method, can offer insight in setting meaningful and appropriate nutrition goals and objectives. SMART is an acronym for objectives that are specific, measurable, achievable, relevant, and time bound (1). As discussed in Chapter 7, a goal is typically not measurable in the strict definition, although in the inpatient setting, the term is used interchangeably with objective in the documentation phase of the NCP. In the documentation in the hospital medical record, the term refers to specific statements that can be measured in order to evaluate the outcome of the nutrition intervention.

The types of goals and objectives and their measurability are dependent on the practice setting. For example, an inpatient intervention of low-sodium nutrition education, an appropriate goal would be "patient to verbalize understanding of low-sodium nutrition education by naming three high sodium foods to avoid." In contrast, a goal that is too vague and not measurable would be "patient understands a low-sodium diet." The monitoring parameter could be "nutrition education understanding" or "knowledge of high-sodium foods." In an inpatient setting, the patient will automatically be compliant with the low-sodium diet ordered, so it's important to ensure the patient has the knowledge needed to make appropriate choices after discharge.

In the outpatient setting, the RD would distinguish between goals and measurable learning objectives, and the learning objectives would be more specific to behavior. Instead of demonstrating knowledge of a low-sodium diet, a learning objective could focus on the client behavior by actually choosing low-sodium foods; for example, "client to limit high-sodium foods to once daily." This is a more specific and measurable objective than "patient to comply with low-sodium diet." Again, specificity will depend on the context and practice setting; an appropriate inpatient goal may be inadequate for outpatient learning objectives, and an appropriate outpatient learning objective may be an unrealistic goal for the inpatient setting.

An outpatient learning objective should be measurable to determine if it is met. Consider the objective "patient to better manage diabetes through diet." It would not be possible without more specific detail to measure if the patient is "managing" their diabetes better. A measurable learning objective would be "patient to consume four carbohydrate choices at three meals daily." And after developing measurable objectives, the RD must ensure that measurement will take place. In this outpatient example, the client can keep a diet diary so that the RD can analyze intake on a subsequent visit.

Goals and objectives should be achievable by the nutrition intervention and/or the patient. A patient with class III obesity is unlikely to lose 100 pounds in six months, and a patient with advanced chronic kidney disease is unlikely to have normal renal laboratory values. Goals such as "gradual weight loss of 1–2 lbs per week" or "renal laboratory values maintained or improved" are more realistic.

A common example in the long-term care setting is pressure injuries, also known as pressure sores or ulcers. Consider the goal "pressure injuries to show signs of healing." Even if the patient is meeting protein needs, perhaps there is inadequate hygiene to facilitate healing. A more suitable goal might be "provide high-calorie, high-protein supplements to support pressure injury healing." The goal can be met with the nutrition intervention without depending on whether the pressure injury actually healed. Consider the goal "patient to achieve normal blood glucose levels." While a patient chooses what they eat, they don't control their blood glucose levels. An achievable goal for the patient might be "patient to consume four carbohydrate choices at meals." The blood glucose level might be affected if the RD prescribes a diabetic diet in the hospital; the goal might be "blood glucose level within normal limits" or "blood glucose levels to improve." It's important to consider that there are other causes of hyperglycemia other than carbohydrate intake, such as medications or infection.

Goals and monitoring parameters should be relevant to the diagnosis and intervention. If the nutrition diagnosis is "inadequate protein-energy intake" and the intervention is to "encourage meal intake and provide high-calorie, high-protein supplement with meals," then the goal and monitoring parameter should directly relate. "Patient to consume >75% of meals and supplements" could be a goal, and "meal and supplement intake" could be a monitoring parameter. Many goals can reflect one diagnosis or intervention.

If appropriate, the RD can set a time limit to the goal and include both short-term and long-term goals. Inpatient goals are typically short term given the temporary nature of hospitalization, although some patients stay for an extended time. In the outpatient or long-term care setting, time limits are more appropriate to include. For example, goals for outpatient weight management counseling may be "patient to limit sugar-sweetened beverages to once daily for the next week" and "patient to eliminate sugar-sweetened beverages in six weeks."

Involve the patient in goal setting and monitoring when possible. One method for patient goal setting is the WHAT model; **W** is what the patient will do, when, and where; **H** is how much or many and how often; **A** is achievable; and **T** is the goal time frame (2).

Consider the goal "patient to record foods and beverages consumed at each meal and snack for four out of the next seven days." This goal specifies what the patient is doing (recording intake), when and how often (at each meal and snack). Perfect adherence may not be achievable, so only four out of seven days is included in the goal; the time frame is seven days. Self-monitoring can promote awareness and behavior change, and tools include written records, web-based records, and mobile tracking devices and wearables (3). Box 8.1 provides an example of a written diet diary. This simple format could be customized to include other pertinent data that informs nutrition care plan modifications, such as blood glucose levels or gastrointestinal symptoms.

BOX 8.1

Example of a Written Diet Diary

Monday

Time: 8:00 am
Cereal with milk, banana, coffee
Time: 10:30 am
Granola bar
Time: 1:00 pm
Bag of chips, energy drink
Time: 6:00 pm
Chicken tenders, fries, diet soda
Time: 10:00 pm
Pretzels, ice cream cone
Comments: I was too busy to eat lunch at work, so I was really hungry after I got home.

Cups of Water: XX
Exercise:

Tuesday

Time: 10:00 am
2 Donuts
Time: 12:30 pm
Bacon cheeseburger, fries, energy drink
Time: 2:00 pm
Big cookie
Time: 7:00 pm
Grilled steak, broccoli, brown rice, salad

Comments: No breakfast, so I ate the donuts from the breakroom at work. I was tired after lunch, but felt better after exercising.

Cups of Water: XXXX
Exercise: Walked on treadmill for 45 min.

Determining Efficacy of Nutrition Interventions

Once the goals and monitoring parameters are set, the RD will follow up to evaluate intervention effectiveness. Organizations may set a standard requirement for a follow-up, such as one week after initial assessment. Outpatient follow-ups are usually determined by the RD and the patient depending on necessity and availability. A complete follow-up typically contains many of the initial elements of the assessment. Sometimes, a brief follow-up is made after the assessment to check on intake, supplement acceptance, or diet advancement. Some patients, such as nutrition support patients in the ICU, require daily monitoring.

An inpatient follow-up might begin with a review of the medical record to determine changes in medical condition, anthropometrics, biochemical data, medical tests, and procedures. The previous nutrition assessment or follow-up note is reviewed. Once again, the RD gathers subjective information from the patient, family, and other health care providers. The physical exam should be repeated if subcutaneous fat or musculoskeletal depletion is suspected since the initial assessment. During outpatient follow-ups, more time is spent counseling the patient instead of reviewing medical records.

The goals set during the assessment are reviewed, and goal progress is noted. If goals are not being met, it is essential to determine the barriers for goal achievement. For example, a goal is set for "patient to consume >75% of meals" but the patient is only consuming 50% of meals. Many things could be causing this, including loss of appetite, early satiety, nausea, weakness, medication side effects, disliking the food choices, or inability to feed oneself. The goal might need revision; if the patient normally eats small amounts, perhaps the meals served are much larger than usually consumed.

Once the barriers to goal achievement are discovered, a new intervention is planned to overcome them if possible. If the patient dislikes the food, liberalizing the diet to offer more choices, encouraging foods from home, or simply stressing the importance of nutrition for healing could be options. If the patient can't feed him- or herself, providing assistance with meals might be effective. Some barriers are outside of the RD's scope of practice. If a patient has persistent loss of appetite, the RD cannot prescribe an appetite-stimulating medication; however, a recommendation to the physician like "consider appetite stimulant" could be included.

The next step is to review the nutrition diagnosis and determine if it is still applicable or has resolved; a new nutrition diagnosis can also be included for new nutrition problems. A patient had an original diagnosis of "inadequate oral intake." On follow-up, the patient is only eating a few bites at each meal and now has subcutaneous fat depletion, musculoskeletal depletion, and edema. A new diagnosis of malnutrition could be made with a corresponding intervention, such as recommending nutrition support.

Alternatively, the patient's appetite is improved with 100% meal intake; the original diagnosis of "inadequate oral intake" is now resolved. However, the patient had a minor surgical procedure since the initial assessment, and now "increased nutrient needs (protein)" could be diagnosed. Providing a high-protein supplement could be the new intervention. New diagnoses, interventions, and goals are not always necessary; if the previous intervention is successful and there is goal progress, continuing the current plan may be the only recommendation.

Putting It into Practice: Writing Goals and Monitoring Parameters

Write goals and monitoring parameters for the following diagnoses and interventions. Remember that appropriate goal setting will depend on the setting, and there can be many possible options.

1. Diagnosis: Increased nutrient needs (energy and protein) related to skin repletion as evidenced by stage 3 pressure injury.

    Intervention: Ordered high-calorie, high-protein shake with meals.

2. Diagnosis: Self-monitoring deficit related to lack of interest as evidenced by noncompliance with home blood glucose testing recommendation.

    Intervention: Instructed patient to test blood glucose three times daily before meals and record result.

3. Diagnosis: Food- and nutrition-related knowledge deficit related to change in medical condition as evidenced by new diagnosis of diverticulitis.

   Interventions: Provided written and verbal nutrition education for low-fiber diet with gradual progression to high-fiber diet; reviewed list of high-fiber foods.

4. Diagnosis: Decreased nutrient needs (sodium) related to cardiac dysfunction as evidenced by edema, diuretics, and new diagnosis of CHF.

   Interventions: Ordered low-sodium diet; provided written and verbal nutrition education for low-sodium diet; reviewed list of high sodium foods.

5. Diagnosis: Biting/chewing (masticatory) difficulty related to poor dentition as evidenced by 50% meal intake because of missing and damaged teeth.

   Interventions: Ordered mechanical soft diet; recommend SLP evaluation.

6. Diagnosis: Inadequate oral intake related to intubation as evidenced by NPO status.

   Intervention: Recommend EN support if NPO expected to continue past 24–48 hrs.

7. Diagnosis: Enteral nutrition composition inconsistent with needs related to endocrine dysfunction as evidenced by hyperglycemia, elevated HbA1c, and history of type 2 diabetes.

   Intervention: Ordered diabetic EN formula, daily blood glucose monitoring, and HbA1c in 3 months.

8. Diagnosis: Unintended weight loss related to GI dysfunction and autoimmunity as evidenced by 10% weight loss in 1 yr., chronic diarrhea, and new diagnosis of celiac disease.

   Interventions: Ordered gluten-free diet; weekly weights; provided written and verbal education for celiac disease nutrition therapy; reviewed gluten-containing grains.

9. Diagnosis: Inconsistent carbohydrate intake related to lack of previous nutrition education as evidenced by hyperglycemia,

hypoglycemia, reported frequent missed meals and consumption of large meals, and history of type 2 diabetes.

Interventions: Provided written and verbal education for type 2 diabetes nutrition therapy; recommended 4 carbohydrate choices at 3 meals daily; encouraged meals and snacks every 4–5 hrs.; encouraged recording intake in diet diary.

10. Diagnosis: Chronic disease or injury related malnutrition related to pulmonary dysfunction and increased protein-energy needs as evidenced by severe subcutaneous fat and musculoskeletal depletion, 22% weight loss with decreased appetite and 75% normal intake over 1 yr., BMI 18.2, moderate edema, stage 2 pressure injury, and admission for acute exacerbation of chronic COPD.

Interventions: Ordered weekly weights; high-calorie, high-protein supplements with meals; encouraged protein intake, such as meat, eggs, and dairy; provided written and verbal nutrition education for high-calorie, high-protein diet.

Answers in Appendix B

ADIME DOCUMENTATION

In 1966, the American Dietetic Association (ADA), now the Academy of Nutrition and Dietetics (AND), and the American Hospital Association issued guidelines for documenting nutrition care in medical records (4). Documenting nutrition care is important for several reasons. A patient's medical record is a legal document showing what care was provided. It is a communication tool between each discipline, allowing assessment of the patient's overall medical status and treatment course. The RD presents the nutrition care plan with supporting rationale to others, while also using it to monitor and evaluate the effectiveness of the interventions. The medical record can also provide data for research and support reimbursement for health care provided (4).

Format

The documentation format of the NCP varies depending on the health care facility, but the ADIME format closely models the NCP steps. Other formats, such as the subjective, objective, assessment, and plan (SOAP) format may also be used in medical record documentation. Since 2014, facilities are required to use electronic health records (EHRs) to document health care, but auxiliary paper records may also be used (4). Regardless of format, documentation should effectively communicate the nutrition problem and care plan. Some RDs will begin documenting when gathering data from the medical record; others may only take a few brief notes before the patient interview. Once the assessment information is collected, the RD can complete documentation.

Typically, a nutrition assessment note has a header that includes some basic patient information, such as name, sex, age, medical record number (MRN), and length of stay (LOS). The assessment section of the ADIME format includes the patient history, food- and nutrition-related history, anthropometric measurements, biochemical data, and nutrition-focused physical findings. The RD consult reason, history of present illness (HPI), and subjective patient interview data should be included. The assessment section is followed by the diagnosis, intervention, monitoring, and evaluation sections. A nutrition assessment note might end with recommendations to other disciplines, the writer's name, credentials, and contact information. Box 8.2 provides an example of an ADIME nutrition assessment note.

BOX 8.2

Example of ADIME Nutrition Assessment Note

Header

- Name: S.C. Age: 67 Sex: F MRN: 123456 LOS: 1
- Consult Reason: MD consult for assessment and CHF nutrition education
- HPI and Subjective: Patient presented to ED with SOB and +2 bilateral LE edema; admitted for CHF exacerbation. Reports normal appetite with 100% normal intake now and before admission. Had 5-lb fluid-related weight gain in 1 week; this is the first episode of edema since recent diagnosis of CHF. No previous diet education; RN at bedside.

A – Assessment

- Patient History: CHF and cholecystectomy. Former smoker; lives with husband.
- Food- and Nutrition-Related History:
  - Current Diet: Sodium 2 gm (Low Na), Low Fat/Low Cholesterol
  - Intake: 100% of normal
  - Food Allergies and/or Cultural or Religious Food Preferences: None per patient
  - Nutritionally Relevant Medications and Infusions: IV furosemide
- Anthropometric Measurements:
  - Height: 157.48 cm Weight: 58.9 kg BMI: 23.8 BMI Classification: Adequate
  - IBW: 50 kg %IBW: 117.8% UBW: 56.7 kg %UBW: 103.9%
  - Weight History: 2.2 kg/3.9% fluid-related weight gain in 1 week
- Biochemical Data, Medical Tests, and Procedures:
  - Na 134 (L)
- Nutrition-Focused Physical Findings:
  - Appetite: Normal Oral: No chewing or swallowing difficulty
  - GI: No nausea, vomiting, diarrhea, or constipation
  - Skin Integrity: WNL per RN admission assessment
  - Edema: +2 bilateral LE per RN flowsheets
  - Subcutaneous or Musculoskeletal Depletion: None per RD physical exam

D – Diagnosis

- Decreased nutrient needs (sodium) related to cardiac dysfunction as evidenced by 2.2 kg/3.9% weight gain in 1 week before admission, edema, hyponatremia, and admission for CHF exacerbation
- Food- and nutrition-related knowledge deficit related to change in medical condition as evidenced by recent diagnosis of CHF and admission for CHF exacerbation

I – Intervention

- Estimated Nutrition Needs:

- o Energy: 1250–1500 kcal (Based on 25–30 kcal/kg IBW 50 kg for maintenance/fluid retention)
- o Protein: 50–62 gm protein (Based on 1.0–1.25 gm/kg IBW 50 kg for older adult maintenance/fluid retention)
- o Fluid: 1500 ml (Based on 30 ml/kg IBW 50 kg) or per medical management; edema present/on furosemide/hyponatremia
- Nutrition Prescription: Continue Sodium 2 gm (Low Na), Low Fat/Low Cholesterol Diet
- Interventions:
  - o Encouraged intake
  - o Noted daily weights already ordered
  - o Provided verbal and written nutrition education for low-sodium nutrition therapy
  - o Provided Outpatient Nutrition Counseling brochure and RD contact information
  - o Discussed with RN

M & E – Monitoring and Evaluation
- Goals:
  - o Patient to consume >75% of meals
  - o Edema and hyponatremia to improve as medically feasible
  - o Weight loss to UBW as fluid retention resolves
  - o Patient to verbalize understanding of low-sodium nutrition therapy and name 3 high-sodium foods to avoid
- Monitoring parameters: Intake, edema, laboratory values, weight, and nutrition education understanding

Recommendations:
- Continue Sodium 2 gm (Low Na), Low Fat/Low Cholesterol Diet
- Referral to Outpatient Nutrition Counseling at discharge

Name, Credentials, and Contact Information:
Thank you for the consult; please contact with any questions.
Registered Dietitian Nutritionist
(123) 456–7890

Information included in the nutrition assessment note will vary depending on the assessment purpose. For example, a patient's skin condition or physical exam may be excluded in an outpatient counseling setting; the subjective patient information and counseling would be the focus. Content of follow-up notes can also vary. Boxes 8.3 and 8.4 provide examples of a brief nutrition follow-up note and a complete ADIME nutrition follow-up note.

BOX 8.3

Example of Brief Nutrition Follow-up Note

Header

- Name: S.C. Age: 67 Sex: F MRN: 123456 LOS: 3
- Reason for Visit: Check oral intake and nutrition education understanding
- Subjective: Patient reports appetite remains normal with 100% meal intake since admission. Had questions about low-sodium snacks; reviewed low-sodium handouts and suggested appropriate snack options.

Name, Credentials, and Contact Information:
RD following per protocol; please contact with any questions.
Registered Dietitian Nutritionist
(123) 456-7890

BOX 8.4

Example of ADIME Nutrition Follow-up Note

Header

Name: S.C. Age: 67 Sex: F MRN: 123456 LOS: 7

- Reason for Visit: Review nutrition care plan
- Subjective: Patient reports appetite is the same, but now with ~50% meal intake because she is "tired of the bland menu." She ate

½ oatmeal, eggs, and toast for breakfast; ate "most of" meatloaf and mashed potatoes for dinner last night. Emphasized importance of nutrition, reviewed benefits of low-sodium diet, encouraged intake, and suggested taste might improve as low-sodium diet is followed long-term. Provided additional handout on low-sodium seasoning options; she has no questions about previous nutrition education material; she named 3 high-sodium foods to avoid (bacon, canned beans, tomato juice). Patient agreeable to strawberry protein shake with dinner to supplement intake.

A – Assessment

- Food- and Nutrition-Related History:
- Current Diet: Sodium 2 gm (Low Na), Low Fat/Low Cholesterol Diet
    - o   Intake: ~50% of meals per patient
    - o   Nutritionally Relevant Medications and Infusions: Oral furosemide
- Anthropometric Measurements:
    - o   Admission Weight: 58.9 kg
    - o   Current Weight: 57.6 kg
    - o   Weight Trend: 1.3 kg/2.2% weight loss in 1 week; noted on furosemide; edema improved
- Biochemical Data, Medical Tests, and Procedures:
    - o   Na 137
- Nutrition-Focused Physical Findings:
    - o   Appetite: Normal
    - o   GI: No nausea, vomiting, diarrhea, or constipation
    - o   Skin Integrity: Redness to coccyx per RN flowsheets
    - o   Edema: +1 bilateral LE per RN flowsheets

D – Diagnosis

- Decreased nutrient needs (sodium) related to cardiac dysfunction as evidenced by 2.2 kg/3.9% weight gain in 1 week before admission, edema, and admission for CHF exacerbation; *updated; remains active*
- Food- and nutrition-related knowledge deficit related to change in medical condition as evidenced by recent diagnosis of CHF and admission for CHF exacerbation; *resolved*

I – Intervention

- Nutrition Prescription: Liberalize to Sodium 2 gm (Low Na) Diet to encourage intake with strawberry protein shake once daily
- Interventions:
  - Ordered supplement; encouraged intake
  - Provided verbal and written nutrition education for low-sodium seasonings
  - Discussed with RN

M & E – Monitoring and Evaluation

- Previous Goals:
  - Patient to consume >75% of meals; *goal not met, discontinued*
  - Edema and hyponatremia to improve as medically feasible; *progressing*
  - Weight loss to UBW as fluid retention resolves; *progressing*
  - Patient to verbalize understanding of low-sodium nutrition therapy and name 3 high-sodium foods to avoid; *goal met; ongoing*
- New Goal:
  - Patient to consume >50% of meals and 100% of supplement
- Monitoring parameters: Intake, supplement acceptance, edema, laboratory values, weight, and nutrition education understanding

Recommendations:

- Liberalize to Sodium 2 gm (Low Na) Diet to encourage intake with strawberry protein shake once daily
- Referral to Outpatient Nutrition Counseling at discharge

Name, Credentials, and Contact Information:
RD following per protocol; please contact with any questions.
Registered Dietitian Nutritionist
(123) 456–7890

Specificity during documentation, such as including food pref-erences, can be very useful and save time during follow-ups. If the patient is unavailable for an interview and a supplement needs to be ordered, it is helpful if previously noted that the patient doesn't like chocolate. If a patient is seen for nutrition counseling and it was already noted the patient doesn't cook at home, the RD can target future interventions and suggestions on convenience food or eating out. In many situations, a follow-up must be done on a patient who was initially assessed by another RD. Having detailed documentation can make it much easier to follow up on an unfamiliar patient.

Include reasoning for a decision when appropriate to make it easier to understand. For example, a patient with chronic kidney disease (CKD) stage 2 is admitted for acute kidney injury (AKI). The renal laboratory values are extremely abnormal, and the physician notes that dialysis might be necessary if the laboratory values don't improve. The patient also has a stage 4 pressure injury. The pressure injury requires increased protein for healing, but minimizing renal stress to avoid dialysis takes initial precedence. A high-protein supplement isn't included in the initial intervention, but the RD will monitor the renal laboratory values and order one if they improve or dialysis is started.

The RD, thinking that it is obvious why a protein supplement wasn't ordered, doesn't include the reasoning in the documentation. Another health care provider, who is unfamiliar with protein's effect on the kidneys, is confounded that a patient with a stage 4 pressure injury isn't on a protein supplement. The provider questions the com-petency of the RD and orders high-protein supplements with each meal. This could have been avoided by including the following in the subjective: "Noted patient with stage 4 pressure injury and increased protein needs; was admitted for AKI on CKD and physician trying to avoid dialysis; will minimize renal stress by avoiding high-protein supplements until renal laboratory values improve or dialysis started."

Documenting reasoning can also help health care providers and families make educated decisions about nutrition care, particularly when ethics are involved. A patient with severe dementia stops eating; the RD knows if nutrition support isn't initiated, the patient will become malnourished. The RD also knows that enteral nutrition (EN) has risks for patients with severe dementia and may not improve the patient's survival time (5). The RD provides this information from the AND's practice paper to show why EN isn't being recommended. The physician can now have a meaningful and educated dialogue with the patient's family about the nutrition care plan.

Style

The AND began developing a standardized language for dietetics in 2003, known as the International Dietetics and Nutrition Terminology, to provide consistency in describing nutrition care (4). This standardized language is continually updated and is now referred to as the Nutrition Care Process Terminology (NCPT). Other professions, such as nursing, physical therapy, and occupational therapy, also use standardized language to describe care provided. Using the standardized language can improve data comparison between organizations, facilitate nutrition informatics, and simplify research. Subscriptions to the NCPT are available online (called the eNCPT) at https://www.ncpro.org (6). The difficulty collecting and combining nutrition data from EHRs is a major barrier to showing the impact of nutrition interventions on patient outcomes. The AND funds the Academy of Nutrition and Dietetics Health Informatics Infrastructure (ANDHII), which facilitates standardized data collection and analysis (7).

Abbreviations are commonly used in medical records, but their meaning can vary with the user. Organizations may adopt a list of acceptable abbreviations for use, ensuring compliance with the organization's list. The Joint Commission (TJC), a nonprofit health care accreditation organization, maintains a list of banned abbreviations that could result in confusion and error, and the list is available on TJC's website (8, 9).

Narrative documentation should be clear and concise. It is important to consider the main purpose of documentation, which is communication to other health care providers. The information should be easy to understand and quickly accessible; avoid esoteric and verbose language. Complete sentences aren't necessary, but proper punctuation, spelling, and grammar should be used, and one should avoid writing in the first person.

Avoid unnecessary words, like compound constructions and idioms (10). "Prior to admission" becomes "before admission." "The patient reports no nausea or vomiting at this time" becomes "the patient reports no nausea or vomiting." The phrase "at this time" does not add additional meaning.

Use the active voice by stating the actor, the action, and the object of the action (10). "There was no chewing or swallowing difficulty reported by the patient" becomes "the patient (*actor*) reports (*action*) no chewing or swallowing difficulty (*object*)." Avoid turning verbs into nouns (10). "The patient made an assumption her medication caused diarrhea" becomes "the patient assumed her medication caused diarrhea."

Include only relevant information in each section to avoid redundancy. If a patient reports no nausea or vomiting, include that under the gastrointestinal symptoms section, not in the subjective. However, if a patient reports extensive nausea and vomiting causing inadequate oral intake, it may be appropriate in the subjective.

Documentation efficiency can be improved by increasing typing speed and accuracy, and documentation software may have functions that enable shortcuts to frequently used phrases. For example, it may be possible to set a standard goal list that will automatically populate using a keyboard shortcut. Instead of typing out each goal individually, the RD can simply remove the goals that aren't needed. Software may also have functions that auto-populate information into the nutrition note, such as patient history, current medications, and weight. Be sure to take advantage of any tool or skill that will reduce documentation time without sacrificing quality.

Financial Implications

Documentation of certain nutrition diagnoses, like malnutrition, can have significant financial implications. Disease-related malnutrition costs an estimated $157 billion yearly in the United States; it is associated with delayed wound healing, immune dysfunction, infection, and prolonged length of stay (11). Medicare reimburses the same dollar amount for each patient with a specific diagnosis under the Medicare Severity Diagnosis Related Group (DRG) system (11). If the patient has a qualifying secondary diagnosis, either comorbidities already present or complications that occur during admission (CCs), it will increase reimbursement (11). More severe CCs are classified as major comorbidities or complications (MCCs). To provide billable data, CCs and MCCs must be documented under the International Classification of Disease 10th Revision (ICD-10) coding system (11).

Malnutrition qualifies as a CC or MCC depending on the severity, and may increase reimbursement in certain situations (11). In order to be coded for reimbursement, it must be documented by a provider, such as a physician, physician assistant, or nurse practitioner (11). The RD's documentation informs providers of the nutrition diagnosis so they can document this diagnosis for proper coding (11). Some institutions use additional communication measures, such as directly alerting providers, to ensure documentation.

This highlights the financial value of the RD to the health care system and helps secure additional resources for nutrition care (11). If the provider includes the malnutrition diagnosis because of the RD's documentation and it is coded as the sole CC or MCC that provides additional reimbursement, the RD is responsible for the financial benefit. If the provider did not include the malnutrition diagnosis and it was not coded properly, the reimbursement would go unclaimed (11). These unclaimed reimbursements may result in losses of tens of thousands of dollars (11).

Put It into Practice: Writing the Subjective

Make the following statements more concise and appropriate for a medical record:

1. The patient reports that because of the fact he was nauseated while in rehab, he was only eating about half of his normal intake at that point in time.

2. An order has been made by the patient's physician for a CT scan for the reason that the patient was complaining of having neck pain.

3. The patient gave a report that he was in such intense pain that he was unable to prepare his own meals at home.

4. The patient's nurse is going to administer a laxative medication to help the patient have a bowel movement.

5. I spent time encouraging the patient to choose more appropriate carbohydrates, like those that are higher in fiber.

6. A report from the patient's primary care provider indicated that the patient is not in compliance with her current insulin regimen.

7. The patient was seen today in the emergency department because he was having shortness of breath, and had also developed edema in his right and left legs.

8. In the past 3 months, the patient has experienced a weight loss of 15 pounds because he was only eating about 30% of his meals.

9. I tried to speak with the patient, but she was out of the room at that time for a medical procedure, and there were no family members there either.

10. The patient first came in to the hospital because she fell and broke her hip. The orthopedic doctor was able to fix the hip fracture with a surgical procedure. She reports she hasn't really been eating well for about 6 months. She could not explain why her appetite was less than normal, and she has been eating approximately 50% of her normal intake. She also has lost a lot of weight over the past 6 months. She thinks it was 25 pounds, but she isn't really sure how much she normally weighs. She drinks protein shakes at home and would like to get one with each of her meals. She likes either strawberry or vanilla flavor.

Answers in Appendix B

To Sum It Up

- Monitoring and evaluation measures the efficacy of the nutrition intervention.
- Nutrition goals should be specific, measurable, achievable, relevant, and time-bound if possible.
- Nutrition follow-ups should determine relevance of previous diagnoses, new diagnoses, goal achievement or barriers, and necessity of additional interventions.
- The ADIME model and the IDNT provide a standard format and language to document the NCP.

- Documentation of the nutrition care plan demonstrates the care provided, communicates it to other health providers, and functions as a tool for monitoring and evaluation.
- Documentation should be clear and concise to effectively communicate the nutrition care plan.
- Proper documentation of certain nutrition diagnoses has significant financial implications and can highlight the value of RDs and nutrition care.

Check for Understanding

1. SMART goals are:
   a. Stated, measurable, achievable, realistic, and time-bound
   b. Specific, maintainable, achievable, relevant, and time-bound
   c. Specific, measurable, achievable, relevant, and time-bound
   d. Specific, measurable, accurate, realistic, and time-bound

2. Which of the following goals is achievable by the patient?
   a. Patient to lose 1-2 lbs in the next week
   b. Patient's skin integrity maintained
   c. Patient's potassium level to improve
   d. Patient to consume protein supplement daily

3. Goal setting should:
   a. Involve the patient
   b. Reflect the perfect or ideal outcome
   c. Be the same in every situation
   d. All of the above

4. Abbreviations can be used in the medical record if:
   a. They are approved by the organization
   b. They are not included in TJC's banned abbreviation list and are used by physicians at the organization, even if the organization doesn't specifically approve them
   c. They are common knowledge
   d. They are approved by the organization and are not included in TJC's banned abbreviation list

5. Proper malnutrition documentation by the RD is important because:

   a. It always increases Medicare reimbursement

   b. It can inform providers for proper coding

   c. RDs can get insurance reimbursement directly

   d. It can help prevent comorbidities and complications

Answers in Appendix B

References

1. HR at MIT: Performance Development: SMART Goals. Available at: http://hrweb.mit.edu/performance-development/goal-setting-developmental-planning/smart-goals. Accessed September 27, 2017.

2. Cunningham, E. (2014). How can I support my clients in setting realistic weight loss goals? *J Acad Nutr Diet, 114*(1): 176.

3. Yu, Z., Sealy-Potts, C., & Rodriguez, J. (2015). Dietary self-monitoring in weight management: Current evidence on efficacy and adherence. *J Acad Nutr Diet, 115*(12): 1931–1933, 1934–1938.

4. The Writing Group of the Nutrition Care Process/Standardized Language Committee. (2008). Nutrition care process part II: Using the international dietetics and nutrition terminology to document the nutrition care process. *J Acad Nutr Diet, 108*(8): 1287–1293.

5. Practice paper of the Academy of Nutrition and Dietetics: Ethical and legal issues in feeding and hydration. (2013). *J Acad Nutr Diet, 113*(6): 828–833.

6. Academy of Nutrition and Dietetics. Nutrition Terminology Reference Manual (eNCPT): Dietetics Language for Nutrition Care. http://www.ncpro.org. Accessed February 28, 2018.

7. ANDHII. Available at: http://www.eatrightpro.org/resources/research/projects-tools-and-initiatives/andhii. Accessed September 30, 2017.

8. About the Joint Commission. Available at: https://www.jointcommission.org/about_us/about_the_joint_commission_main.aspx. Accessed September 16, 2017.

9. Facts about the Official "Do Not Use" List. https://www.jointcommission.org/facts_about_do_not_use_list/. Accessed September 16, 2017.

10. Wydick, R. C. (2005). *Plain English for lawyers,* 5th ed. Durham, NC: Carolina Academic Press.

11. Dobak, S., Peterson, S. J., Corrigan, M. L., & Lefton, J. (2017). Current practices and perceived barriers to diagnosing, documenting, and coding to malnutrition: A survey of the dietitians in nutrition support dietetic practice group. Available at: http://jandonline.org/article/S2212-2672(17)30230-7/fulltext. Accessed September 9, 2017.

CHAPTER 9

Case Studies

PRACTICING THE NUTRITION CARE PROCESS

Elise Kowalski, RDN

Dear Registered Dietitian Nutritionist,

Congratulations on passing your exam, and welcome to our team! We are so excited to have a new graduate join us here at Star General Hospital and Medical Center. Since you will be working a few days on the general medical floor before your full orientation and training next week, I wanted to give you some basic information for your assessments.

I included an abbreviated list of diets and supplements we carry and our nutrition assessment template to get you started. I also left some generic business cards to give to your patients until yours arrive. A variety of education materials and Outpatient Nutrition Counseling brochures are available on our website; we have Outpatient Nutrition Counseling and a Weight Management Center in the medical office building.

You can order assistance with meals, automatic trays, weights, and supplements for your patients. You can recommend diets, multivitamins, and tests to the doctors. Please page a doctor alerting them to any patients who are severely malnourished or are NPO/Clear Liquids for five days.

We are looking forward to working with you! Don't hesitate to ask any of the other RDNs if you have any questions. Remember, there is never only one "right" nutrition diagnosis!

Sincerely,
Clinical Nutrition Manager

BOX 9.1

Star General Hospital and Medical Center Diets and Supplements

Diets

- Regular
- Mechanical Soft
- GI Soft (Low Fiber)
- 3–4 gram Sodium/No Added Salt
- Cardiac (Low Fat/Low Cholesterol/3–4 gram Sodium)
- Diabetic (1300–1500, 1600–1800, 1900–2100, 2200–2400)
- 2 gram Sodium (Low Na)
- 2 gram Potassium (Low K)
- Low Fat/Low Cholesterol
- Renal
- Renal with Dialysis
- Full Liquid
- Clear Liquid

Supplements

- Chocolate, Vanilla, and Strawberry Protein Shakes
- Clear Liquid Protein Supplement
- Sugar-Free Protein Supplement
- High-Protein Ice Cream

BOX 9.2

Nutrition Assessment Template

Nutrition Assessment			
Name:	LOS:	Age:	Sex:
Reason for Consult:			
HPI:			
Subjective:			
Patient History			
Medical History:			
Surgical History:			
Social History:			
Food- and Nutrition-Related History			
Current Diet:			
Intake:			
Food Allergies:			
Cultural or Religious Food Preferences:			
Nutritionally Relevant Medications and Infusions:			

Anthropometric Measurements			
Height:	Weight:	BMI:	BMI Classification:
IBW:	%IBW:	UBW:	%UBW:
Weight History and Change:			

Biochemical Data, Medical Tests, and Procedures

Nutrition-Focused Physical Findings
Appetite:
Oral:
GI:
Skin:
Edema:
Subcutaneous Fat Depletion:
Musculoskeletal Depletion:

Nutrition Diagnosis

Nutrition Intervention
Estimated Nutrition Needs
Calories:
Protein:
Fluid:
Nutrition Prescription and Interventions

Nutrition Prescription:
Interventions:
Nutrition Monitoring and Evaluation
Goals:
Monitoring:
Recommendations

CASE 1: L.S.'S FALL

Admission Sheet

Name	LOS	Age	Sex	Marital Status	Race/Ethnicity
L.S.	2	78	F	Widowed	Caucasian

Primary Language	Interpreter Needed	Next of Kin	Attending
English	No	Son (123) 555-1417	McClane, J., MD

Allergies	Chief Complaint	Admitting Diagnosis
No known allergies	Hip pain after fall, lethargy, lower abdominal pain, loose stools, nausea, poor oral intake	Left hip fracture, acute diarrhea, urinary tract infection without hematuria, altered mental status, hyponatremia

Patient History

Medical and Surgical History	Social History	Weight History	
GERD HTN CAD Arthritis Anemia Osteoporosis Constipation Alzheimer's dementia	Smoking Status: Never smoker Alcohol Use: No Drug Use: No Residence: ECF	3 months ago	51.9 kg
		10 months ago	50.7 kg
		1 year, 7 months ago	55.1 kg

Nursing Admission Assessment

Height	Weight	BMI	A&O	Glasgow	Braden
152.4 cm Estimate	48.6 kg Bed scale	20.9	To person x 1 To place x 1	13	17

Skin Integrity	Malnutrition Universal Screening Tool	
Blanchable erythema to center coccyx Abrasion to left knee Bruising and swelling to left hip	Decrease in appetite or intake? (Yes = 1, No = 0)	1

Weight loss >10 lbs in 3 months? (Yes = 1, No = 0)	1
BMI score (<18.5 = 2, 18.5–20.0 = 1, >20.0 = 0)	0
Total Score (2 or more triggers dietitian consult)	2

Active Orders

Consults	**Nursing**
CONSULT TO PHYSCIAN—left non-displaced femoral neck fracture CONSULT TO PHYSCIAN—occult + stools and fatigue CONSULT DIETITIAN FROM NURSING REFERRAL—*weight loss and decreased appetite* CONSULT DIETITIAN—*nutrition assessment* PT EVAL/TREATMENT OT EVAL/TREATMENT	PRESSURE INJURY PRECAUTIONS HIGH-RISK FALL PRECAUTIONS PNEUMATIC COMPRESSION DEVICE, CALVES INTAKE AND OUTPUT MEASURE WEIGHT—*on admission*

Laboratory/Imaging	**Medications/Infusions**
C. DIFFICILE TOXIN CULTURE, URINE COMPLETE BLOOD COUNT BASIC METABOLIC PANEL	Ceftriaxone—*intravenous* Donepezil—*oral* Famotidine—*oral* Metoprolol—*oral* Acetaminophen-codeine—*PRN* Sodium chloride 0.9% at 50 ml/hr

DIET: Cardiac (Low Fat/Low Cholesterol/3–4 gram Sodium)

Physician H & P

History of Present Illness: Patient is a 78-year-old female who presents with hip pain after falling at her nursing home. She is a poor historian. Nursing home staff reports patient had increased lethargy, lower abdominal pain, loose stools, nausea, and poor oral intake for approximately 3 days before falling. She has also lost weight over the past few months. ED workup showed left femoral fracture and UTI.

Temp	BP	Heart Rate	Resp	SpO2	O2 (L/min)
37.0°C	104/53 mmHg	70	18	97%	RA

Review of Systems and Physical Exam		
Constitutional	HEENT	Neck
Awake and alert; no distress	Normal	Normal
Pulmonary/Chest	Cardiovascular	Gastrointestinal
Clear to auscultation	No palpitations	Soft, non-tender; no ascites
Extremities	Skin	Neurological
Swelling to left hip; no edema	Bruising	Oriented x1

Assessment	Plan
Principal Problem: Non-displaced left femoral neck fracture Generalized weakness and lethargy Diarrhea UTI Hyponatremia Dementia DVT prophylaxis	Orthopedic surgery and GI consulted Continue IV fluids; urine culture; stool studies Monitor electrolytes Strict input and output Dietitian consulted for weight loss and poor intake
J. McClane, MD	

Flowsheets

Date	Hospital Day 1			Hospital Day 2		
Time	**0800**	**1200**	**1600**	**0800**	**1200**	
Meal Intake		0%	25%	15%	5%	
Outputs						
Urine Occurrences	1	2	1	1		
Stool Occurrences	2		1	1	2	
Edema						
RUE	None			None		
LUE	None			None		
RLE	None			None		
LLE	None			None		

Laboratory Results

	Ref. Range	
WBC	3.5–10.1 bil/L	6.9
Sodium	135–145 mmol/L	129 (L)
Potassium	3.5–5.2 mmol/L	4.2
Glucose	60–99 mg/dL	164 (H)
BUN	8–22 mg/dL	23 (H)
Creatinine	0.60–1.40 mg/dL	0.86
GFR Non-African American	>59 mL/min/1.73m2	61
GFR African American	>59 mL/min/1.73m2	70

Dietitian Interview and Physical

Your patient seems confused; she is unable to give you her name or birthday.

Appetite and intake: "My appetite is fine; I always eat. Unless it's a sandwich, I hate it when they give me a sandwich, but they serve the best meatloaf."

Weight loss and UBW: "I don't know."

Food allergies: "I don't think so."

Cultural or religious food preference: "I'm Catholic."

Difficulty chewing or swallowing: "No."

Nausea, vomiting, constipation, or diarrhea: "No."

Preferences: "I like chocolate shakes."

Musculoskeletal Depletion: None
Subcutaneous Fat Depletion: None

You call the next of kin listed in the medical record, her son.

"I don't really know how she eats; you would have to call the nursing home. I sometimes visit during lunch on the weekends, she usually eats about half her plate. I don't really know if she's lost weight, but I did have to buy her some smaller pants, so I guess she has. She doesn't have any food allergies that I know of."

You talk to her nurse.

"She isn't really eating much, and we've been ordering trays for her. I think she just forgets that she's eating and stops. She swallows fine. She's been having diarrhea; we just sent out a sample for C. difficile."

CASE 2: A.A.'S BACK PAIN

Admission Sheet

Name	LOS	Age	Sex	Marital Status	Race/Ethnicity
A.A.	1	67	M	Married	Hispanic

Primary Language	Interpreter Needed	Next of Kin	Attending
English	No	Wife (123) 555-1417	Plissken, S., MD

Allergies	Chief Complaint	Admitting Diagnosis
Bee stings, Demerol HCl	Multiple infected sacral decubitus ulcers, worsening chronic back pain, and lethargy	Decubitus ulcer of left buttock, stage 4; decubitus ulcer of right heel, stage 3; acute exacerbation of chronic back pain

Patient History

Medical and Surgical History	Social History	Weight History	
DM type 2 CKD stage 3, GFR 30–59 CAD Ischemic cardiomyopathy MI Hypothyroid Chronic pain CABG Implantable cardiac defibrillator	Smoking Status: Former smoker; quit 7 years ago Alcohol Use: 2–3 beers/week Drug Use: No Residence: Lives with wife	1 month ago	122.1 kg
		2 months ago	125.2 kg
		3 months ago	124.9 kg

Nursing Admission Assessment

Height	Weight	BMI	A&O	Glasgow	Braden
170.2 cm Pt estimate	118.6 kg Bed scale	40.9	To person x 3 To place x 3	15	12

Skin Integrity	Malnutrition Universal Screening Tool	
Stage 4 pressure injury to left buttock Stage 3 pressure injury to right heel Unstageable pressure injury to right buttock	Decrease in appetite or intake? (Yes = 1, No = 0)	0

	Weight loss >10 lbs in 3 months? (Yes = 1, No = 0)	1
	BMI score (<18.5 = 2, 18.5–20.0 = 1, >20.0 = 0)	0
	Total Score (2 or more triggers dietitian consult)	1

Active Orders

Consults	Nursing
CONSULT TO PHYSCIAN—pressure injuries not healing CONSULT TO PHYSCIAN—infected pressure injuries CONSULT TO PHYSCIAN—*back pain* WOUND/OSTOMY/CONTINENCE NURSE—*pressure injuries* CONSULT DIETITIAN—worsening pressure injuries, wound healing recommendations PT EVAL/TREATMENT OT EVAL/TREATMENT	PRESSURE INJURY WOUND CARE GLUCOSE, POINT OF CARE URINARY CATHETER HIGH-RISK FALL PRECAUTIONS MEASURE WEIGHT—*on admission*
Laboratory/Imaging	**Medications/Infusions**
CULTURE, WOUND DEEP COMPLETE BLOOD COUNT W DIFF COMPREHENSIVE METABOLIC PANEL LUMBOSACRAL SPINE IMAGING—*minimum 4 views*	Acetaminophen—*oral* Aspirin—*oral* Atorvastatin—*oral* Carvedilol—*oral* Cefepime—*intravenous* Docusate—*oral* Heparin injection—*subcutaneous* Hydrocerin—*topical* Insulin glargine—*subcutaneous* Insulin lispro—*subcutaneous* Levothyroxine—*oral* Losartan—*oral* Metronidazole—*intravenous* Miconazole—*oral* Omeprazole—*oral* Wound Cleanser—*topical*
DIET: Cardiac (Low Fat/Low Cholesterol, 3–4 gram Sodium)	

Physician H & P

History of Present Illness: Patient is a 67-year-old male who presents with multiple pressure ulcers, lethargy, and worsening chronic back pain. He first developed the ulcers during hospitalization 2 months ago for pneumonia. He was then discharged to rehab. He has chronic back pain for about 6 or 7 years, but it has markedly increased over the past 2 weeks.

Temp	BP	Heart Rate	Resp	SpO2	O2 (L/min)
36.3°C	107/55 mmHg	62	18	99%	RA

Review of Systems and Physical Exam

Constitutional	HEENT	Neck
Well nourished	Sclera white, oral mucosa pink	Supple, no masses
Pulmonary/Chest	Cardiovascular	Gastrointestinal
No dyspnea	No murmur	Non-tender
Extremities	Skin	Neurological
Good muscle tone	4 cm pressure ulcer to the left buttock with yellow sloughing; 3.5 cm pressure ulcer to the right buttock; 1.5 cm pressure ulcer to the right heel with overlying eschar. Foley in place.	A & O x 3

Assessment	Plan
Primary Problem: Decubitus ulcer of left buttock, stage 4 Decubitus ulcer of right heel, stage 3 Acute exacerbation of chronic back pain Diabetes mellitus Foley catheter in place CAD CKD stage 3, GFR 30–59	Wound care and infectious disease consulted Foley catheter Wound cultures X-ray for acute on chronic back pain Dietitian consulted for wound healing recommendations

S. Plissken, MD

Flowsheets

Date	Day 1					
Time	0800	1200	1800			
Meal Intake	100%	100%	100%			
Outputs						
Stool Occurrences						
Foley Catheter	450 ml	375 ml	475 ml			
Edema						
RUE	None	None	None			
LUE	None	None	None			
RLE	Trace	Trace	Trace			
LLE	Trace	Trace	Trace			

Laboratory Results

	Ref. Range	Day 1 0351
WBC	3.5–10.1 bil/L	6.3
Sodium	135–145 mmol/L	135
Potassium	3.5–5.2 mmol/L	4.7
Glucose	60–99 mg/dL	270 (H)
BUN	8–22 mg/dL	38 (H)
Creatinine	0.60–1.40 mg/dL	1.57 (H)
Phosphorus	2.3–4.3 mg/dL	4.2
GFR Non-African American	>59 mL/min/1.73m2	40 (L)
GFR African American	>59 mL/min/1.73m2	47 (L)

Glucose, Point of Care

Day 1 0743	Day 1 1139	Day 1 1748	Day 2 0747
226 (H)	218 (H)	282 (H)	165 (H)

Dietitian Interview and Physical

Your patient is waiting for his breakfast to arrive.

Appetite and intake: "My appetite is okay I guess; yeah, it's pretty much normal. I eat everything they give me, but I'm not crazy about the food. I ate fine at the rehab, even though I don't like the food there either. My wife brings me what I like. I know I'm supposed to watch my sugars, but it's too hard. My doctor gave me a bunch of pamphlets about food; I don't need any more information."

Weight loss and UBW: "I don't know if I've lost weight; I am usually about 275 pounds."

Food allergies: "None that I know of."

Cultural or religious food preference: "No."

Difficulty chewing or swallowing: "No."

Nausea, vomiting, constipation, or diarrhea: "I'm constipated. I don't remember when my last bowel movement was."

Preferences: "The foods my wife makes; spaghetti, meatloaf, tacos, baked potatoes, and chicken."

Musculoskeletal Depletion: None

Subcutaneous Fat Depletion: None

You talk to his nurse.

"He's eating all of his meals. I think his wife brings him snacks, too. I told him he needs to watch what he is eating because his blood sugar has been so high."

CASE 3: C.P.'S UPSET STOMACH

Admission Sheet					
Name	**LOS**	**Age**	**Sex**	**Marital Status**	**Race/Ethnicity**
C.P.	1	23	F	Single	Indian
Primary Language	**Interpreter Needed**		**Next of Kin**		**Attending**
English	No		Mother (123)555-1417		Dallas, K., MD
Allergies	**Chief Complaint**			**Admitting Diagnosis**	
No known allergies	Nausea, vomiting, weight loss, abdominal pain			Diabetic ketoacidosis without coma	

Patient History

Medical and Surgical History	Social History	Weight History
No medical or surgical history on file	Smoking Status: Current smoker; 1 pack/day for 6 years Alcohol Use: 2–3 drinks/week Drug Use: None Residence: Lives with roommate	No weight history on file

Nursing Admission Assessment

Height	Weight	BMI	A&O	Glasgow	Braden
170.2 cm Pt estimate	54.5 kg Pt estimate	18.8	To person x 3 To place x 3	15	22

Skin Integrity	Malnutrition Universal Screening Tool	
Intact	Decrease in appetite or intake? (Yes = 1, No = 0)	1
	Weight loss >10 lbs in 3 months? (Yes = 1, No = 0)	1
	BMI score (<18.5 = 2, 18.5–20.0 = 1, >20.0 = 0)	1
	Total Score (2 or more triggers dietitian consult)	3

Active Orders

Consults	Nursing
CONSULT TO PHYSCIAN—*stomach pain* CONSULT TO PHYSCIAN—*new onset DM; DKA* CONSULT DIETITIAN FROM NURSING REFERRAL—decreased appetite, N/V, unplanned weight loss CONSULT DIETITIAN—new type 1 diabetic instruction CONSULT CARE MANAGEMENT—glucometer for home use, on insulin CONSULT SOCIAL WORK—*substance abuse*	INTAKE AND OUTPUT GLUCOSE, POINT OF CARE TEACH DIABETIC CARE MEASURE WEIGHT—*on admission*

Laboratory/Imaging	Medications/Infusions
COMPLETE BLOOD COUNT W DIFF COMPREHENSIVE METABOLIC PANEL ELECTROLYTES PANEL EVERY 4 HOURS MAGNESIUM EVERY 4 HOURS PHOSPHORUS EVERY 4 HOURS LIPID PANEL	Insulin lispro—*subcutaneous* Insulin NPH—*subcutaneous* Insulin regular human—*subcutaneous* Pantoprazole—*intravenous* Zofran—*PRN* Bismuth subsalicylate—*PRN* Insulin regular human 100 units in sodium chloride 0.9% at 2 units/hr Sodium chloride 0.9% at 75 ml/hr

DIET: Clear Liquid, Advance as Tolerated

Physician H & P

History of Present Illness: Patient is a 23-year-old female who presents with nausea, vomiting, and abdominal pain for 5 days. She also has lost weight over the last week. She denies fever, chills, or sweating. No personal or family history of diabetes. She admits to daily marijuana use and drinks socially. ER workup showed DKA and insulin was started.

Temp	BP	Heart Rate	Resp	SpO2	O2 (L/min)
36.8°C	145/79 mmHg	67	20	100%	RA

Review of Systems and Physical Exam

Constitutional	HEENT	Neck
Appears tired	Pupils reactive, moist MM	Supple, no thyromegaly
Pulmonary/Chest	Cardiovascular	Gastrointestinal
Clear to auscultation	Regular rate and rhythm	No hepatosplenomegaly
Extremities	Skin	Neurological
No cyanosis	No skin rash	Cranial nerves intact

Assessment	Plan
Principal Problem: DKA Dehydration Nausea and vomiting	Endocrinology and GI consulted Monitor electrolytes Input and output Continue IV insulin and fluids
K. Dallas, MD	

Flowsheets

Date	Day 1					
Time	0800					
Meal Intake	10%					
Outputs						
Urine Occurrences						
Stool Occurrences						
Edema						
RUE	None					
LUE	None					
RLE	None					
LLE	None					

Laboratory Results

	Ref. Range	Day 1 0134	Day 1 0526
WBC	3.5–10.1 bil/L	19.5	
Sodium	135–145 mmol/L	133 (L)	137
Potassium	3.5–5.2 mmol/L	5.3 (H)	4.6
Glucose	60–99 mg/dL	448 (H)	198 (H)
BUN	8–22 mg/dL	15	
Creatinine	0.60–1.40 mg/dL	2.12	
Phosphorus	2.3–4.3 mg/dL		5.0 (H)
Magnesium	1.6–2.4 mg/dL	2.4	2.0
GFR Non-African American	>59 mL/min/1.73m2	42 (L)	
GFR African American	>59 mL/min/1.73m2	48 (L)	
Beta Hydroxybutyrate	0.02–0.27 mmol/L	12.15 (H)	
HbA1c	4.0–5.6%	11.9 (H)	
Estimated Average Glucose		295	

| Urinalysis, Glucose | Negative mg/dL | >=1000 (!) | |
| Urinalysis, Ketones | Negative mg/dL | >=80 (!!) | |

Glucose, Point of Care			
Day 1 0229	Day 1 0332	Day 1 0437	Day 1 0718
333 (H)	282 (H)	182 (H)	209 (H)

Dietitian Interview and Physical

Your patient is sleeping, but her mother is at bedside.

"Oh, I am so glad you are here, you are just the person I want to speak with about my daughter!"

Appetite and intake: "She hasn't been able to keep anything down for 5 days! Maybe just a few sips of water or pop here and there. We thought it was a stomach bug she picked up at school. She's been staying with me the last few days, and I brought her in last night because she just wasn't getting any better. Well, come to find out, she has diabetes. We are shocked; no one else in our family has diabetes. I have a lot of questions about how she has to eat now. I think she was eating fine before this started, but she's been at school, so I don't know for sure."

Weight loss and UBW: "She's always been on the thin side, but she's lost like 10 pounds in the past week, week and half. She's normally around 130 pounds."

Food allergies: "She gets hives whenever she eats tomatoes."

Cultural or religious food preferences: "She doesn't eat meat; but she eats eggs and dairy."

Difficulty chewing or swallowing: "No."

Nausea, vomiting, constipation, or diarrhea: "She was having bad stomach pains and vomiting for 5 days before we brought her in. She hasn't vomited yet today. She just had a few sips of juice not too long ago."

Preferences: "She's a light eater. She loves fruit and drinks a lot of smoothies. I always try to get her to eat more at dinner. Lately she's been doing the gluten-free thing. Do you think this has something to do with what happened?"

Musculoskeletal Depletion: You don't complete the physical exam because she is sleeping under the covers.

Subcutaneous Fat Depletion:

You talk to her nurse.

"She has been very sleepy since she came up to the floor. The doctor said to keep her on clear liquids to make sure the vomiting has stopped. We might put her on full liquids later if it goes well. Her mom is very worried about the whole thing; I'm glad you came right away."

CASE 4: B.F.'S SHORTNESS OF BREATH

Admission Sheet

Name	LOS	Age	Sex	Marital Status	Race/Ethnicity
B.F.	2	59	M	Married	Arabic

Primary Language	Interpreter Needed	Next of Kin	Attending
Arabic	Yes	Wife (123)555-2272	Powers, K.,MD

Allergies	Chief Complaint	Admitting Diagnosis
Ativan	Shortness of breath, foot wound	Acute COPD exacerbation, diabetic foot ulcer

Patient History

Medical and Surgical History	Social History	Weight History	
DM type 2 Diabetic neuropathy CAD COPD Hyperlipidemia Hypercholesterolemia PAD Cardiac catheterization	Smoking Status: Current smoker; 2 packs/day for 40 years Alcohol Use: 1 drink/day Drug Use: None Residence: Lives with wife	4 months ago	79.8 kg
		1 year, 2 months ago	75.8 kg
		2 years ago	70.3 kg

Nursing Admission Assessment

Height	Weight	BMI	A&O	Glasgow	Braden
172.7 cm Pt estimate	83.5 kg Standing scale	28.0	To person x 3 To place x 3	15	17

Skin Integrity	Malnutrition Universal Screening Tool	
Left foot ulcer s/p debridement and wound vac placement Abrasions to right and left feet	Decrease in appetite or intake? (Yes = 1, No = 0)	0
	Weight loss >10 lbs in 3 months? (Yes = 1, No = 0)	0
	BMI score (<18.5 = 2, 18.5–20.0 = 1, >20.0 = 0)	0
	Total Score (2 or more triggers dietitian consult)	0

Active Orders	
Consults	**Nursing**
CONSULT TO PHYSCIAN—candidate for proximal amputation left foot CONSULT TO PHYSCIAN—*diabetic foot ulcer* CONSULT TO PHYSCIAN—SOB, COPD CONSULT DIETITIAN—nutritional needs for wound healing and diabetic diet education WOUND/OSTOMY/CONTINENCE NURSE—*wound vac left foot* PT EVAL/TREATMENT	ALTERNATIVE SPLINT AND/OR FOAM BOOTS WITH SCDs GLUCOSE, POINT OF CARE WOUND VAC ONGOING WOUND CARE MEASURE WEIGHT—*on admission*
Laboratory/Imaging	**Medications/Infusions**
CULTURE, BLOOD CULTURE, WOUND DEEP CULTURE, TISSUE COMPLETE BLOOD COUNT W DIFF COMPREHENSIVE METABOLIC PANEL C REACTIVE PROTEIN LIPID PANEL	Aspirin—*oral* Atorvastatin—*oral* Carvedilol—*oral* Cefazolin—*intravenous* Clopidogrel—*oral* Fluticasone-vilanterol—*inhalation* Heparin injection—*subcutaneous* Insulin lispro—*subcutaneous* Linagliptin—*oral* Lisinopril—*oral* Acetaminophen—*PRN* Bisacodyl—*PRN* Docusate—*PRN* Melatonin—*PRN* Polyethylene glycol 3350—*PRN*
DIET: Diabetic 1600–1800	

Physician H & P

History of Present Illness: Patient is a 59-year-old male who presents with shortness of breath. Patient does not speak English, and family is providing history. He is a current smoker and has a history of COPD. He started having shortness of breath when walking upstairs earlier today. It did not improve much with rest, so he came into the ED. He also has a chronic diabetic ulcer on his left foot that is worsening. He denies fever, chills, chest pain, nausea, and vomiting. ED chest X-rays showed stable cardiomegaly with no sizable pleural effusion or pneumothorax.

Temp	BP	Heart Rate	Resp	SpO2	O2 (L/min)
36.6°C	114/74 mmHg	92	20	95%	RA

Review of Systems and Physical Exam		
Constitutional	HEENT	Neck
Nontoxic, oriented	PERRLA, no jaundice	No carotid bruits
Pulmonary/Chest	Cardiovascular	Gastrointestinal
No wheezing, no crackles	Regular rate and rhythm	No masses felt; non-tender
Extremities	Skin	Neurological
No edema	Diabetic ulcer to left foot	No focal motor deficits

Assessment	**Plan**
Principal Problem: Acute COPD exacerbation Diabetic foot ulcer Diabetes mellitus, type 2 Suspected lower extremity peripheral vascular disease	Pulmonary, wound care, and infectious disease consulted Ulcer debridement and wound vac placement Wound and blood cultures Continue antibiotics Dietitian consulted for wound healing recommendations and diabetic diet instruction
K. Powers, MD	

Flowsheets

Date	Day 1			Day 2		
Time	0800	1200	1600	0800		
Meal Intake						
Outputs						
Urine Occurrences	1	1	1	1		
Stool Occurrences			1			

Negative Pressure Wound Therapy	Left foot, placed day 1 at 1342						
			0 ml	Scant			
Edema							
RUE	None			None			
LUE	None			None			
RLE	None			None			
LLE	None			None			

Laboratory Results

	Ref. Range	Day 1 0934
WBC	3.5–10.1 bil/L	21.1 (H)
Sodium	135–145 mmol/L	136
Potassium	3.5–5.2 mmol/L	4.6
Glucose	60–99 mg/dL	178 (H)
BUN	8–22 mg/dL	26 (H)
Creatinine	0.60–1.40 mg/dL	1.28
GFR Non-African American	>59 mL/min/1.73m2	61
GFR African American	>59 mL/min/1.73m2	71
HbA1c	4.0–5.6%	7.0 (H)
Estimated Average Glucose		154

Glucose, Point of Care

Day 1 1209	Day 1 1457	Day 1 2012	Day 2 0732
199 (H)	123 (H)	207 (H)	162 (H)

Dietitian Interview and Physical

Your patient does not speak English and no family is at bedside. You use a translation computer to communicate.

Appetite and intake: "My appetite is good. Yes, it was good at home, and I am eating all my meals. I've had diabetes for a few years, but I don't know what to eat; my doctor never told me. I just eat what my family cooks."

Weight loss and UBW: "I don't know."

Food allergies: "None."

Cultural or religious food preference: "I don't eat pork."

Difficulty chewing or swallowing: "No."

Nausea, vomiting, constipation, or diarrhea: "No."

Preferences: "I like shish taouk, tabbouleh, shawarma, labneh, hummus, baba ghanouj, kibbeh, and kofta. I eat one or two pitas and a plate of rice with almost every meal."

Musculoskeletal Depletion: None

Subcutaneous Fat Depletion: None

You talk to his nurse.

"His family is bringing in food that looks really high in carbs. I just don't think they know much about diabetes or how to count carbohydrates."

CASE 5: R.D.'S FATIGUE

Admission Sheet					
Name	**LOS**	**Age**	**Sex**	**Marital Status**	**Race/Ethnicity**
R.D.	1	76	M	Divorced	African American
Primary Language	**Interpreter Needed**		**Next of Kin**		**Attending**
English	No		Niece (123) 555-8071		Shultz, K., MD
Allergies	**Chief Complaint**			**Admitting Diagnosis**	
No known allergies	Low hemoglobin, fatigue, and decreased appetite			Anemia	

Patient History			
Medical and Surgical History	**Social History**	**Weight History**	
CVA COPD Hyperlipidemia Hearing loss CAD Pneumonia Arthritis Lung cancer	Smoking Status: Current smoker; 1 pack/day for 50 years Alcohol Use: No Drug Use: No Residence: Assisted living	4 months ago	51.2 kg
		5 months ago	50.7 kg
		9 months ago	52.3 kg

Nursing Admission Assessment

Height	Weight	BMI	A&O	Glasgow	Braden
165.1 cm Pt estimate	45.6 kg Standing scale	16.7	To person x 3 To place x 3	15	17

Skin Integrity	Malnutrition Universal Screening Tool	
Intact	Decrease in appetite or intake? (Yes = 1, No = 0)	1
	Weight loss >10 lbs in 3 months? (Yes = 1, No = 0)	1
	BMI score (<18.5 = 2, 18.5–20.0 = 1, >20.0 = 0)	2
	Total Score (2 or more triggers dietitian consult)	4

Active Orders

Consults	Nursing
CONSULT TO PHYSCIAN—*anemia* CONSULT DIETITIAN FROM NURSING REFERRAL—*low weight* PT EVAL/TREATMENT OT EVAL/TREATMENT	PRESSURE INJURY PRECAUTIONS HIGH-RISK FALL PRECAUTIONS BLEEDING PRECAUTIONS MEASURE WEIGHT—*on admission*

Laboratory/Imaging	Medications/Infusions
COMPLETE BLOOD COUNT W DIFF COMPREHENSIVE METABOLIC PANEL HEMOGLOBIN AND HEMATOCRIT	Aspirin—*oral* Atorvastatin—*oral* Clopidogrel—*oral* Dexamethasone—*oral* Labetalol—*oral* Omeprazole—*oral* Albuterol-ipratropium—*PRN* Diphenhydramine—*PRN* Prochlorperazine—*PRN* Sodium chloride 0.9% at 75 ml/hr

DIET: Cardiac (Low Fat/Low Cholesterol/3–4 gram Sodium)

Physician H & P

History of Present Illness: Patient is a 76-year-old male who presents with hemoglobin of 7. He was seen at his PCP earlier today for fatigue and was sent here for a transfusion. He just completed chemotherapy treatment last week for lung cancer. He reports a poor appetite and nausea since starting chemotherapy 6 weeks ago.

Temp	BP	Heart Rate	Resp	SpO2	O2 (L/min)
36.7°C	119/63 mmHg	84	18	97%	RA

Review of Systems and Physical Exam

Constitutional	HEENT	Neck
Appears ill; no acute distress	PERRLA, no jaundice	No masses or carotid bruits
Pulmonary/Chest	Cardiovascular	Gastrointestinal
No wheezing or crackles	Regular rate and rhythm	Abdomen soft, non-tender
Extremities	Skin	Neurological
No edema	No rash, no palpable nodules	Appropriate mood and affect

Assessment	Plan
Principal Problem: Anemia Guaiac negative stool Fatigue Lung cancer s/p chemotherapy CT head negative for acute hemorrhage Nicotine addiction	Hematology consulted Monitor H&H, transfuse PRN

K. Shultz, MD

Flowsheets

Date	Day 1					
Time	0800	1200				
Meal Intake		5%				
Outputs						
Urine Occurrences						

Stool Occurrences						
Edema						
RUE		None				
LUE		None				
RLE		None				
LLE		None				

Laboratory Results			
	Ref. Range	**Day 1 0940**	**Day 1 1309**
WBC	3.5–10.1 bil/L	6.7	8.4
RBC	3.87–5.08 tril/L	2.14 (L)	2.84 (L)
Hemoglobin	12.1–15.0 g/dL	6.6 (L)	8.9 (L)
Hematocrit	35.4–44.2%	21.8 (L)	27.6 (L)
MCV	80–100 fL	102 (H)	97
MCH	28–33 pg	31	31
MCHC	32–35 g/dL	30 (L)	32
Sodium	135–145 mmol/L	143	
Potassium	3.5–5.2 mmol/L	3.6	
Glucose	60–99 mg/dL	72	
BUN	8–22 mg/dL	11	
Creatinine	0.60–1.40 mg/dL	0.43	
GFR Non-African American	>59 mL/min/1.73m2	103	
GFR African American	>59 mL/min/1.73m2	119	
Iron	30–160 mcg/dL		63
Total Iron Binding Capacity	228–417 mcg/dL		204 (L)
Ferritin	12–207 ng/mL		416 (H)
Folate	>5.4 ng/mL		12.0
Vitamin B12	271–870 pg/mL		474

Dietitian Interview and Physical

Your patient is watching TV in bed.

Appetite and intake: "I've haven't been eating much since the chemo started about 6 or 7 weeks ago. I get really nauseous and things just don't taste the same. I've been eating probably a quarter of what I normally do. Some days I don't even eat a whole meal. I know I should eat more. My doctor wants me to drink those protein shakes, but I don't like them."

Weight loss and UBW: "I was 110 pounds for the past 3 to 4 years before the chemo started, and they said I was only 100 when they weighed me here. I used to be 140 when I was younger; I was never a big guy. Over the past 10 years or so I've gotten a lot thinner. I just don't eat as much as I used to."

Food allergies: "None."

Cultural or religious food preference: "None."

Difficulty chewing or swallowing: "I have dentures, but they don't fit very good anymore since losing this weight. It's harder for me to chew with them in, so I've been eating softer foods."

Nausea, vomiting, constipation, or diarrhea: "I have a lot of nausea from the chemo. Sometimes I throw up a few times a day. The last time I threw up was a couple days ago, but I still have my usual nausea. My bowel movements are pretty normal, I had one yesterday."

Preferences: "I used to eat anything, but nothing really appeals to me now. I've been eating a ton of ice cream because it's all I can stand sometimes."

Musculoskeletal Depletion: Severe to temple, clavicle, deltoid, hand, thigh, patella, and calf

Subcutaneous Fat Depletion: Severe to orbital and triceps

You call his nurse, but he is with another patient and can't talk.

CASE 6: C.B.'S CONFUSION

Admission Sheet					
Name	**LOS**	**Age**	**Sex**	**Marital Status**	**Race/Ethnicity**
C.B.	3	73	F	Married	Chinese
Primary Language	**Interpreter Needed**		**Next of Kin**		**Attending**
English	No		Husband (123)555-3365		Connor, S., MD

Allergies	Chief Complaint	Admitting Diagnosis
Cats, pollen, lactose intolerance	Slurred speech, left-sided facial droop, increased confusion	Cerebrovascular accident

Patient History

Medical and Surgical History	Social History	Weight History	
Hypothyroid Hyperlipidemia GERD Gout HTN Cholecystectomy CAD MI	Smoking Status: Former smoker; quit 25 years ago Alcohol Use: None Drug Use: None Residence: Lives with husband	2 years ago	58.5 kg

Nursing Admission Assessment

Height	Weight	BMI	A&O	Glasgow	Braden
154.9 cm Estimate	57.3 kg Bed scale	23.9	To person x 1 To place x 1	10	12

Skin Integrity	Malnutrition Universal Screening Tool	
Bruising to right arm Redness to coccyx	Decrease in appetite or intake? (Yes = 1, No = 0)	1
	Weight loss >10 lbs in 3 months? (Yes = 1, No = 0)	0
	BMI score (<18.5 = 2, 18.5–20.0 = 1, >20.0 = 0)	0
	Total Score (2 or more triggers dietitian consult)	1

Active Orders

Consults	Nursing
CONSULT TO PHYSCIAN—*stroke, aphasia* CONSULT DIETITIAN—nutrition assessment, supplements PT EVAL/TREATMENT OT EVAL/TREATMENT CONSULT CARE MANAGEMENT—*ECF placement*	PRESSURE INJURY PRECAUTIONS HIGH-RISK FALL PRECAUTIONS ASPIRATION PRECAUTIONS NEUROLOGICAL ASSESSMENT EVERY 2 HOURS PNEUMATIC COMPRESSION DEVICE, CALVES STRICT BED REST MEASURE WEIGHT—*on admission*
Laboratory/Imaging	**Medications/Infusions**
CULTURE, URINE CULTURE, BLOOD BASIC METABOLIC PANEL COMPLETE BLOOD COUNT W DIFF THYROID STIMULATING HORMONE	Aspirin—*oral* Atorvastatin—*oral* Famotidine—*intravenous* Labetalol—*intravenous* Lisinopril—*oral* Acetaminophen—*PRN* Albuterol-ipratropium—*PRN* Ondansetron—*PRN*

DIET: Cardiac (Low Fat/Low Cholesterol/3–4 gram Sodium)

Physician H & P

History of Present Illness: Patient is a 73-year-old female who presents with stroke symptoms and increased confusion in the past 24 hours. Her husband brought her into the ED after noticing she had a left-sided facial droop and slurred speech. He says that she hadn't "been herself" all day. She has no history of CVA. CT scan shows area of stroke.

Temp	BP	Heart Rate	Resp	SpO2	O2 (L/min)
37.1°C	178/89 mmHg	73	16	94%	4L NC

Review of Systems and Physical Exam

Constitutional	HEENT	Neck
Lethargic	Normal	Thyroid not palpable
Pulmonary/Chest	Cardiovascular	Gastrointestinal
No cough	Regular rate with flow murmur	No abdominal pain

Extremities	Skin	Neurological
No edema	No rash	Left facial droop

Assessment	**Plan**
Principal Problem: CVA with confusion CAD HTN GERD	Neurology consulted Speech language pathologist and dietitian consulted Repeat CT scan IV labetalol for BP Check TSH
S. Connor, MD	

Speech Language Pathologist Note

Patient is awake and alert. Accepts range of PO, but not able to feed herself. Oral phase is intact with timely swallow. No overt signs of airway compromise. Recommend regular texture diet with thin liquids; 1:1 feed.

A. Stark, MA, CCC-SLP

Flowsheets

Date	Day 2			Day 3		
Time	**0800**	**1200**	**1600**	**0800**	**1200**	
Meal Intake	0%	0%	100%	90%		
Outputs						
Urine Occurrences	1	1		1	1	
Stool Occurrences		1		1		
Edema						
RUE	None			None		
LUE	None			None		
RLE	None			None		
LLE	None			None		

Laboratory Results

	Ref. Range	Day 3 0455
WBC	3.5–10.1 bil/L	13.8 (H)
Sodium	135–145 mmol/L	140
Potassium	3.5–5.2 mmol/L	3.8
Glucose	60–99 mg/dL	93
BUN	8–22 mg/dL	24 (H)
Creatinine	0.60–1.40 mg/dL	0.64
Phosphorus	2.3–4.3 mg/dL	2.7
GFR Non-African American	>59 mL/min/1.73m2	85
GFR African American	>59 mL/min/1.73m2	98

Dietitian Interview and Physical

Your patient is awake but is unresponsive to interview questions.

Musculoskeletal Depletion: You don't do the physical exam because the patient is unable to consent; she appears well nourished

Subcutaneous Fat Depletion:

You call the next of kin listed in the medical record, her husband.

Appetite and intake: "She can't feed herself since the stroke, but she ate all her dinner last night when I was feeding her. She was eating just fine before this happened. We always liked to go out to dinner together, and she would order a big meal and dessert. Is someone helping her eat when I'm not there?"

Weight loss and UBW: "She wouldn't ever tell me how much she weighed. I don't think she's lost weight, but I'm not sure."

Food allergies: "None that I know of, but she doesn't drink milk because it hurts her stomach."

Cultural or religious food preference: "No."

Difficulty chewing or swallowing: "I don't think so."

Nausea, vomiting, constipation, or diarrhea: "I don't know, I haven't been up there today yet."

Preferences: "She usually isn't very picky. She loves eating eggs and bacon for breakfast, and usually has a yogurt at lunch. She is always eating little chocolates when she watches her programs."

You talk to her nurse.
"Yeah, she isn't really with it; she's A&O x 1. She will eat if you hold it up to her mouth; I know her husband was here last night feeding her dinner. The nursing aides are ordering meals for her when he's not here. She's not having any vomiting or diarrhea."

CASE 7: B.K.'S SYNCOPE

Admission Sheet					
Name	**LOS**	**Age**	**Sex**	**Marital Status**	**Race/Ethnicity**
B.K.	3	53	M	Divorced	Caucasian
Primary Language	**Interpreter Needed**		**Next of Kin**		**Attending**
English	No		Brother (123) 555-7625		White, W., MD
Allergies		**Chief Complaint**		**Admitting Diagnosis**	
No known allergies		Vomiting, syncope		STEMI	

Patient History Medical and Surgical History	Smoking Status: Never smoker Alcohol Use: No Drug Use: No Residence: Lives alone	4 months ago	96.4 kg
		Weight History	
	Social History		

Nursing Admission Assessment					
Height	**Weight**	**BMI**	**A&O**	**Glasgow**	**Braden**
188.0 cm Pt Estimate	101.9 kg Standing Scale	28.8	To person x 3 To place x 3	15	20
Skin Integrity			**Malnutrition Universal Screening Tool**		

Incision to left chest Procedure site to right wrist Puncture to right groin	Decrease in appetite or intake? (Yes = 1, No = 0)	0
	Weight loss >10 lbs in 3 months? (Yes = 1, No = 0)	0
	BMI score (<18.5 = 2, 18.5–20.0 = 1, >20.0 = 0)	0
	Total Score (2 or more triggers dietitian consult)	0

Active Orders

Consults	Nursing
CONSULT TO PHYSCIAN—IM consult for medical management and transfer service CONSULT TO PHYSCIAN—CKD stage 4 s/p cardiac cath CONSULT DIETITIAN—nutrition assessment and education PT EVAL/TREATMENT OT EVAL/TREATMENT CARDIAC REHABILITATION—outpatient phase II and phase III CONSULT CARE MANAGEMENT—*ECF placement*	NEUROVASCULAR ASSESSMENT EVERY 4 HOURS INCISION CARE STRICT BED REST BLEEDING PRECAUTIONS STAT ECG—if chest pain, hypotension, or dyspnea occurs HIGH-RISK FALL PRECAUTIONS PRESSURE INJURY PRECAUTIONS ENCOURAGE FLUIDS INTAKE AND OUTPUT MEASURE WEIGHT—*on admission*
Laboratory/Imaging	**Medications/Infusions**
COMPLETE BLOOD COUNT RENAL FUNCTION PANEL CHEST SINGLE VIEW FRONTAL INSPIRATION—*s/p ICD implant*	Amlodipine—*oral* Aspirin—*oral* Atorvastatin—*oral* Clopidogrel—*oral* Docusate—*oral* Ferrous sulfate—*oral* Finasteride—*oral* Heparin injection—*subcutaneous* Hydralazine—*oral* Levothyroxine—*oral* Metoprolol—*oral* Oxybutynin—*oral* Sodium bicarbonate—*oral* Acetaminophen—*PRN*

	Alum & mag hydroxide-simeth—*PRN*
	Ondansetron—*PRN*
	Sodium chloride 0.9% at 20 ml/hr

DIET: Sodium 2 gm (Low Na), Low Fat/Low Cholesterol

Physician H & P

History of Present Illness: Patient is a 53-year-old male who presents with vomiting and syncope. He was eating breakfast with his brother at a restaurant and became nauseated. He vomited once, and then became unresponsive. EMS transported him to the ED, and EKG showed ST elevation at V2/V3. He denies chest pain.

Temp	BP	Heart Rate	Resp	SpO2	O2 (L/min)
36.8°C	165/80	55	16	98%	RA

Review of Systems and Physical Exam

Constitutional	HEENT	Neck
Negative for fever	Negative for discharge	No carotid bruits
Pulmonary/Chest	Cardiovascular	Gastrointestinal
Negative for SOB	Negative for chest pain	Positive for vomiting
Extremities	Skin	Neurological
No edema	Negative for rash	Positive for syncope

Assessment	Plan
Principal Problem: STEMI History of CAD CKD stage 4 HTN Hyperlipidemia Arrhythmia	ASA/heparin bolus given Start IV fluids Active emergency cath team
W. White, MD	

Physician Progress Note

History of Present Illness: Patient presented 2 days ago with STEMI s/p cardiac cath with PCI and stent on admission. VT s/p ICD placement yesterday. He is resting comfortably. No chest pain or SOB.

Assessment	Plan
Principal Problem: STEMI s/p cardiac catheterization and coronary artery stent VT s/p implantable cardiac defibrillator History of CAD and hyperlipidemia CKD stage 4 HTN Arrhythmia	Nephrology and internal medicine consulted Chest X-ray s/p ICD Continue IV fluids, amlodipine, atorvastatin, aspirin, clopidogrel, hydralazine, and metoprolol Dietitian consulted for nutrition assessment and low-sodium nutrition education

W. White, MD

Flowsheets

Date	Day 2			Day 3		
Time	0800	1200	1600	0800		
Meal Intake	NPO	NPO	50%	70%		
Outputs						
Urine Occurrences		2	1	1		
Stool Occurrences						
Edema						
RUE	None			None		
LUE	None			None		
RLE	None			None		
LLE	None			None		

Laboratory Results

	Ref. Range	Day 2 1234	Day 3 0631
WBC	3.5–10.1 bil/L	4.6	5.3
Sodium	135–145 mmol/L	139	139
Potassium	3.5–5.2 mmol/L	4.9	4.8
Glucose	60–99 mg/dL	86	127 (H)
BUN	8–22 mg/dL	49 (H)	48 (H)
Creatinine	0.60–1.40 mg/dL	2.65 (H)	2.68 (H)
Phosphorus	2.3–4.3 mg/dL		2.9
Magnesium	1.6–2.4 mg/dL		1.8
GFR Non-African American	>59 mL/min/1.73m2	23 (L)	22 (L)
GFR African American	>59 mL/min/1.73m2	26 (L)	26 (L)
Cholesterol	70–199 mg/dL		97
Triglycerides	30–149 mg/dL		43
HDL Cholesterol	40–90 mg/dL		44
LDL Cholesterol	50–129 mg/dL		45 (L)
Cholesterol/HDL Ratio	1.8–4.9		2.2
Troponin I	0.00–0.05 ng/mL	<0.03	

Dietitian Interview and Physical

Your patient is resting in bed, watching TV.

Appetite and intake: "I've never had a problem with my appetite. I was eating my favorite pancake breakfast when this all happened. I don't like the food here; it's so bland. I'm hungry! They won't let me order what I want! They said I couldn't have any sausage for breakfast. I didn't finish dinner last night or breakfast this morning because I didn't like it; I ate about half. I would eat healthy if it tastes better than this."

Weight loss and UBW: "No, I haven't lost any weight. I don't know how much I weigh; I don't have a scale at home. I think they weighed me here, but I don't remember what it was."

Food allergies: "Not that I know of."

Cultural or religious food preference: "No."

Difficulty chewing or swallowing: "No."

Nausea, vomiting, constipation, or diarrhea: "I haven't vomited since I came in. I'm pretty backed up though; I think the last time I went to the bathroom was 4 days ago. They've been giving me something for it."

Preferences: "The food here is terrible. My brother is bringing me in a sandwich for lunch."

Musculoskeletal Depletion: None
Subcutaneous Fat Depletion: None

You talk to his nurse.

"He hates the food here. I tried to explain to him that he has to eat better if he doesn't want to end back up in here again."

CASE 8: Y.D.'S BITE OF MEATLOAF

Admission Sheet					
Name	**LOS**	**Age**	**Sex**	**Marital Status**	**Race/Ethnicity**
Y.D.	1	69	F	Married	African American
Primary Language	**Interpreter Needed**		**Next of Kin**		**Attending**
English	No		Husband (123)555-8271		Ripley, E., MD
Allergies		**Chief Complaint**		**Admitting Diagnosis**	

Patient History			
Medical and Surgical History	**Social History**	**Weight History**	
Parkinson's disease HTN	Smoking Status: Former smoker; quit 30 years ago Alcohol Use: No Drug Use: No Residence: Lives with husband	2 months ago	70.6 kg
		5 months ago	69.7 kg
		8 months ago	71.1 kg

Nursing Admission Assessment

Height	Weight	BMI	A&O		Glasgow	Braden
157.5 cm Estimate	67.4 kg Bed scale	27.2	To person x 1 To place x 1		15	14

Skin Integrity	Malnutrition Universal Screening Tool	
Abrasion to right arm	Decrease in appetite or intake? (Yes = 1, No = 0)	1
	Weight loss >10 lbs in 3 months? (Yes = 1, No = 0)	0
	BMI score (<18.5 = 2, 18.5–20.0 = 1, >20.0 = 0)	0
	Total Score (2 or more triggers dietitian consult)	1

Active Orders

Consults	Nursing
CONSULT TO PHYSCIAN—*acute kidney injury* CONSULT TO PHYSCIAN—*Parkinson's disease* CONSULT DIETITIAN—*nutrition assessment* PT EVAL/TREATMENT OT EVAL/TREATMENT CONSULT PALLIATIVE CARE—*family request*	PRESSURE INJURY PRECAUTIONS HIGH-RISK FALL PRECAUTIONS NEUROLOGICAL ASSESSMENT PNEUMATIC COMPRESSION DEVICE, CALVES INTAKE AND OUTPUT URINARY CATHETER MEASURE WEIGHT—*on admission*

Laboratory/Imaging	Medications/Infusions
CULTURE, URINE CULTURE, RESPIRATORY COMPLETE BLOOD COUNT W DIFF COMPREHENSIVE METABOLIC PANEL CT HEAD/BRAIN W/O IV CONTRAST—*hallucinations*	Aspirin—*oral* Carbidopa-levodopa—*oral* Metoprolol—*oral* Rivastigmine—*transdermal* Fluticasone—*PRN* Menthol-zinc oxide—*PRN* Sodium chloride at 75 ml/hr

DIET: Mechanical Soft/Honey Thick Liquids

Physician H & P

History of Present Illness: Patient is a 69-year-old female who presents with swallowed foreign body. Her husband reports she started coughing violently and choking on a bite of meatloaf, but was breathing normally with no cough by the time they arrived at the ED. She also has been hallucinating, ambulating less, urinating less, and not eating well for the past 4 days. ED workup showed creatinine of 11; chest X-ray and renal US were negative.

Temp	BP	Heart Rate	Resp	SpO2	O2 (L/min)
36.2°C	120/68	76	18	94%	RA

Review of Systems and Physical Exam

Constitutional	HEENT	Neck
Well developed, well nourished	Normocephalic, pupils equal	No tracheal deviation
Pulmonary/Chest	Cardiovascular	Gastrointestinal
No respiratory distress	Normal rate and rhythm	Normal bowel sounds
Extremities	Skin	Neurological
3+ BLE edema, limited ROM	Not diaphoretic	Alert, cogwheel rigidity

Assessment	Plan
Principal Problem: AKI Dysphagia Hallucinations Urine retention Decreased appetite Parkinson's disease	Neurology and nephrology consulted Speech language pathologist and dietitian consulted Foley catheter Continue IV fluids; urine culture Strict input and output

E. Ripley, MD

Speech Language Pathologist Note

Patient is alert. Swallow and throat clearing not consistently effective. Prolonged mastication and oral manipulation; delayed swallow initiation. Cough post-swallow with thin liquids; increased vocal wetness with nectar thick; no change in vocal quality with honey thick. Recommend mechanical soft diet with honey thick liquids by tsp only; oral suction PRN for secretions; 1:1 feed.

Will follow up for diet tolerance and need for MBSS.

S. Tarly, MA, CCC-SLP

Flowsheets

Date	Day 1					
Time	**0800**					
Meal Intake	5%					
Outputs						
Foley Output	800 ml					
Stool Occurrences						
Edema						
RUE	None					
LUE	None					
RLE	+3					
LLE	+3					

Laboratory Results

	Ref. Range	ED 1728	Day 1 0604
WBC	3.5–10.1 bil/L	8.2	6.7
Sodium	135–145 mmol/L	143	149 (H)
Potassium	3.5–5.2 mmol/L	4.8	4.1
Glucose	60–99 mg/dL	97	89
BUN	8–22 mg/dL	164 (H)	116 (H)
Creatinine	0.60–1.40 mg/dL	11.81 (H)	6.04 (H)
Magnesium	1.6–2.4 mg/dL	2.8 (H)	
GFR Non-African American	>59 mL/min/1.73m2	<5 (L)	8 (L)
GFR African American	>59 mL/min/1.73m2	<5 (L)	10 (L)

Dietitian Interview and Physical

Your patient is unable to give you her name or birthday; her husband is at bedside.

Appetite and intake: "She normally is a good eater, but she's been really off for about the last 4 to 5 days. I can hardly get a couple bites into her. I was trying to get her to eat some meatloaf and she started choking on it; that's why I had to bring her in. She took a few spoons of pudding and apple juice this morning, but that's it. I'll be here to order her meals and help her eat."

Weight loss and UBW: "I don't think she's lost weight. She is usually about 155 pounds when they weigh her at the doctor's; she was just there about a month ago."

Food allergies: "She swells up if she eats shellfish."

Cultural or religious food preference: "None."

Difficulty chewing or swallowing: "She usually eats soft foods; she's never had to have that thickened stuff before."

Nausea, vomiting, constipation, or diarrhea: "No, but she's had loose stools for the past couple days. They've been really small."

Preferences: "She likes oatmeal in the morning; she loves apple juice. I usually give her a vanilla protein shake at home. She's not real big into lunch; usually just some soup and crackers or a muffin. Our daughter cooks a lot, and she brings the leftovers over for dinner. She loves pasta; we eat that a few times a week."

Musculoskeletal Depletion: None
Subcutaneous Fat Depletion: None

You talk to her nurse.

"She is hardly eating; she had maybe a bite or two of pudding this morning. She's a one-to-one feed; her husband was helping her this morning. Apparently, she was feeding herself at home, but she's really out of it now. SLP went in earlier and put her on honey thick liquids. She hasn't had any bowel movements today."

CASE 9: D.V.'S ABDOMINAL PAIN

Admission Sheet					
Name	**LOS**	**Age**	**Sex**	**Marital Status**	**Race/Ethnicity**
D.V.	5	49	M	Widower	Indian
Primary Language	**Interpreter Needed**		**Next of Kin**		**Attending**
English	No		Daughter (123)555-5408		O'Brian, M., MD

Allergies	Chief Complaint	Admitting Diagnosis
No known allergies	Abdominal pain, nausea, cramping, constipation, vomiting	SBO

Patient History

Medical and Surgical History	Social History	Weight History	
GERD	Smoking Status: Never smoker	2 months ago	104.9 kg
Elevated cholesterol	Alcohol Use: 2 drinks/week	5 months ago	106.8 kg
HTN	Drug Use: No		
	Residence: Lives with daughter	7 months ago	105.2 kg

Nursing Admission Assessment

Height	Weight	BMI	A&O	Glasgow	Braden
170.2 cm Pt estimate	108.5 kg Standing scale	37.5	To person x 3 To place x 3	15	16

Skin Integrity	Malnutrition Universal Screening Tool	
Redness to groin	Decrease in appetite or intake? (Yes = 1, No = 0)	0
	Weight loss >10 lbs in 3 months? (Yes = 1, No = 0)	0
	BMI score (<18.5 = 2, 18.5–20.0 = 1, >20.0 = 0)	0
	Total Score (2 or more triggers dietitian consult)	0

Active Orders

Consults	Nursing
CONSULT TO PHYSCIAN—*SBO*	NASOGASTRIC TUBE, INSERT/MAINTAIN PROGRESSIVE ACTIVITY MEASURE WEIGHT—*on admission*
Laboratory/Imaging	**Medications/Infusions**

COMPLETE BLOOD COUNT W DIFF COMPREHENSIVE METABOLIC PANEL	Clonidine—*transdermal* Docusate—*oral* Furosemide—*intravenous* Heparin—subcutaneous Morphine—*PRN* Ondansetron—*PRN*
DIET: Clear Liquids	

General Surgery Physician Consult

History of Present Illness: Patient is a 49-year-old male who presented last night to the ED with abdominal pain, nausea, and cramping that started around 4 pm. He had 1 episode of emesis before arriving, and had a bowel movement after admission. He has not passed flatus since. CT showed a dilated small bowel with what appears to be a small bowel obstruction in the lower midline pelvis.

Temp	BP	Heart Rate	Resp	SpO2	O2 (L/min)
36.7°C	152/85 mmHg	110	22	94%	2L NC

Review of Systems and Physical Exam

Constitutional	HEENT	Neck
Negative	PERRLA	No lymphadenopathy
Pulmonary/Chest	Cardiovascular	Gastrointestinal
Chest clear	Regular rate and rhythm	Abdomen soft, tender
Extremities	Skin	Neurological
No edema	Negative	No deficits

Assessment	Plan
Principal Problem: Partial small bowel obstruction	Acute abdominal series tomorrow IV fluids; analgesics Monitor electrolytes Activity as tolerated; encourage walking If no improvement in the next 24–48 hours, will consider laparotomy for obstruction
B. Crusher, MD	

General Surgery Physician Progress Note—Day 5

Patient is feeling better; large loose bowel movement today; less abdominal pain. Initial acute abdominal series showed contrast moved into the colon with gas in the rectum.

Plan:
Continue non-operative management for partial SBO
Clamp NG tube and trial clear liquid diet
Increase activity
If tolerating clears, may discontinue NG tube tomorrow and advance diet

B. Crusher, MD

Flowsheets

Date	Day 4			Day 5		
Time	0800	1200	1600	0800		
Meal Intake	NPO	NPO	NPO	100%		
Outputs						
Urine Occurrences	1	2	1	1		
Stool Occurrences				1		
NG/OG Tube	0 ml	0 ml	0 ml	Clamped		
Edema						
RUE	None			None		
LUE	None			None		
RLE	None			None		
LLE	None			None		

Laboratory Results

	Ref. Range	Day 5 0641
WBC	3.5–10.1 bil/L	11.3 (H)
Sodium	135–145 mmol/L	142
Potassium	3.5–5.2 mmol/L	3.5
Glucose	60–99 mg/dL	103 (H)
BUN	8–22 mg/dL	25 (H)

Creatinine	0.60–1.40 mg/dL	0.86
GFR Non-African American	>59 mL/min/1.73m2	66
GFR African American	>59 mL/min/1.73m2	76

Imaging Results

Acute Abdomen Series, Day 3   0841
Comparison:
Prior studies earlier this month. Correlation is also made to CT scan during this admission.

Impression:
Nasogastric tube tip retracted into the distal esophagus. Air and stool are seen along the descending colon. Gaseous distention of small bowel loops is increased with proximal small bowel distention to 3.3 cm in the left upper abdomen. Differential air-fluid levels are noted in the small bowel. There is no free air.

Dietitian Interview and Physical

Your dietitian assistant alerts you that this patient has been NPO/Clear Liquids for 5 days and must be assessed. Your patient is sitting in a chair. He has a clamped NG tube; a tray with an empty Jell-O and juice cup is on the bedside table.

Appetite and intake: "Well, the only thing I've had since I've been here is that Jell-O and apple juice. I didn't even want it, but the doctor wanted me to try it. My stomach still feels weird. I wish they would pull this tube out! My appetite was fine and I was eating normally before this all started."

Weight loss and UBW: "I'm sure I've lost weight since I've been here since I haven't eaten anything. I'm usually about 230 pounds."

Food allergies: "None."

Cultural or religious food preference: "None."

Difficulty chewing or swallowing: "It's hard to swallow with this tube in."

Nausea, vomiting, constipation, or diarrhea: "I'm feeling sorta nauseous right now, but I haven't thrown up since before I got here. I had a big bowel movement this morning; it wasn't really diarrhea, but it wasn't normal."

Preferences: "I don't want anything right now; nothing sounds good."

Musculoskeletal Depletion: None
Subcutaneous Fat Depletion: None

You talk to his nurse.

"The doctor came by this morning and started him on clears; we also clamped the NG tube. He didn't want to order anything, but we got him to try some Jell-O and juice. He hasn't been vomiting or anything, but he told me he was a little nauseous afterwards. I am going to give him some meds for it. If he does okay, I think the doctor will advance him to fulls tomorrow."

CASE 10: H.S.'S ALCOHOL ABUSE

Admission Sheet

Name	LOS	Age	Sex	Marital Status	Race/Ethnicity
H.S.	1	37	F	Single	Hispanic

Primary Language	Interpreter Needed		Next of Kin	Attending
English	No		None listed	Schaeffer, A., MD

Allergies	Chief Complaint	Admitting Diagnosis
No known allergies	Abdominal pain and distention, shortness of breath	Ascites due to alcoholic cirrhosis, ETOH abuse, ETOH dependence, elevated LFTs

Patient History

Medical and Surgical History	Social History	Weight History	
Anxiety Depression Acute alcoholic pancreatitis ETOH abuse ETOH dependence Hepatitis Cirrhosis	Smoking Status: Current smoker; 1 pack/day for 20 years Alcohol Use: 5–6 liquor drinks/day Drug Use: Smokes marijuana daily; occasional cocaine use; no IV drug use Residence: Lives alone	3 months ago	58.9 kg
		1 year, 7 months ago	68.2 kg

Nursing Admission Assessment

Height	Weight	BMI	A&O	Glasgow	Braden
165.1 cm Pt Estimate	62.5 kg Standing Scale	22.9	To person x 3 To place x 3	15	21

Skin Integrity	Malnutrition Universal Screening Tool	
Intact, jaundice, bruising	Decrease in appetite or intake? (Yes = 1, No = 0)	1
	Weight loss >10 lbs in 3 months? (Yes = 1, No = 0)	1

	BMI score (<18.5 = 2, 18.5–20.0 = 1, >20.0 = 0)	0
	Total Score (2 or more triggers dietitian consult)	2

Active Orders

Consults	Nursing
CONSULT TO PHYSCIAN—*ascites, jaundice* CONSULT DIETITIAN FROM NURSING REFERRAL—*decreased appetite* CONSULT SOCIAL WORK—substance abuse, provide alcohol recovery education materials	ALCOHOL WITHDRAWAL BPA COMPLETION ORDER ALCOHOL WITHDRAWAL ASSESSMENT UTILIZING CIWA SCALE ASPIRATION PRECAUTIONS SEIZURE PRECAUTIONS NEUROVASCULAR ASSESSMENT TRANSFUSE PLASMA/FFP PNEUMATIC COMPRESSION DEVICE MEASURE WEIGHT—*daily*

Laboratory/Imaging	Medications/Infusions
COMPLETE BLOOD COUNT W DIFF COMPREHENSIVE METABOLIC PANEL ACUTE HEPATITIS PANEL ALBUMIN, PERITONEAL FLUID PROTEIN TOTAL, PERITONEAL FLUID LACTATE DEHYDROGENASE, PERITONEAL FLUID CULTURE, ANAEROBIC, FUNGUS, PERITONEAL FLUID CELL COUNT, PERITONEAL FLUID STAIN, GRAM, PERITONEAL FLUID ALPHA FETOPROTEIN, NONPREGNANT	Folic acid—*oral* Lactulose—*oral* Multivitamin—*oral* Calcium carbonate—*oral* Melatonin—*oral* Omeprazole—*oral* Lorazepam—*PRN* Thiamine 100 mg in sodium chloride 0.9% 50 ml infusion

DIET: Cardiac (Low Fat/Low Cholesterol/3–4 gram Sodium)

Physician H & P

History of Present Illness: Patient is a 37-year-old female who presents with abdominal pain, distention, and shortness of breath. She drinks alcohol every day and has a poor appetite. She reports she quit drinking for 2 months, but started again 1 month ago.

Temp	BP	Heart Rate	Resp	SpO2	O2 (L/min)
36.8°C	121/79 mmHg	98	18	96%	RA

Review of Systems and Physical Exam

Constitutional	HEENT	Neck
Cachectic appearance	Pupils reactive, normocephalic	Supple, no masses
Pulmonary/Chest	Cardiovascular	Gastrointestinal
Crackles in the base	Regular rate and rhythm	Abdomen distended, fluid thrill present, splenomegaly
Extremities	Skin	Neurological
No cyanosis	Spider angiomata, jaundice	Cranial nerves intact

Assessment	Plan
Principal Problem: Ascites due to alcoholic cirrhosis ETOH abuse ETOH dependence Elevated LFTs	GI consulted Fresh frozen plasma before therapeutic and diagnostic paracentesis CIWA pathway DVT prophylaxis with SCDs Potassium replacement Lactulose for constipation

A. Schaeffer, MD

Flowsheets

Date	Day 1			
Time	0800			
Meal Intake	75%			
Outputs				

Urine Occurrences	1					
Stool Occurrences	0					
Edema						
RUE	None					
LUE	None					
RLE	None					
LLE	None					

Laboratory Results

	Ref. Range	EC 1051	Day 1 0626
WBC	3.5–10.1 bil/L	4.5	4.2
Sodium	135–145 mmol/L	134 (L)	133 (L)
Potassium	3.5–5.2 mmol/L	3.2 (L)	3.5
Glucose	60–99 mg/dL	106 (H)	92
Blood Urea Nitrogen (BUN)	8–22 mg/dL	<5 (L)	<5 (L)
Creatinine	0.60–1.40 mg/dL	0.54 (L)	0.45 (L)
Alkaline Phosphatase	30–110 U/L	174 (H)	138 (H)
Aspartate Aminotransferase	10–37 U/L	93 (H)	75 (H)
Alanine Aminotransferase	9–47 U/L	30	31
Ethanol	< = 10.0	<10	
GFR Non-African American	>59 mL/min/1.73m2	>120	>120
GFR African American	>59 mL/min/1.73m2	>120	>120

Dietitian Interview and Physical

Your patient is resting in bed; she is waiting for her lunch to be delivered.

Appetite and intake: "My appetite is starting to come back; I ate almost all of my breakfast this morning. I haven't been eating much at home because of the drinking. I guess it's been about a month. I was doing real good for a while and didn't drink for like 2 months, and I was eating better, too. But then I started drinking again, and I just didn't feel like eating. I was probably eating less than a quarter of what I normally eat, like 1 meal a day."

Weight loss and UBW: "I haven't really lost weight because of all the fluid in my stomach; they already drained some out. But my arms and legs seem a lot skinnier than they were a few months ago. I'm usually right around 138 pounds, but I used to be 150 a couple years ago before the drinking got bad."

Food allergies: "None."

Cultural or religious food preference: "None."

Difficulty chewing or swallowing: "None."

Nausea, vomiting, constipation, or diarrhea: "I have nausea and vomiting that sorta comes and goes, I mean it depends on how much I drink. Nothing today. They are giving me something for constipation now, but I haven't gone yet. I'm not sure when I last went. Sometimes I get diarrhea if I drink a lot."

Preferences: "I like to cook at home, but I don't do it when I'm drinking. I usually go through the drive-through and grab a burger and a strawberry shake."

Musculoskeletal Depletion: Severe to temple, clavicle, deltoid, hand, thigh, patella, and calf

Subcutaneous Fat Depletion: Severe to triceps

You note her abdomen is very distended.

You talk to her nurse.

"They took about 4.5 liters of fluid off in the paracentesis. She wasn't drunk when she got here, but it sounds like she drinks quite a bit at home. She ate most of her breakfast this morning."

APPENDIX A:
ANSWERS TO "CASE STUDIES: PRACTICING
THE NUTRITION CARE PROCESS"

CASE 1: L.S.'S FALL

Nutrition Assessment

Name: L.S. **LOS:** 2 **Age:** 78 **Sex:** F

Reason for Consult: MD consult for assessment; nursing referral for decreased appetite/intake and weight loss.

HPI: Patient presented to the ED with hip pain after fall, lethargy, lower abdominal pain, loose stools, nausea, and poor oral intake for 3 days; admitted for left hip fracture, acute diarrhea, urinary tract infection without hematuria, altered mental status, hyponatremia; orthopedic surgery and GI consulted.

Subjective: Patient unable to give name or birthday during interview attempt; noted history of Alzheimer's dementia; A&O x 1 per RN flowsheets. She reports her appetite is "fine"; she doesn't like sandwiches, but likes meatloaf and chocolate shakes. She is unsure of weight loss or UBW. Called patient's son; he reports intake of 50% of meals when he visits her at the ECF on the weekends; he is unsure of weight loss or UBW, but had to buy her smaller clothes. RN reports minimal intake; they have been ordering meals for her; she suspects patient forgets she is eating.

Patient History

Medical History: GERD, HTN, CAD, osteoporosis, constipation, Alzheimer's dementia

Surgical History: None on file

Social History: Never smoker; no alcohol or drug use; lives at ECF

Food- and Nutrition-Related History

Current Diet: Cardiac (Low Fat/Low Cholesterol/3–4 gram Sodium)

Intake: Minimal per RN; 0–25% of meals per flowsheets; poor intake for 3 days before admission

Nutrition Assessment

Food Allergies: None per patient, family member, and chart review.
Cultural or Religious Food Preferences: None per patient.

Nutritionally Relevant Medications and Infusions: Famotidine, metoprolol, NaCl 0.9% at 50 ml/hr

Anthropometric Measurements

Height: 152.4 cm **Weight:** 48.6 kg **BMI:** 20.9 **BMI Classification:** Adequate
IBW: 45.5 kg **%IBW:** 106.8% **UBW:** 50.7–51.9 kg in the past year per chart review
%UBW: 95.9%
Weight History and Change: Weight of 51.9 kg 3 months ago; −3.3 kg/6.4%

Biochemical Data, Medical Tests, and Procedures

Laboratory Results: Na 129 (L), Glu 164 (H), BUN 23 (H), Cr 0.86
Microbiology Results: C. difficile in process

Nutrition-Focused Physical Findings

Appetite: Suspected decrease based on reported intake and recent weight loss
Oral: No difficulty chewing or swallowing
GI: No nausea or vomiting; diarrhea per RN with 4 bowel movements in the past 24 hours; abdominal pain and nausea 3 days before admission

Skin: Blanchable erythema to center coccyx, abrasion to left knee, bruising and swelling to left hip per RN admission assessment
Edema: None per RN flowsheets

Subcutaneous Fat Depletion: None per RDN physical exam
Musculoskeletal Depletion: None per RDN physical exam; some losses anticipated with advanced age

Nutrition Diagnosis

Inadequate oral intake related to suspected loss of appetite from cognitive/GI dysfunction and increased nutrient needs as evidenced by reported intake of 0–25% of meals during admission, 3.3 kg/6.4% weight loss over 3 months, diarrhea, history of Alzheimer's dementia, and admission for left hip fracture s/p fall

Nutrition Intervention

Estimated Nutrition Needs

Calories: 1361–1604 kcal (based on 28–33 kcal/kg actual weight 48.6 kg for maintenance/fracture healing)

Protein: 58–63 gm (based on 1.2–1.3 kcal/kg actual weight 48.6 kg for maintenance/fracture healing)

Fluid: 1458 ml (based on 30 ml/kg actual weight 48.6 kg)

Nutrition Prescription and Interventions

Nutrition Prescription: Regular Diet to encourage intake with chocolate protein shakes twice daily

Interventions:

- Ordered supplements, assistance with meals, automatic trays, and weekly weights
- Encouraged intake
- Provided RDN contact information to patient and family member
- Discussed with RN

Nutrition Monitoring and Evaluation

Goals:

- Patient to consume >25% of meals and supplements
- Provide high–calorie, high–protein supplements to support healing
- Avoid weight loss from 48.6 kg/gradual weight gain during admission

Monitoring: Intake, supplement acceptance, and weight

Recommendations

1. Liberalize to Regular Diet to encourage intake with chocolate protein shakes twice daily
2. Monitor sodium levels
3. Assistance and encouragement with meals; automatic meal trays

CASE 2: A.A.'S BACK PAIN

Nutrition Assessment

Name: A.A. **LOS:** 1 **Age:** 67 **Sex:** M

Reason for Consult: MD consult for worsening pressure injuries and wound healing recommendations.

HPI: Patient presented to the ED with multiple infected sacral decubitus ulcers, worsening chronic back pain, and lethargy; admitted for decubitus ulcer of left buttock, stage 4; decubitus ulcer of right heel, stage 3; acute exacerbation of chronic back pain; wound care and infectious disease consulted.

Subjective: Patient reports normal appetite now and before admission with intake of 100% of meals; he is unsure of weight loss. He doesn't like the food here, and his wife is bringing in food from outside. He doesn't follow a diabetic diet at home; he likes spaghetti, meatloaf, tacos, baked potatoes, and chicken. He has information on diabetic diet and declines further education.

Patient History

Medical History: DM type 2, CKD stage 3, CAD, MI, hypothyroid
Surgical History: CABG, implantable cardiac defibrillator
Social History: Former smoker; drinks 2–3 beers/week; no drug use; lives with wife

Food- and Nutrition-Related History

Current Diet: Cardiac (Low Fat/Low Cholesterol/3–4 gram Sodium)
Intake: 100% of meals now and before admission per patient

Food Allergies: None per patient
Cultural or Religious Food Preferences: None per patient

Nutritionally Relevant Medications and Infusions: Atorvastatin, docusate, insulin glargine, insulin lispro, levothyroxine, omeprazole

Anthropometric Measurements

Height: 170.2 cm **Weight:** 118.6 kg **BMI:** 40.9 **BMI Classification:** Morbidly Obese
IBW: 67.3 kg **%IBW:** 176.2% **UBW:** 125 kg per patient **%UBW:** 94.9%
Weight History and Change: Weight of 125.2 kg 2 months ago per chart review; -6.6 kg/5.3%

Nutrition Assessment

Biochemical Data, Medical Tests, and Procedures

Laboratory Results: Glu 165–282 (H), BUN 38 (H), Cr 1.57 (H), GFR 40 (L)

Nutrition-Focused Physical Findings

Appetite: Normal now and before admission
Oral: No difficulty chewing or swallowing
GI: No nausea or vomiting; constipation; patient unsure of last bowel movement; noted on docusate

Skin: Wound care RN consulted; stage 4 pressure injury to left buttock, stage 3 pressure injury to right heel, unstageable pressure injury to right buttock per RN admission assessment
Edema: Trace to RLE/LLE per RN flowsheets

Subcutaneous Fat Depletion: None per RDN physical exam
Musculoskeletal Depletion: None per RDN physical exam; losses may be obscured by adiposity

Nutrition Diagnosis

Increased nutrient needs (protein and energy) related to skin repletion as evidenced by unstageable, stage 4, and stage 3 pressure injuries

Limited adherence to nutrition-related recommendations related to lack of interest/motivation as evidenced by hyperglycemia, history of DM type 2, and previous nutrition education

Nutrition Intervention

Estimated Nutrition Needs

Calories: 2019–2356 kcal (based on 30–35 kcal/kg IBW 67.3 kg for obesity/pressure injury healing)
Protein: 101–135 gm (based on 1.5–2.0 kcal/kg IBW 67.3 kg for obesity/pressure injury healing; noted patient with CKD; will monitor renal laboratory values and adjust protein as appropriate)
Fluid: 2019–2356 ml (based on 1 ml/kcal)

Nutrition Intervention

Nutrition Prescription and Interventions

Nutrition Prescription: Diabetic 1900–2100, Cardiac (Low Fat/Low Cholesterol/3–4 gram Sodium) Diet with sugar-free protein supplement twice daily

Interventions:
- Ordered supplements
- Offered nutrition education; patient declined
- Encouraged supplement and protein intake, such as meat, eggs, and dairy
- Provided RDN contact information
- Discussed with RN

Nutrition Monitoring and Evaluation

Goals:
- Patient to consume >75% of meals and supplements
- Provide high-protein supplements to support pressure injury healing
- Blood glucose to improve

Monitoring: Intake, supplement acceptance, pressure injury healing, and laboratory values

Recommendations

1. Diabetic 1900–2100, Cardiac (Low Fat/Low Cholesterol/3–4 gram Sodium) Diet to improve hyperglycemia with sugar-free protein supplement twice daily
2. Multivitamin to support wound healing
3. HbA1c level
4. Continue stool softener until bowel movement produced
5. Referral to Weight Management Program and Outpatient Nutrition Counseling at discharge
6. Patient meets criteria for Morbid Obesity

CASE 3: C.P.'S UPSET STOMACH

Nutrition Assessment

Name: C.P. **LOS:** 1 **Age:** 23 **Sex:** F

Reason for Consult: MD consult for new type 1 diabetic instruction; nursing referral for decreased appetite, nausea, vomiting, and weight loss.

HPI: Patient presented to the ED with nausea, vomiting, weight loss, and abdominal pain for 5 days; admitted for diabetic ketoacidosis without coma; endocrinology and GI consulted.

Subjective: Patient sleeping during interview attempt; mother at bedside. Reports patient has vomited all intake for 5 days before admission; she has also lost 10 pounds in the past 1–1.5 weeks. She drank sips of juice earlier and hasn't vomited today. No family history of diabetes; she follows an ovo-lacto vegetarian diet at home. Reviewed nutrition education materials with patient's mother; will follow up as appropriate to review with patient. RN reports MD may advance to full liquids today if patient tolerates clears.

Patient History

Medical History: None on file
Surgical History: None on file
Social History: Current smoker; 2–3 drinks/week; no drug use; lives with roommate

Food- and Nutrition-Related History

Current Diet: Clear Liquid, Advance as Tolerated
Intake: Sips of juice today; vomiting all intake for 5 days before admission

Food Allergies: Tomatoes cause hives per patient's mother
Cultural or Religious Food Preferences: Ovo-lacto vegetarian

Nutritionally Relevant Medications and Infusions: Insulin lispro, insulin NPH, insulin regular human, pantoprazole, Zofran, bismuth subsalicylate, NaCl 0.9% at 75 ml/hr

Anthropometric Measurements

Height: 170.2 cm **Weight:** 54.5 kg **BMI:** 18.8 **BMI Classification:** Adequate
IBW: 61.4 kg **%IBW:** 88.8% **UBW:** 59.1 kg per patient's mother 1–1.5 weeks ago
%UBW: 92.2%
Weight History and Change: Noted admission weight is patient estimate; -4.6 kg/7.8% over the past 1–1.5 weeks

Nutrition Assessment

Biochemical Data, Medical Tests, and Procedures

Laboratory Results: Na 137, K 4.6, Glu 182–448 (H), P 5.0 (H), Mg 2.0, HbA1c 11.9 (H)

Nutrition-Focused Physical Findings

Appetite: Decreased for 5 days before admission
Oral: No difficulty chewing or swallowing
GI: No vomiting today; no constipation or diarrhea; nausea, vomiting, and abdominal pain for 5 days before admission

Skin: Intact per RN admission assessment
Edema: None per RN flowsheets

Subcutaneous Fat Depletion: RDN physical exam not completed because patient was sleeping
Musculoskeletal Depletion: NA (see above)

Nutrition Diagnosis

Inadequate oral intake related to endocrine/GI dysfunction as evidenced by reported nausea, vomiting, and abdominal pain, minimal intake for 5 days, 4.6 kg/7.8% weight loss over the past 1–1.5 weeks, admission for diabetic ketoacidosis, and new diagnosis of DM type 1

Food- and nutrition-related knowledge deficit related to change in medical condition as evidenced by hyperglycemia, elevated HbA1c, admission for diabetic ketoacidosis, and new diagnosis of DM type 1

Nutrition Intervention

Estimated Nutrition Needs

Calories: 1635–1908 kcal (based on 30–35 kcal/kg actual weight 54.5 kg for repletion/ weight gain)
Protein: 55–65 gm (based on 1.0–1.2 kcal/kg actual weight 54.5 kg for repletion)
Fluid: 1908 ml (based on 35 ml/kg actual weight 54.5 kg)

Nutrition Intervention

Nutrition Prescription and Interventions

Nutrition Prescription: Advance diet as tolerated to goal Diabetic 1600–1800 Diet

Interventions:

- Ordered current and weekly weights
- Discussed with RN
- Reported food allergy to RN and Nutrition Services
- Provided verbal and written nutrition education for Vegetarian/Type 1 Diabetes Nutrition Therapy
- Provided Outpatient Nutrition Counseling brochure and RDN contact information
- RDN to follow up for physical exam, subjective, and education with patient as appropriate

Nutrition Monitoring and Evaluation

Goals:

- Diet advanced past Clear Liquids in the next 24–48 hours
- Patient to tolerate oral diet and consume >50% of meals
- Avoid weight loss/gradual weight gain during admission once measured weight obtained
- Blood glucose to improve
- Patient and family to verbalize understanding of Vegetarian/Type 1 Diabetes Nutrition Therapy

Monitoring: Diet advancement and tolerance, intake, weight, laboratory values, and nutrition education understanding

Recommendations

1. Advance diet as tolerated to goal Diabetic 1600–1800 Diet
2. Referral to Outpatient Nutrition Counseling at discharge
3. Monitor electrolytes

CASE 4: B.F.'S SHORTNESS OF BREATH

Nutrition Assessment

Name: B.F. **LOS:** 2 **Age:** 59 **Sex:** M

Reason for Consult: MD consult for nutritional needs for wound healing and diabetic diet education.

HPI: Patient presented to the ED with shortness of breath and worsening chronic diabetic foot wound; admitted for acute COPD exacerbation and diabetic foot ulcer; pulmonary, wound care, and infectious disease consulted; patient s/p wound debridement and wound vac placement.

Subjective: Patient doesn't speak English; no family at bedside; translation computer used for interview and education. Patient reports normal appetite with intake of 100% of meals now and before admission; he is unsure of weight loss or UBW. He was diagnosed with diabetes "a few years ago," but doesn't follow a diabetic diet at home; no previous nutrition education. He eats traditional foods with his family like shish taouk, tabbouleh, shawarma, labneh, hummus, baba ghanouj, kibbeh, kofta, pita, and rice. RN reports family is bringing in high-carbohydrate meals from home.

Patient History

Medical History: DM type 2, diabetic neuropathy, CAD, COPD, hyperlipidemia, hypercholesterolemia, PAD

Surgical History: Cardiac catheterization

Social History: Current smoker; 1 alcohol drink/day; no drug use; lives with wife

Food- and Nutrition-Related History

Current Diet: Diabetic 1600–1800 Diet

Intake: 100% of meals per patient; family bringing in meals

Food Allergies: None per patient

Cultural or Religious Food Preferences: Patient doesn't eat pork

Nutritionally Relevant Medications and Infusions: Atorvastatin, clopidogrel, insulin lispro, linagliptin, lisinopril, bisacodyl, docusate, polyethylene glycol 3350

Nutrition Assessment

Anthropometric Measurements

Height: 172.7 cm **Weight:** 83.5 kg **BMI:** 28.0 **BMI Classification:** Overweight
IBW: 70.0 kg **%IBW:** 119.3% **UBW:** 70.3–79.8 kg in the past 2 years per chart review
%UBW: 118.8%
Weight History and Change: +13.2 kg/18.8% over the past 2 years

Biochemical Data, Medical Tests, and Procedures

Laboratory Results: WBC 21.1 (H), Glu 123–207 (H), BUN 26 (H), Cr 1.28, HbA1c 7.0 (H)

Nutrition-Focused Physical Findings

Appetite: Normal now and before admission
Oral: No difficulty chewing or swallowing
GI: No nausea, vomiting, constipation, or diarrhea

Skin: Left foot ulcer s/p debridement and wound vac placement, abrasions to right and left feet per RN admission assessment
Edema: None per RN flowsheets

Subcutaneous Fat Depletion: None per RDN physical exam
Musculoskeletal Depletion: None per RDN physical exam

Nutrition Diagnosis

Excessive carbohydrate intake related to endocrine dysfunction and lack of previous nutrition education as evidenced by hyperglycemia, elevated HbA1c, reported intake of high-carbohydrate meals, admission for diabetic foot ulcer, and history of DM type 2

Nutrition Intervention

Estimated Nutrition Needs

Calories: 2100–2450 kcal (based on 30–35 kcal/kg IBW 70.0 kg for wound healing/overweight)
Protein: 84–105 gm (based on 1.2–1.5 kcal/kg IBW 70.0 kg for wound healing/overweight)
Fluid: 2505 ml (based on 30 ml/kg actual weight 83.5 kg)

Nutrition Intervention

Nutrition Prescription and Interventions

Nutrition Prescription: Diabetic 1900–2100, No Pork Diet to meet estimated nutrition needs with sugar-free protein supplement once daily

Interventions:
- Ordered weekly weights
- Encouraged supplement and protein intake, such as meat, eggs, and dairy
- Discussed with RN
- Provided verbal and written nutrition education for Basic Diabetic Dietary Guidelines, 4–5 Carbohydrate Choice Meals, and Carbohydrate Portions of Arabic Foods
- Provided Outpatient Nutrition Counseling brochure and RDN contact information
- RDN to follow up for diet education questions and to review education material with family if possible

Nutrition Monitoring and Evaluation

Goals:
- Patient to consume >75% of meals
- Provide high-protein supplement to support wound healing
- Blood glucose improved
- Patient to verbalize understanding of Arabic Foods, Basic Diabetic Dietary Guidelines, and Carbohydrate Meal Portions
- Patient to consume 4–5 carbohydrate choices when eating meals with family

Monitoring: Intake, wound healing, laboratory values, carbohydrate portion compliance, and nutrition education understanding

Recommendations

1. Diabetic 1900–2100, No Pork Diet to meet estimated nutrition needs with sugar-free protein supplement once daily
2. Multivitamin to support wound healing
3. Referral to Outpatient Nutrition Counseling at discharge

CASE 5: R.D.'S FATIGUE

Nutrition Assessment

Name: R.D. **LOS:** 1 **Age:** 76 **Sex:** M

Reason for Consult: Nursing referral for low weight, decreased appetite/intake, weight loss, and BMI 16.7

HPI: Patient presented to the ED with low hemoglobin, fatigue, nausea, and decreased appetite; admitted for anemia and received blood transfusion; hematology consulted; completed 6 weeks of chemotherapy for lung cancer 1 week ago.

Subjective: Patient reports decreased appetite with intake of 25% and 10-lb weight loss over the past 7 weeks; he relates it to nausea and taste changes during chemotherapy. His dentures don't fit well since losing weight, so he eats soft foods; he tried protein shakes at home, but doesn't like them. He also reports gradual weight loss from his UBW of 140 lbs over the past 10 years from eating less.

Patient History

Medical History: CVA, COPD, hyperlipidemia, CAD, lung cancer s/p chemotherapy

Surgical History: None on file

Social History: Current smoker; no alcohol or drug use; lives at assisted living

Food- and Nutrition-Related History

Current Diet: Cardiac (Low Fat/Low Cholesterol/3–4 gram Sodium)

Intake: <25% of normal for 6 weeks

Food Allergies: None per patient

Cultural or Religious Food Preferences: None per patient

Nutritionally Relevant Medications and Infusions: Atorvastatin, clopidogrel, dexamethasone, omeprazole, prochlorperazine, NaCl 0.9% at 75 ml/hr

Anthropometric Measurements

Height: 165.1 cm **Weight:** 45.6 kg **BMI:** 16.7 **BMI Classification:** Underweight

IBW: 61.8 kg **%IBW:** 73.8% **UBW:** 50 kg 7 weeks ago per patient **%UBW:** 91.2%

Weight History and Change: -4.4 kg/8.8% over the past 7 weeks

Biochemical Data, Medical Tests, and Procedures

Nutrition Assessment

Laboratory Results: RBC 2.84 (L), Hgb 8.9 (L), Hct 27.6 (L), MCV 97, MCHC 32, Iron 63, Folate 12.0, Vitamin B12 474

Nutrition-Focused Physical Findings

Appetite: Decreased for 7 weeks
Oral: Difficulty chewing because of ill-fitting dentures; no difficulty swallowing
GI: Nausea; intermittent vomiting with last episode 2 days ago; no constipation or diarrhea

Skin: Intact per RN admission assessment
Edema: None per RN flowsheets

Subcutaneous Fat Depletion: Severe to temple, clavicle, deltoid, hand, thigh, patella, and calf per RDN physical exam
Musculoskeletal Depletion: Severe to orbital and triceps per RDN physical exam

Nutrition Diagnosis

Inadequate protein-energy intake related to increased protein-energy needs, altered GI function, and medical treatment as evidenced by severe musculoskeletal and subcutaneous fat depletion, 4.4 kg/8.8% weight loss over the past 7 weeks, reported intake of <25% of normal with nausea, vomiting, and taste changes, BMI 16.7, and history of lung cancer s/p chemotherapy

Severe protein-calorie malnutrition in the context of acute illness related to inadequate protein-energy intake, increased protein-energy needs, altered GI function, and medical treatment as evidenced by severe musculoskeletal and subcutaneous fat depletion, 4.4 kg/8.8% weight loss over the past 7 weeks, reported intake of <25% of normal with nausea, vomiting, and taste changes, BMI 16.7, and history of lung cancer s/p chemotherapy

Nutrition Intervention

Estimated Nutrition Needs

Calories: 1596–1824 kcal (based on 35–40 kcal/kg actual weight 45.6 kg for repletion/weight gain/oncology)
Protein: 55–68 gm (based on 1.2–1.5 gm/kg actual weight 45.6 kg for repletion/oncology)
Fluid: 1596–1824 ml (based on 1 ml/kcal actual weight 45.6 kg)

Nutrition Intervention

Nutrition Prescription and Interventions

Nutrition Prescription: Regular, Mechanical Soft Diet to encourage intake with high-protein ice cream 3 times daily

Interventions:
- Ordered supplements and weekly weights
- Encouraged supplement and protein intake, such as meat, eggs, and dairy
- Attempted to contact RN
- Paged attending MD with malnutrition alert and supplement plan
- Provided verbal and written nutrition education for High-Protein, High-Calorie/Chemotherapy Nutrition Therapy
- Provided Outpatient Nutrition Counseling brochure and RDN contact information

Nutrition Monitoring and Evaluation

Goals:
- Patient to safely consume >50% of meals and supplements
- Provide high-calorie, high-protein supplements to support healing
- Avoid weight loss from 45.6 kg/gradual weight gain during admission
- BMI to increase
- Patient to verbalize understanding of High-Protein, High-Calorie/Chemotherapy Nutrition Therapy

Monitoring: Intake, supplement acceptance, weight, BMI, and nutrition education understanding

Recommendations

1. Regular, Mechanical Soft Diet to encourage intake with high-protein ice cream 3 times daily
2. Referral to Outpatient Nutrition Counseling at discharge
3. Continue medical intervention to reduce nausea
4. Patient meets criteria for severe protein-calorie malnutrition

CASE 6: C.B.'S CONFUSION

Nutrition Assessment

Name: C.B. **LOS:** 3 **Age:** 73 **Sex:** F
Reason for Consult: MD consult for nutrition assessment and supplements

HPI: Patient presented to the ED with slurred speech, left-sided facial droop, increased confusion; admitted for CVA with confusion; neurology consulted.

Subjective: Patient unresponsive to interview questions; A&O x 1 per RN; husband interviewed via telephone. Reports normal intake before admission, but she isn't able to feed herself since the CVA. He's been helping at some meals; expresses concern about patient getting meals and assistance when he isn't here. He is unsure of weight loss or UBW. She likes eggs, bacon, yogurt, and chocolates.

Patient History

Medical History: Hypothyroid, hyperlipidemia, GERD, gout, HTN, CAD, MI
Surgical History: Cholecystectomy
Social History: Former smoker; no alcohol or drug use; lives with husband

Food- and Nutrition-Related History

Current Diet: Cardiac (Low Fat/Low Cholesterol/3–4 gram Sodium)
Intake: 100% intake of dinner last night; 90% of breakfast this morning; 100% of normal before admission

Food Allergies: None per patient's husband, but is lactose intolerant; she doesn't drink milk, but eats yogurt
Cultural or Religious Food Preferences: None per patient's husband

Nutritionally Relevant Medications and Infusions: Atorvastatin, famotidine, lisinopril, ondansetron

Anthropometric Measurements

Height: 154.9 cm **Weight:** 57.3 kg **BMI:** 23.9 **BMI Classification:** Adequate
IBW: 47.7 kg **%IBW:** 120.1% **UBW:** 58.5 kg 2 years ago per chart review
%UBW: 97.9%
Weight History and Change: No evidence of recent weight loss

Nutrition Assessment

Biochemical Data, Medical Tests, and Procedures

Laboratory Results: WBC 13.8 (H), BUN 24 (H), Cr 0.64

Nutrition-Focused Physical Findings

Appetite: Normal now and before admission
Oral: SLP following; recommends regular texture with thin liquids; noted patient unable to feed herself
GI: No nausea or vomiting per RN; 1 bowel movement this morning per RN flowsheets

Skin: Bruising to right arm and redness to coccyx per RN admission assessment
Edema: None per RN flowsheets

Subcutaneous Fat Depletion: RDN physical exam not completed because patient unable to consent; she appears well nourished
Musculoskeletal Depletion:

Nutrition Diagnosis

Self-feeding difficulty related to cognitive dysfunction as evidenced by SLP recommendation for 1:1 feed and admission for CVA

Nutrition Intervention

Estimated Nutrition Needs

Calories: 1433–1719 kcal (based on 25–30 kcal/kg actual weight 57.3 kg for weight maintenance)
Protein: 57–72 gm (based on 1.0–1.25 gm/kg actual weight 57.3 kg for older adult maintenance)
Fluid: 1719 ml (based on 30 ml/kcal actual weight 57.3 kg)

Nutrition Prescription and Interventions

Nutrition Prescription: 3–4 gram Sodium/No Added Salt Diet to encourage intake with yogurt at lunch

Nutrition Intervention

Interventions:
- Ordered assistance with meals, automatic meal trays, and weekly weights
- Reported food preferences and lactose intolerance to Nutrition Services
- Provided RDN contact information
- Discussed with RN

Nutrition Monitoring and Evaluation

Goals:
- Patient to safely consume >75% of meals
- Avoid weight loss from 57.3 kg during admission

Monitoring: Intake and weight

Recommendations

1. Liberalize to 3–4 gram Sodium/No Added Salt Diet to encourage intake with yogurt at lunch
2. Assistance and encouragement with meals; automatic meal trays
3. Continue SLP evaluation

CASE 7: B.K.'S SYNCOPE

Nutrition Assessment

Name: B.K. **LOS:** 3 **Age:** 53 **Sex:** M

Reason for Consult: MD consult for nutrition assessment and low-sodium nutrition education

HPI: Patient presented to the ED with vomiting and syncope; admitted for STEMI; had cardiac catheterization, coronary artery stent, and ICD placed; nephrology and internal medicine consulted.

Subjective: Patient reports normal appetite and intake before admission; he ate 50% of dinner yesterday and breakfast this morning because he doesn't like the food; was NPO before that. His brother is bringing in a sandwich for lunch today. He denies recent weight loss, but is unsure of UBW. He follows a regular diet at home.

Nutrition Assessment

Patient History

Medical History: CAD, CKD stage 4, HTN, hyperlipidemia, hyperparathyroidism, hypothyroidism
Surgical History: None on file
Social History: Never smoker; no alcohol or drug use; lives alone

Food- and Nutrition-Related History

Current Diet: Sodium 2 gm (Low Na), Low Fat/Low Cholesterol
Intake: 50% of last 2 meals; 100% of normal before admission

Food Allergies: None per patient
Cultural or Religious Food Preferences: None per patient

Nutritionally Relevant Medications and Infusions: Atorvastatin, clopidogrel, docusate, ferrous sulfate, levothyroxine, metoprolol, alum & mag hydroxide-simeth, ondansetron, NaCl 0.9% at 20 ml/hr

Anthropometric Measurements

Height: 188.0 cm **Weight:** 101.9 kg **BMI:** 28.8 **BMI Classification:** Overweight
IBW: 86.4 kg **%IBW:** 117.9% **UBW:** 96.4 kg per chart review 4 months ago
%UBW: 105.7%
Weight History and Change: 5.5 kg/5.7% weight gain over the past 4 months

Biochemical Data, Medical Tests, and Procedures

Laboratory Results: Potassium 4.8, Glu 127 (H), BUN 48 (H), Cr 2.68 (H), P 2.9, Mg 1.8, GFR 22 (L)

Nutrition-Focused Physical Findings

Appetite: Normal appetite now and before admission
Oral: No difficulty chewing or swallowing
GI: No nausea or vomiting since admission; constipation with last bowel movement 4 days ago per patient; on stool softener

Nutrition Assessment

Skin: Incision to left chest, procedure site to right wrist, puncture to right groin per RN admission assessment

Edema: None per RN flowsheets

Subcutaneous Fat Depletion: None per RDN physical exam
Musculoskeletal Depletion: None per RDN physical exam

Nutrition Diagnosis

Decreased nutrient needs (sodium, protein) related to cardiac and renal dysfunction as evidenced by 2-gram sodium diet, history of CKD stage 4 and HTN, and admission for STEMI

Food- and nutrition-related knowledge deficit related to change in medical condition as evidence by admission for STEMI s/p cardiac catheterization, coronary artery stent, and ICD

Nutrition Intervention

Estimated Nutrition Needs

Calories: 2038–2547 kcal (based on 20–25 kcal/kg actual weight 101.9 kg for weight loss)
Protein: 61 gm (based on 0.6 gm/kg actual weight 101.9 kg for CKD stage 4)
Fluid: Per nephrology MD

Nutrition Prescription and Interventions

Nutrition Prescription: Continue Sodium 2 gm (Low Na), Low Fat/Low Cholesterol Diet as tolerated

Interventions:
- Encouraged diet compliance and intake
- Discussed with RN
- Provided verbal and written nutrition education for Low-Sodium/Heart Healthy Nutrition Therapy
- Provided Outpatient Nutrition Counseling brochure and RDN contact information

Nutrition Monitoring and Evaluation

Goals:

- Patient to consume >50% of meals
- Patient to verbalize understanding of Low-Sodium/Heart Healthy Nutrition Therapy and name 3 high-sodium foods to avoid

Monitoring: Intake and nutrition education understanding

Recommendations

1. Continue Sodium 2 gm (Low Na), Low Fat/Low Cholesterol Diet as tolerated
2. Referral to Outpatient Nutrition Counseling at discharge

CASE 8: Y.D.'S BITE OF MEATLOAF

Nutrition Assessment

Name: Y.D. **LOS:** 1 **Age:** 69 **Sex:** F
Reason for Consult: MD consult for nutrition assessment

HPI: Patient presented to the ED after choking on a bite of meatloaf with hallucinations, poor intake for 4 days, urinary retention, and decreased ambulation; admitted for AKI, AMS, and choking; neurology and nephrology consulted.

Subjective: Patient unable to provide name or birthday; A&O x 1 per chart review; husband at bedside answering interview questions. Reports decreased appetite with minimal intake of bites at meals now and 4 days before admission; had normal appetite and intake before then. Denies recent weight loss. She likes oatmeal, apple juice, vanilla protein shakes, soup, crackers, muffins, and pasta; she eats soft foods at home with no history of thickened liquids. He is ordering meals and helping her eat.

Patient History

Medical History: Parkinson's disease, HTN
Surgical History: None on file
Social History: Former smoker; no drugs or alcohol use; lives with husband

Nutrition Assessment

Food- and Nutrition-Related History

Current Diet: Mechanical Soft/Honey Thick Liquids
Intake: Minimal intake/bites at meals now and 4 days before admission

Food Allergies: Shellfish causes swelling per patient's husband
Cultural or Religious Food Preferences: None per patient's husband

Nutritionally Relevant Medications and Infusions: Carbidopa-levodopa, metoprolol, sodium chloride at 75 ml/hr

Anthropometric Measurements

Height: 157.5 cm **Weight:** 67.4 kg **BMI:** 27.2 **BMI Classification:** Overweight
IBW: 50 kg **%IBW:** 134.8% **UBW:** 70.5 kg per patient's husband 1 month ago **%UBW:** 95.6%
Weight History and Change: 3.1 kg/4.4% weight loss over 1 month

Biochemical Data, Medical Tests, and Procedures

Laboratory Results: Na 149 (H), BUN 116 (H), Cr 6.04 (H), Mg 2.8 (H), GFR 10 (L)

Nutrition-Focused Physical Findings

Appetite: Decreased now and 4 days before admission
Oral: SLP following; recommends mechanical soft diet with honey thick liquids by tsp only; 1:1 feed
GI: No vomiting; small loose stools for the past 2 days per patient's husband; no bowel movement today per RN

Skin: Abrasion to right arm per RN admission assessment
Edema: +3 to RLE/LLE per RN flowsheets

Subcutaneous Fat Depletion: None per RDN physical exam
Musculoskeletal Depletion: None per RDN physical exam

Nutrition Diagnosis

Inadequate oral intake related to dysphagia and cognitive dysfunction as evidenced by reported minimal intake of bites at meals now and 4 days before admission, 3.1 kg/4.4% weight loss over 1 month, mechanical soft diet with honey thickened liquids per SLP, history of Parkinson's disease, and admission for AMS.

Nutrition Intervention

Estimated Nutrition Needs

Calories: 1685–2022 kcal (based on 25–30 kcal/kg actual weight 67.4 kg for weight maintenance)

Protein: 67–84 gm (based on 1.0–1.25 gm/kg actual weight 67.4 kg for older adult maintenance)

Fluid: Per nephrology MD

Nutrition Prescription and Interventions

Nutrition Prescription: Continue Mechanical Soft Diet with Honey Thick Liquids per SLP with honey thick vanilla protein shakes 3 times daily

Interventions:
- Ordered supplements and weekly weights
- Discussed importance of supplement and protein intake, such as meat, eggs, and dairy, with husband
- Discussed with RN
- Provided RDN contact information

Nutrition Monitoring and Evaluation

Goals:
- Patient to safely consume >50% of meals and supplements
- Provide high-calorie, high-protein supplements to support healing
- Maintain weight during admission once edema resolves
- Edema to improve as medically feasible

Monitoring: Intake, supplement acceptance, laboratory values, weight, and edema

Recommendations
1. Continue Mechanical Soft Diet with Honey Thick Liquids per SLP with honey thick vanilla protein shakes 3 times daily
2. Continue SLP evaluation

CASE 9: D.V.'S ABDOMINAL PAIN

Nutrition Assessment
Name: D.V. **LOS:** 5 **Age:** 49 **Sex:** M
Reason for Consult: Dietitian referral for NPO/Clear Liquids for 5 days
HPI: Patient presented to the ED with abdominal pain, nausea, cramping, constipation, and vomiting; admitted for SBO; general surgery consulted; plan to continue non-operative management of partial SBO; clamped NG tube and is trialing clear liquid diet today; may discontinue NG tube and advance diet tomorrow if tolerates clears per MD progress note.
Subjective: Diet advanced to clear liquids today; patient reports no appetite, but tried Jell-O and apple juice this morning; has nausea, but no vomiting; had large bowel movement this morning. Suspects weight loss during admission; current weight shows gain from reported UBW. RN about to give anti-nausea medication.

Patient History
Medical History: GERD, elevated cholesterol, HTN
Surgical History: None on file
Social History: Never smoker; 2 alcohol drinks/week; lives with daughter

Food- and Nutrition-Related History
Current Diet: Clear Liquids
Intake: NPO/Clear Liquids/1 Jell-O and 1 apple juice for 5 days
Food Allergies: None per patient
Cultural or Religious Food Preferences: None per patient
Nutritionally Relevant Medications and Infusions: Clonidine, docusate, furosemide, ondansetron PRN

Nutrition Assessment

Anthropometric Measurements

Height: 170.2 cm **Weight:** 108.5 kg **BMI:** 37.5 **BMI Classification:** Obese
IBW: 67.3 kg **%IBW:** 161.2% **UBW:** 104.5 kg per patient **%UBW:** 103.8%
Weight History and Change: 4.0 kg/3.8% weight gain from reported UBW; weight of 104.9 kg 2 months ago per chart review

Biochemical Data, Medical Tests, and Procedures

Laboratory Results: WBC 11.3 (H), Glu 103 (H), BUN 25 (H)
Imaging Results:
Acute Abdomen Series, Day 3 0841
Impression:
Nasogastric tube tip retracted into the distal esophagus. Air and stool are seen along the descending colon. Gaseous distention of small bowel loops is increased with proximal small bowel distention to 3.3 cm in the left upper abdomen. Differential air-fluid levels are noted in the small bowel. There is no free air.

Nutrition-Focused Physical Findings

Appetite: None now; normal before admission
Oral: Some swallowing difficulty because of NG tube
GI: Clamped NG tube; nausea, but no vomiting; large loose bowel movement today per patient; improved abdominal pain per MD progress note

Skin: Redness to groin per RN admission assessment
Edema: None per RN flowsheets

Subcutaneous Fat Depletion: None per RDN physical exam
Musculoskeletal Depletion: None per RDN physical exam; musculoskeletal depletion may be obscured by adiposity

Nutrition Diagnosis

Inadequate oral intake related to GI dysfunction as evidenced by NPO/Clear Liquids for 5 days, nausea, abdominal pain, and admission for partial SBO

Nutrition Intervention

Estimated Nutrition Needs

Calories: 1682–2019 kcal (based on 25–30 kcal/kg IBW 67.3 kg for maintenance/obesity)

Protein: 54–81 gm (based on 0.8–1.2 gm/kg IBW 67.3 kg for maintenance/repletion/obesity)

Fluid: 1682–2019 ml (based on 1 ml/kcal)

Nutrition Prescription and Interventions

Nutrition Prescription: Advance diet as tolerated past Clear Liquids in the next 24–48 hours with clear liquid protein supplement 3 times daily; goal GI Soft (Low-Fiber) Diet

Interventions:
- Ordered supplements and weekly weights
- Encouraged supplement intake
- Paged general surgery MD with NPO/Clear Liquid alert and supplement plan
- Discussed with RN
- Provided RDN contact information

Nutrition Monitoring and Evaluation

Goals:
- Diet advanced past Clear Liquids and tolerated in the next 24–48 hours
- Provide high-calorie, high-protein supplements to support healing

Monitoring: Diet advancement, tolerance, and supplement acceptance

Recommendations

1. Advance diet as tolerated past Clear Liquids in the next 24–48 hours with clear liquid protein supplement 3 times daily; goal GI Soft (Low-Fiber) Diet

CASE 10: H.S.'S ALCOHOL ABUSE

Name: H.S. **LOS:** 1 **Age:** 37 **Sex:** F

Reason for Consult: Nursing referral for decreased appetite/intake and weight loss.

HPI: Patient presented to the ED with abdominal pain, abdominal distention, and SOB; admitted for ascites due to alcoholic cirrhosis s/p paracentesis, ETOH abuse, ETOH dependence, and elevated LFTs; GI consulted.

Subjective: Patient reports poor appetite and intake of <25% of normal/1 meal daily for the past month; she relates it to alcohol abuse; her appetite and intake were improved for a couple months before that because of sobriety. Her appetite is improved since admission with intake of ~75% of breakfast this morning. Patient denies recent weight loss because of fluid retention, but notes some musculoskeletal losses in her arms and legs.

Patient History

Medical History: Acute alcoholic pancreatitis, ETOH abuse, ETOH dependence, hepatitis, cirrhosis

Surgical History: None on file

Social History: Current pack/day smoker for 20 years; 5–6 liquor drinks/day; marijuana and cocaine use; lives alone

Food- and Nutrition-Related History

Current Diet: Cardiac (Low Fat/Low Cholesterol/3–4 gram Sodium)

Intake: <25% of normal 1 month before admission; improving with 75% intake of breakfast this morning

Food Allergies: None per patient

Cultural or Religious Food Preferences: None per patient

Nutritionally Relevant Medications and Infusions: Folic acid, lactulose, multivitamin, calcium carbonate, omeprazole, thiamine 100 mg infusion

Anthropometric Measurements

Height: 165.1 cm **Weight:** 62.5 kg **BMI:** 22.9 **BMI Classification:** Adequate

IBW: 56.8 kg **%IBW:** 110.0% **UBW:** 62.7 kg; was 68.2 kg 2 years ago per patient **%UBW:** 99.7%

Weight History and Change: Weight of 68.2 kg 1 year, 7 months ago per chart review; 5.7 kg/8.4% weight loss

Nutrition Assessment

Biochemical Data, Medical Tests, and Procedures

Laboratory Results: Sodium 133 (L), BUN <5 (L), Cr 0.45 (L), ALP 138 (H), AST 75 (H), ALT 31, Ethanol <10

Nutrition-Focused Physical Findings

Appetite: Improving; decreased for 1 month before admission
Oral: No difficulty chewing or swallowing
GI: Abdominal distention; no nausea or vomiting; constipation per patient; on lactulose; history of intermittent nausea, vomiting, and diarrhea related to alcohol use

Skin: Intact, jaundice, bruising per RN admission assessment
Edema: None per RN flowsheets

Subcutaneous Fat Depletion: Severe to triceps per RDN physical exam
Musculoskeletal Depletion: Severe to temple, clavicle, shoulder, hand, knee, thigh, and calf per RDN physical exam

Nutrition Diagnosis

Inadequate protein-energy intake related to loss of appetite from alcohol consumption, GI/hepatic dysfunction, and increased protein needs as evidenced by reported intake of <25% of normal for 1 month, severe subcutaneous fat and musculoskeletal depletion, intermittent nausea, vomiting, and diarrhea, elevated LFTs, and admission for ascites due to alcoholic cirrhosis

Severe protein-calorie malnutrition in the context of acute illness related to inadequate protein—energy intake, loss of appetite from alcohol consumption, GI/hepatic dysfunction, and increased protein needs as evidenced by reported intake of <25% of normal for 1 month, severe subcutaneous fat and musculoskeletal depletion, intermittent nausea, vomiting, and diarrhea, elevated LFTs, and admission for ascites due to alcoholic cirrhosis

Nutrition Intervention

Estimated Nutrition Needs

Calories: 1704–1988 kcal (based on 30–35 kcal/kg IBW 56.8 kg for fluid retention/weight gain)
Protein: 68–85 gm (based on 1.2–1.5 gm/kg IBW 56.8 kg for fluid retention/cirrhosis)
Fluid: Per MD considering fluid retention

Nutrition Intervention

Nutrition Prescription and Interventions

Nutrition Prescription: 3–4 gram Sodium/No Added Salt Diet to encourage intake with strawberry protein shakes twice daily

Interventions:
- Ordered supplements; daily weights already ordered
- Encouraged supplement and protein intake, such as meat, eggs, and dairy
- Paged attending MD with malnutrition alert and supplement plan
- Discussed with RN
- Provided verbal and written nutrition education for High-Calorie, High-Protein/Cirrhosis Nutrition Therapy
- Provided Outpatient Nutrition Counseling brochure and RDN contact information

Nutrition Monitoring and Evaluation

Goals:
- Patient to consume >75% of meals and supplements
- Provide high-calorie, high-protein supplements to support healing
- Avoid weight loss during admission once fluid retention/ascites resolves
- Patient to verbalize understanding of High-Calorie, High-Protein/Cirrhosis Nutrition Therapy

Monitoring: Intake, supplement acceptance, weight, fluid retention/ascites, and nutrition education understanding

Recommendations

1. Liberalize to 3–4 gram Sodium/No Added Salt Diet to encourage intake with strawberry protein shakes twice daily
2. Continue multivitamin, folic acid, and thiamine supplementation
3. Referral to Outpatient Nutrition Counseling at discharge
4. Patient meets criteria for severe protein-calorie malnutrition

APPENDIX B:
ANSWERS TO "CHECK FOR UNDERSTANDING" AND "PUT IT INTO PRACTICE"

ANSWERS TO "CHECK FOR UNDERSTANDING"

Chapter 1: 1) A; 2) B; 3) A; 4) A; 5) A

Chapter 2: 1) D; 2) C; 3) B; 4) D; 5) A

Chapter 3: 1) C; 2) B; 3) D; 4) C; 5) D

Chapter 4: 1) A; 2) A; 3) C; 4) A; 5) B;

Chapter 5: 1) D; 2) A; 3) B; 4) B; 5) A

Chapter 6: 1) B; 2) D; 3) A; 4) B; 5) C

Chapter 7: 1) B; 2) D; 3) A; 4) C; 5) B

Chapter 8: 1) C; 2) D; 3) A; 4) D; 5) B

ANSWERS TO "PUT IT INTO PRACTICE"

Put It into Practice Answers: Writing Goals and Monitoring Parameters

1. Goals: Patient to consume protein shake with meals; provide-high calorie, high-protein supplements to support pressure injury healing
    Monitoring: Supplement acceptance and intake; pressure injury healing
2. Goal: Patient to measure and record blood glucose 3 times daily before meals for 3 out of the next 7 days
    Monitoring: Patient's blood glucose records

3. Goals: Patient to verbalize understanding of low-fiber diet with gradual progression to high-fiber diet and name 3 high-fiber foods to initially avoid

   Monitoring: Nutrition education understanding

4. Goals: Edema to improve as medically feasible; patient to verbalize understanding of low-sodium nutrition therapy and name 3 high-sodium foods to avoid

   Monitoring: Edema; nutrition education understanding

5. Goal: Patient to safely consume >50% of meals

   Monitoring: Intake, diet tolerance, and SLP evaluation

6. Goal: Feeding modality determined in the next 24–48 hours

   Monitoring: Oral diet or EN support initiation

7. Goals: Blood glucose improved/WNL; HbA1c improved

   Monitoring: Blood glucose and HbA1c levels

8. Goals: Avoid further weight loss during admission; patient to verbalize understanding of celiac disease nutrition therapy and name gluten-containing grains to avoid; diarrhea to improve

   Monitoring: Weight, nutrition education understanding, and bowel movements

9. Goals: Patient to record all meals and snacks for 10 out of the next 14 days in diet diary; patient to consume meals or snacks every 4–5 hours; patient to consume 4 carbohydrate choices at 3 meals daily

   Monitoring: Diet diary recording compliance, meal and snack timing, carbohydrate consumption at meals

10. Goals: Avoid further weight loss/gradual weight gain during admission once edema resolves; patient to consume >75% of meals and supplements; BMI to increase; edema to improve as medically feasible; provide high-calorie, high-protein supplements to promote pressure injury healing; patient to verbalize understanding of high-calorie, high-protein nutrition therapy

    Monitoring: Weight, intake, supplement acceptance, BMI, edema, pressure injury healing, and nutrition education understanding

Put it Into Practice Answers: Writing the Subjective

1. The patient reports ~50% intake of normal during rehab because of nausea.
2. The MD ordered a CT scan because of the patient's neck pain.
3. The patient was unable to prepare home meals because of intense pain.
4. The RN will administer a laxative to help stimulate a bowel movement.
5. Writer encouraged high-fiber carbohydrate choices.
6. Patient noncompliant with insulin regimen per PCP.
7. Patient presented to ED today with SOB and bilateral LE edema.
8. Patient had 15-lb weight loss in 3 months from 30% meal intake.
9. Patient at procedure during interview attempt; no family at bedside.
10. Patient presented with hip fracture after falling s/p surgical repair. Reports decreased appetite with ~50% normal intake and 25-lb weight loss over 6 months; she is unsure the reason or UBW. She drinks strawberry or vanilla protein shakes at home and requests them with meals.

APPENDIX C:
EVIDENCE-BASED DIETETIC PRACTICE:
UNDERSTANDING SCIENTIFIC RESEARCH

EVIDENCE-BASED DIETETIC PRACTICE

The dietitian must use evidence-based dietetic practice (EBDP) in order to provide effective and proven nutrition care to patients and clients. The Academy defines EBDP as "the process of asking questions, systematically finding research evidence, and assessing its validity, applicability and importance to food and nutrition practice decisions; and includes applying relevant evidence in the context of the practice situation and the values of clients, customers and communities to achieve positive outcomes" (1). This requires an understanding of scientific research.

Basic Points About Research

Research can be defined as a systematic study to answer questions posed (hypotheses). Researchers begin with the null hypothesis, which states that study observations arise from only chance. The alternative hypothesis states that the study observations arise from a cause that is not random or due to chance. Research also should follow the scientific method, as follows, as it relates to epidemiological research, which typifies most nutritional research:

1. Observe
2. Count cases/events (vital statistics)
3. Relate cases/events to population at risk
4. Make comparisons (statistical associations)
5. Develop the hypothesis
6. Test the hypothesis
7. Draw scientific inferences
8. Conduct experimental study (clinical trial)
9. Replicate results of study

10. Intervene and evaluate

11. Formulate dietary recommendations, if appropriate strength of association

Types of Studies

Controlled (Experimental) Study: Study conducted to evaluate the effect of specific intervention, in which one or more independent variables are selected and controlled. It is artificial, planned, and results can suggest cause and effect. This type of study is placebo controlled, and can be randomized or nonrandomized, and double-blind, all of which are important to validity. An example of this type of study in humans is a human intervention or clinical trial.

Ecological (Correlational): Comparison of the frequency of events in different populations with consumption of a dietary factor. Represents natural observation, no manipulation, not randomized.

Cross-Sectional (Prevalence): Examination of relationship between intake, disease, or variable within a population at a specific time point. Represents a "snapshot" of the population, with the study time frame being when the study is being conducted. Defines prevalence but can't establish cause and effect. The National Health and Nutrition Examination Survey (NHANES) is of this type.

Cohort (Incidence): A disease-free group is tracked within a specific time period with assessment of dietary intake, which avoids selection bias at the outset. At the endpoint, the group is evaluated as to the number who developed the disease, and a comparison is made between the dietary intakes of disease-free group and the group with the disease. It is prospective (looks into the future), with some ability to confirm cause and effect, and it establishes incidence.

Case-Control: Disease-free group (controls) is compared to a group with the disease (cases) at the outset and their dietary intake, based on recall of past eating, is compared. Cases and controls must be closely matched, and this represents a retrospective study (looking at the past).

Meta-Analysis: Statistical analysis combining results of several studies, which address a set of related research hypotheses. Results are observational, even if individual studies are clinical trials. The higher the number of studies considered and the greater the similarity in their methodologies, the stronger and higher the validity of the meta-analysis.

MOOSE: Meta-analysis of only observational studies in epidemiology.

Epidemiologic AL Studies

Most studies in nutritional science are epidemiological. The National Institutes of Health defines epidemiology as "the branch of medical science that investigates all the factors that determine the presence or absence of diseases and disorders. Epidemiological research helps us to understand how many people have a disease or disorder, if those numbers are changing".[1]

Nutritional epidemiology, in turn, is "a subdiscipline of epidemiology and provides specific knowledge to nutritional science,"[2] focusing on how diet influences the development of disease.

Key points about epidemiological studies:

- Compares disease in various populations
- Mortality, morbidity for specific diseases
- Is concerned with etiology, treatment, prevention
- Forms the basis for further studies (more controlled)

Questions to Ask: How to Critically Analyze a Study

1. Source: Credentials of researchers; what was their previous research (any conflicts of interest)?
2. Do results fit the existing body of research?
3. Have results been replicated, or is this the first report of these findings?
4. Subjects: Selection process, sample size?

---

1   U.S. Department of Health & Human Services. National Institutes of Health. What is Epidemiology? https://www.nidcd.nih.gov/health/statistics/what-epidemiology

2   Boeing, H. (2013). Nutritional epidemiology: New perspectives for understanding the diet-disease relationship? *EJCN, 67*: 424–429.

5. Study design: Observational/experimental: If experimental, was it randomized and controlled?

6. Can results be generalized to other groups (animal versus human; if human, sex, age)?

Research and Statistical Terms

Bias: A systematic error arising in a study,[3] which occurs when there is no real association between X and Y, but one is manufactured because of the way the study was conducted. Several types of bias may occur (74 types). Two major types of bias:

- *Selection Bias:* Selection of certain study subjects which may be associated with another variable.

- *Information Bias:* Some aspect of collecting or measuring a specific variable may be associated with an effect.

Biologic Plausibility: The basis in scientific theory that would support the results from a study indicating cause and effect. In epidemiological studies, although results do not immediately suggest biologic plausibility, it may be identified or described at a later date.

Case: Incident of disease in an individual; also called an "event."

Cohort: A group of people possessing a common trait.

Confounding: Occurs when there is an association between the two variables being studied, but the magnitude of the association is influenced by a previously unknown third variable.[4]

Correlation (Correlation Coefficient R): A measure of the strength and direction of the linear association between two variables. The correlation may be positive or negative (inverse).

Determinants: Causes or factors associated with risk for disease.

Disease frequency: Measure of the amount of disease in a population.

Distribution: Relationship between disease and the population; who gets it (age, gender, etc.).

---

3   The Association for Qualitative Research. Bias. https://www.aqr.org.uk/glossary/bias

4   Skelly, A. C., Dettori, J. R., & Brodt, E. D. (2012). Assessing bias: The importance of considering confounding. *Evid Based Spine Care J, 3*(1): 9–12.

Dose-Response Relationship: Results of study showing a relationship in which a variation in the amount, intensity, or duration of exposure causes a change in risk of disease.

Environmental factors: Factors affecting disease risk that arise from the environment; examples include passive smoke, water supply, soil contaminants.

Host factors: Relate to characteristics of the person with the disease; examples include body weight and gender.

Incidence: A measure of the risk of developing a new condition within a specified time period. Represents the rate of occurrence of new cases and the risk of contracting the disease.

Null Hypothesis: Premise in research that states that no effect, or statistically significant difference, exists from study observations.

Odds Ratio: A measure of the association that exists between exposure to a variable and the outcome (for example, a disease) compared to the outcome without exposure to the variable.

Placebo: An inert treatment from which the subject (or patient) reports experiencing an actual effect, a phenomenon called the placebo effect. In research, a study that is placebo controlled refers to providing the control group an inert treatment (placebo) to mimic the actual treatment in an effort to prevent the placebo effect.

Prevalence: All events/cases of disease in a specific time period. Rather than the rate of occurrence of new cases, prevalence indicates how widespread the disease is rather than the risk of contracting the disease (incidence).

Randomized: The assignment of subjects in a study to either the control group or the treatment group in a randomized manner to prevent bias. Randomization increases study validity.

Random Variation (Chance): In any study, the possibility exists that a result may occur which is not associated with the controlled variables. Estimates of study results arising from chance: Up to 33% of statistically significant findings are false positives purely by random chance, and this assumes that there is no bias in the studies.

Reliability: The reproducibility of the findings of a specific study, which reflects how closely the findings would be replicated in another study using similar materials and methods.

Umbrella Review: Professional group makes an overview of meta-analyses across the literature. It includes systematic reviews, meta-analyses (epidemiologic and clinical trials).

Risk: Likelihood of disease.

Risk factor: A sign associated with risk for developing a disease (a statistical association) until proven to be a cause (cause and effect) from experimental studies.

Relative Risk (RR): The probability that a member of an exposed group will develop disease relative to the probability that a member of an unexposed group will develop disease.[5] An important consideration is the strength of the association. The National Cancer Institute stated that "RR of less than 2 (< 100%) is not strong enough to use for public policy pronouncements," and should be viewed with skepticism.

Reverse Causality (Protopathic Bias): When study results indicate an association between two factors (X and Y), researchers must consider that it's equally likely that Y caused X as it is that X caused Y. Researchers can mistake what came first in the order of causation.

Validity (External and Internal): Extent to which a study is able to measure what it was intended to measure and scientifically answer the questions it is intended to answer. Internal validity refers to validity within the study itself. High internal validity arises from tightly controlled experiment conditions; for example, highly homogeneous subjects (rats of the same species, age, etc.). External validity refers to the validity of the study when applying the results beyond the subjects and variables of the study. High external validity arises from applicability to other groups and situations (e.g., gender, age, ethnicity). Internal validity and external validity oppose each other; i.e., the higher the internal validity, the lower the external.

Sources of Evidence-Based Analysis of Research

- Academy of Nutrition and Dietetics Evidence Analysis Library: https://www.andeal.org/. Available free to members or for subscription.

---

5   National Institutes of Health. National Cancer Institute. NCI Dictionary of Cancer Terms. Relative risk. https://www.cancer.gov/publications/dictionaries/cancer-terms/def/relative-risk

- Cochrane Library: http://www.cochranelibrary.org/
- Food and Agriculture Organization of the United Nations: www.fao.org/agris/search/search.do
- The Global Resource for Nutrition Practice: http://www.pen-nutrition.com/index.aspx. Available for subscription.
- National Institutes of Health. National Center for Biotechnology Information. U.S. National Library of Medicine. PubMed: https://www.ncbi.nlm.nih.gov/pubmed
- U.S. Department of Agriculture. Center for Nutrition Policy and Promotion. National Evidence Library: https://www.cnpp.usda.gov/nutritionevidencelibrary/
- U.S. Department of Health and Human Services. Agency for Healthcare Research and Quality. National Guideline Clearinghouse: https://www.ngc.gov/

References

1. Academy of Nutrition and Dietetics. Scope of Practice. Academy Definition of Terms. Available at: http://www.eatrightpro.org/~/media/eatrightpro%20files/practice/scope%20standards%20of%20practice/academydefinitionoftermslist.ashx. Accessed April 15, 2018.
2. National Institutes of Health. U.S. National Library of Medicine. MedlinePlus. Understanding Medical Research. Available at: https://medlineplus.gov/understandingmedicalresearch.html. Accessed April 13, 2018.

The Association for Qualitative Research. Available at: https://www.aqr.org.uk/glossary/validity. Accessed April 14, 2018.

Stat Trek. Statistics Dictionary. Available at: http://stattrek.com/statistics/dictionary.aspx?definition=null%20hypothesis. Accessed April 14, 2018.

Szumilas, M. (2010). Explaining odds ratios. *J Can Acad Child Adolesc Psychiatry, 19*(3): 227–229.

APPENDIX D:
VITAMIN AND MINERAL FACTS

A. Vitamins			
Vitamin	**Functions**	**Deficiency**	**Toxicity**
A	Maintain integrity of cornea, epithelial cells, and mucous membranes; skin and bone and teeth growth; regulate synthesis of reproductive hormones; immune and cancer protection	Anemia Blindness, night Blindness Bone growth deficit Corneal breakdown Diarrhea Joint pain Kidney stones Infection susceptibility	Amenorrhea Anorexia Bone pain Fatigue Headache Nosebleeds Skin rash
D	Maintain bone tissue by regulating the absorption and excretion of calcium and phosphorus	Defective bone growth (bowed legs, joint pain) Muscle spasms	Anorexia Headaches Excessive thirst Hypercalcemia Kidney stones Nausea Weakness
E	Maintains cell membranes; acts as an antioxidant in fighting disease-causing free radicals and in protecting other important compounds from oxidation	Anemia Breast cysts Leg cramps Weakness	Enhances action of anticoagulants Gastrointestinal distress

K	Synthesis of blood-clotting compounds; regulation of calcium levels in blood	Excessive bleeding	Jaundice Interference of anticoagulant drugs
B$_1$ **Thiamin**	Coenzyme in energy metabolism; maintenance of appetite and nervous system function	Abnormal heart beat Cardiomegaly/heart failure Fluid retention Mental confusion Muscle pain, weakness, wasting paralysis	None documented
B$_2$ **Riboflavin**	Coenzyme in energy metabolism; maintenance of skin and visual function	Corneal abnormalities Dry, cracking at corners of mouth Sensitivity to light Skin rash Tongue abnormalities	None documented
B$_3$ **Niacin, Nico-tinamide**	Coenzyme in energy metabolism; maintenance of skin, nervous and digestive systems	Anorexia Diarrhea Skin rash Tongue abnormalities Weakness and dizziness	Diarrhea Dizziness Liver dysfunction Low blood pressure Sweating, flushing
B$_6$ **Pyridoxine**	Coenzyme in protein and fat metabolism; synthesis of red blood cells; synthesis of niacin	Anemia Kidney stones Dermatitis Spastic muscles, convulsions Tongue abnormalities	Fluid retention Depression, memory loss Fatigue Weakness

Folate	Coenzyme in cellular synthesis	Anemia Depression, mental confusion Diarrhea, constipation Infection susceptibility Tongue abnormalities	Mask B_{12} deficiency
B_{12} Cobalamine	Cellular synthesis; maintenance of nervous system function	Anemia Fatigue Paralysis Skin abnormalities Tongue abnormalities	None documented
Pantothenic Acid	Coenzyme in energy metabolism	Fatigue Insomnia Vomiting, other intestinal problems	Fluid retention
Biotin	Coenzyme in energy metabolism; synthesis of fat and glycogen	Alopecia Anorexia Depression Fatigue Heartbeat abnormalities Nausea Skin rash	None documented
Choline	Coenzyme in energy metabolism; synthesis of phospholipids and neurotransmitters	Growth failure Kidney failure Liver dysfunction (fat accumulation) Memory abnormalities	Fishy body odor Low blood pressure

| C Ascorbic Acid | Collagen synthesis; antioxidant; immune function; enhancement of iron absorption; synthesis of thyroid hormone; protein metabolism | Anemia
Bleeding gums, loose teeth
Bone fracture susceptibility
Depression
Infection susceptibility

Joint pain
Muscle pain and wasting
Skin problems
Wound healing delayed | Abdominal cramps, diarrhea
Headache
Nausea
Skin rash

Interferes with interpretation of some laboratory values |

Alpers, D., Taylor, B. E., Bier, D. M., & Klein, S. (2015). *Manual of nutritional therapeutics*, 6th ed. Philadelphia PA: Wolters Kluwer.

B. Vitamin C

Food	Portion Size	Vitamin C (mg)	% Daily Value (DV)
Papaya	1 whole fresh	188	313%
Orange juice	1 cup fresh	124	207%
Brussels sprouts	1 cup cooked	96	160%
Grapefruit juice	1 cup fresh	94	157%
Green pepper	1 whole	90	150%
Strawberries	1 cup fresh	85	142%
Orange	1 fresh medium	80	133%
Broccoli	1 cup cooked	74	123%
Cauliflower	1 cup cooked	72	120%
Cantaloupe	1 cup fresh	68	113%
Mango	1 fresh	57	95%
Pink grapefruit	½ fresh	47	78%
Honeydew melon	1 cup fresh	42	70%
Turnip greens	1 cup cooked	40	67%

Parsley	½ cup chopped	40	67%
Mustard greens	1 cup cooked	36	60%
Tomatoes	1 whole canned	36	60%
Cabbage	1 cup raw	34	57%
Sauerkraut	1 cup canned	34	57%
Tomato juice	6 oz canned	33	55%
Raspberries	1 cup fresh	31	52%
Butternut squash	1 cup boiled	30	50%
Sweet potato	1 baked w/skin	28	47%
Baked potato	1 whole	26	43%
Pineapple chunks	1 cup fresh	24	40%
Asparagus	1 cup cooked	20	33%
Watermelon	1 cup fresh	15	25%
Apple	1 medium fresh	8	13%
Milk	2%, 8 oz	2	3%

Quick Reference for Patient Teaching

- Snacks: Orange, tomato, and grapefruit juices

- Entrée: Stir-fried broccoli, Brussels sprouts, green pepper, and cauliflower

- Mashed, baked, or boiled potatoes

- Fruit salad of strawberries, papaya, mango, watermelon in place of sweets

- Kabob of green peppers, cherry tomatoes, strawberries, and pineapples

C. Riboflavin

			% Dietary Reference Intake (DRI)	
Food	*Portion Size*	*Riboflavin*	*Women*	*Men*
Brewer's yeast	1 Tbs	1.21	110%	93%
Yogurt	1 cup low fat	0.51	46%	39%
Mushrooms	1 cup cooked	0.46	42%	35%

Ricotta cheese	1 cup part skim	0.46	42%	35%
Corn flakes	1 cup	0.43	39%	33%
Cottage cheese	1 cup low fat	0.42	38%	32%
Milk	2%, 8 oz	0.4	36%	31%
Buttermilk	1 cup	0.38	35%	29%
Sirloin steak	3.5 oz broiled	0.29	26%	22%
Peach halves	10 dried	0.28	25%	22%
Pork chop	3.5 oz roasted	0.26	24%	20%
Ground beef	3.5 oz lean baked	0.24	22%	18%
Black-eyed peas	1 cup cooked	0.24	22%	18%
Kidney beans	1 cup canned	0.23	21%	18%
Asparagus	1 cup cooked	0.22	20%	17%
Almonds	1 oz whole dried	0.22	20%	17%
Oysters	3 oz raw	0.2	18%	15%
Ham	3.5 oz cooked	0.19	17%	15%
Turkey	3.5 oz w/o skin	0.18	16%	14%
Broccoli	1 cup cooked	0.16	15%	12%
Green beans	1 cup cooked	0.14	13%	11%
Cheddar cheese	1 oz	0.11	10%	8%
Spinach	1 cup cooked	0.1	9%	8%
Strawberries	1 cup fresh	0.1	9%	8%
Chicken breast	½ breast roasted	0.1	9%	8%
Sole/flounder	3 oz baked	0.07	6%	5%
Orange	1 medium fresh	0.06	5%	5%
Bread	Whole wheat 1 slice	0.05	5%	4%
Bean sprouts	1 cup stir fried	0.04	4%	3%
Cantaloupe	1 cup fresh	0.03	3%	2%
Apple	1 medium fresh	0.02	2%	2%

Quick Reference for Patient Teaching
• A bowl of corn flakes with 8 oz milk provides 75% of DRI for women
• Yogurt as a snack and as a dip for fruits and vegetables
• Mushrooms in pizza, salads, or stir fries
• Low-fat cottage or ricotta cheeses in lasagna, ravioli, or other main dish

D. Vitamin B$_6$

Food	Portion Size	B$_6$ (mg)	% DRI
Beef liver	3.5 oz braised	0.91	70%
Baked potato	1 whole	0.7	54%
Salmon	3 oz cooked	0.7	54%
Banana	1 peeled	0.66	51%
Chicken breast	½ breast w/o skin	0.51	39%
Corn flakes	1 cup	0.5	38%
Avocado	½ average	0.48	37%
Trout	3 oz broiled	0.46	35%
Turkey	3.5 oz w/o skin	0.46	35%
Brewer's yeast	1 oz	0.45	35%
Sirloin steak	3.5 oz broiled	0.45	35%
Pork chop	3.5 oz roasted	0.45	35%
Spinach	1 cup cooked	0.44	34%
Soybeans	1 cup cooked	0.4	31%
Wheat germ	¼ cup	0.38	29%
Tuna, in water	3 oz canned	0.3	23%
Navy beans	1 cup cooked	0.3	23%
Sunflower seeds	¼ cup dry	0.3	23%
Turnip greens	1 cup cooked	0.26	20%
Cauliflower	1 cup cooked	0.26	20%

Broccoli	1 cup cooked	0.24	18%
Green pepper	1 whole	0.24	18%
Watermelon	1 cup fresh	0.23	18%
Ground beef	3.5 oz lean baked	0.22	17%
Asparagus	1 cup cooked	0.22	17%
Figs	5 dried	0.21	16%
Cantaloupe	1 cup fresh	0.18	14%
Sole/flounder	3 oz cooked	0.18	14%
Mustard greens	1 cup cooked	0.16	12%
Zucchini	1 cup cooked	0.14	11%
Milk	2%, 8 oz	0.11	8%

Quick Reference for Patient Teaching

- Baked potato for lunch with Greek yogurt dressing

- Banana with corn flakes for breakfast

- Poach, grill, or broil salmon for a quick meal

E. Vitamin B_{12}

Food	Portion Size	B_{12} (µg)	% DRI
Clams	3 oz cooked	84.1	3,500%
Beef liver	3.5 oz braised	71	3,000%
Oysters	3 oz cooked	32.5	1,350%
Clam chowder	1 cup	10.3	427%
Rabbit	3.5 oz roasted	8.3	346%
Braunschweiger	1 oz, tube type	5.2	216%
Sirloin steak	3.5 oz broiled	2.9	119%
Salmon	3 oz cooked	2.7	113%
Tuna, in water	3 oz canned	2.5	106%
Lamb chop	3.5 oz braised	2.3	95%

Vegetarian burger	½ cup	2	83%
Raisin bran	¾ cup	2	83%
Ground beef	3.5 oz lean baked	1.7	71%
Cottage cheese	1 cup 1% fat	1.4	58%
Sole/flounder	3 oz cooked	1.3	54%
Shrimp	3 oz cooked	1.3	54%
Halibut	3 oz broiled	1.2	50%
Milk	2%, 8 oz	0.89	37%
Frankfurter	1 beef, 2 oz	0.88	37%
Ham	3.5 oz cooked	0.74	29%
Tempeh	½ cup	0.7	29%
Pork chop	3.5 oz roasted	0.6	25%
Buttermilk	8 oz, cultured	0.54	23%
Egg	1 whole fresh	0.5	21%
Turkey	3.5 oz w/o skin	0.37	15%
Canadian bacon	2 slices cooked	0.36	15%
Miso	½ cup	0.29	12%
Chicken breast	½ breast w/o skin	0.29	12%
Yogurt	8 oz low fat	0.24	10%
Cheddar cheese	1 oz	0.23	10%
Goat's milk	8 oz	0.16	7%

Quick Reference for Patient Teaching

- Raisin Bran with low-fat milk for breakfast

- Low-fat cottage cheese with fruit as a snack

- 3 oz of salmon, tuna, or rabbit provides 100% DRI of B_{12}

- Oysters or clams served steamed or in stews and chowders

F. Biotin

Food	Portion Size	Biotin (µg)	% DRI
Egg	1 whole fresh	10	33%
Wheat germ	1/4 cup toasted	7	23%
Ry-Krisp	½ oz	6.8	23%
Granola	¼ cup w/raisins	5	17%
Egg noodles	1 cup cooked	4	13%
Almonds	1 oz whole natural	1	3%
Pistachios	1 oz, red	1	3%
Cornmeal	1 oz yellow	1	3%

Quick Reference for Patient Teaching

- Granola as a cereal or snack, or mixed into yogurt
- Wheat germ in casseroles and breads or on cereal
- Ry-Krisp with peanut butter and jelly for a snack
- Egg noodles with veggies, fat-free Italian dressing
- Scrambled, poached, or hardboiled eggs

G. Choline

Food	Portion Size	Choline (µg)	% DRI Women	Men
Beef liver	3.5 oz	583.1	137%	106%
Cauliflower	1 cup cooked	162	38%	29%
Peanuts	1 oz, dried	127.3	30%	23%
Peanut butter	2 Tbs	124.6	29%	23%
Grape juice	8 oz, canned	120	28%	22%
Potato	1 whole baked	103.2	24%	19%
Iceberg lettuce	1 leaf raw	58.6	14%	11%
Tomato	1 whole raw	52.9	12%	10%

Milk	Whole, 8 oz	36.6	9%	7%
Orange	1 fresh medium	28	7%	5%
Banana	1 whole peeled	27.4	6%	5%
Bread	Whole wheat 1 slice	24.2	6%	4%
Cucumber	½ cup raw	11.3	3%	2%
Beef steak	3.5 oz	7.5	2%	1%
Apple	1 fresh medium	3.7	<1%	<1%
Egg	1 fresh whole	2.1	<1%	<1%
Ginger ale	12 oz	0.73	<1%	<1%
Butter	1 tsp	0.21	<1%	<1%
Margarine	1 tsp, tub type	0.15	<1%	<1%
Corn oil	1 Tbs	0.04	<1%	<1%

Quick Reference for Patient Teaching

- Dinner: 3.5 oz beef liver, 1 cup cauliflower, baked potato, 8 oz grape juice, banana
- Add romaine lettuce to a sandwich
- Swap straight soda for a "choline cocktail"—8 oz grape juice, 12 oz ginger ale
- Snack: 1 oz peanuts and 8 oz milk

H. Folate

Food	Portion Size	Folate (µg)	% DRI
Pinto beans	1 cup cooked	294	74%
Asparagus	1 cup cooked	264	66%
Spinach	1 cup cooked	262	66%
Navy beans	1 cup cooked	255	64%
Beef liver	3.5 oz braised	217	54%
Black-eyed peas	1 cup cooked	209	52%
Great Northern beans	1 cup cooked	181	45%
Turnip greens	1 cup cooked	170	43%

Lima beans	1 cup cooked	156	39%
Kidney beans	1 cup canned	129	32%
Broccoli	1 cup cooked	104	26%
Corn flakes	1 cup	100	25%
Parsley	1 cup chopped	92	23%
Beets	1 cup cooked	90	23%
Wheat germ	¼ cup	82	21%
Romaine lettuce	1 cup chopped	76	19%
Cauliflower	1 cup cooked	64	16%
Pineapple juice	8 oz canned	58	15%
Orange	1 fresh medium	47	12%
Zucchini	1 cup cooked	30	8%
Peanuts	1 oz dried	29	7%
Cantaloupe	1 cup fresh	27	7%
Winter squash	1 cup cooked	26	7%
Strawberries	1 cup fresh	26	7%
Grapefruit juice	1 cup canned	26	7%
Egg	1 whole fresh	23	6%
Green beans	1 cup cooked	22	6%
Tofu	½ cup raw	19	5%
Tomato	1 whole raw	18	5%
Bread, whole wheat	1 slice	14	4%

Quick Reference for Patient Teaching

- Use dry beans in soups or as a main dish salad
- Add spinach to lasagna or serve cooked with lemon juice
- Salad of spinach, romaine lettuce, tomato, broccoli, cauliflower, and beets
- Dinner: 3.5 oz beef liver, 1 cup asparagus, 1 cup lima beans
- Breakfast: Cornflakes in milk; fruit salad of cantaloupe, strawberries, orange

I. Niacin

Food	Portion Size	Niacin (mg)	% DRI Women	Men
Chicken breast	½ roasted w/o skin	11.8	84%	74%
Tuna, in water	3 oz canned	11.3	81%	71%
Beef liver	3.5 oz braised	10.7	76%	67%
Brewer's yeast	1 oz	10.7	76%	67%
Salmon	3 oz broiled	8.6	61%	54%
Mushrooms	1 cup cooked	7	50%	44%
Halibut	3 oz broiled	6.1	44%	38%
Peach halves	10 dried	5.7	41%	36%
Pink salmon	3 oz canned	5.6	40%	35%
Pork chop	3.5 oz roasted	5.5	39%	34%
Lamb chop	3.5 oz braised	5.5	39%	34%
Turkey	3.5 oz w/o skin	5.4	39%	34%
Sirloin steak	3.5 oz broiled	4.3	31%	27%
Ground beef	3.5 oz lean baked	4.2	30%	26%
Peanuts	1 oz dried unsalted	4	29%	25%
Baked potato	1 whole	3.3	24%	21%
Sole/flounder	3 oz baked	2.5	18%	16%
Kidney beans	1 cup canned	2.4	17%	15%
Braunschweiger	1 oz tube-type	2.3	16%	14%
Shrimp	3 oz boiled	2.2	16%	14%
Wheat bran	¼ cup	2	14%	13%
Asparagus	1 cup cooked	2	14%	13%
Oysters	3 oz raw	1.7	12%	11%
Sardines	2 sardines in oil	1.3	9%	8%

Crabmeat	3 oz canned	1.2	9%	8%
Bread, whole wheat	1 slice	1	8%	6%
Summer squash	1 cup cooked	1	8%	6%
Cantaloupe	1 cup fresh	0.9	6%	6%
Peach	1 fresh medium	0.9	6%	6%
Spinach	1 cup cooked	0.9	6%	6%
Broccoli	1 cup cooked	0.8	6%	5%

Quick Reference for Patient Teaching

- Choose tuna, halibut, and salmon instead of red meat
- Add mushrooms to soups and salads and stir fry
- Dinner: Half chicken breast, baked potato, 1 cup asparagus
- Fortified breakfast cereals (contain 25% of the DRI for niacin per serving)

J. Pantothenic Acid

Food	Serving Size	Pantothenic Acid (mg)	% DRI
Beef liver	3.5 oz braised	4.6	91%
Mushrooms	½ cup boiled	1.7	34%
Avocado	1 medium	1.7	34%
Salmon	3 oz cooked	1.4	28%
Lentils	1 cup boiled	1.3	25%
Split peas	1 cup boiled	1.2	23%
Potato	1 whole baked	1.1	22%
Turkey	3.5 oz w/o skin	0.94	19%
Pomegranate	1 medium raw	0.92	18%
Chicken breast	½ roasted w/o skin	0.83	17%
Peanuts	1 oz dried	0.79	16%
Milk	2%, 8 oz	0.78	16%
Sweet potato	1 whole baked	0.74	15%

Chickpeas	1 cup canned	0.72	14%
Wheat germ	¼ cup	0.66	13%
Pork chop	3.5 oz roasted	0.65	13%
Egg	1 whole fresh	0.63	13%
Broccoli	1 cup cooked	0.5	10%
Ham	3.5 oz cooked	0.47	9%
Sole/flounder	3 oz cooked	0.43	9%
Kidney beans	1 cup canned	0.38	8%
Sirloin steak	3.5 oz broiled	0.37	7%
Corn	1 cup boiled	0.36	7%
Orange	1 fresh medium	0.35	7%
Watermelon	1 cup fresh	0.34	7%
Ground beef	3.5 oz baked lean	0.27	5%
Spinach	1 cup cooked	0.26	5%
Bread, whole wheat	1 slice	0.18	4%
Tuna, in water	3 oz canned	0.18	4%
Macaroni	1 cup cooked, enriched	0.16	3%
Cheddar cheese	1 oz	0.12	2%

Quick Reference for Patient Teaching

- Avocado sliced in a salad or in guacamole dip
- Dinner: 3 oz salmon, 1 baked potato, 8 oz milk, 1 cup broccoli
- Soups with lentils or split peas
- Salad: Chicken breast, avocado, spinach, mushrooms, broccoli

K. Thiamin

| | | | % DRI | |
Food	Portion Size	Thiamin (mg)	Women	Men
Brewer's yeast	1 oz	4.43	403%	369%

Pork chop	3.5 oz roasted	0.91	83%	76%
Ham	3.5 oz cooked	0.78	71%	65%
Green peas	1 cup cooked	0.42	38%	35%
Canadian bacon	2 pieces cooked	0.38	35%	32%
Cornflakes	1 cup	0.38	35%	32%
Split peas	1 cup cooked	0.37	34%	31%
Macaroni, enriched	1 cup cooked	0.29	26%	24%
Kidney beans	1 cup canned	0.27	25%	23%
Oatmeal	1 cup cooked	0.26	24%	22%
Millet	1 cup cooked	0.25	23%	21%
Acorn squash	1 cup boiled	0.24	22%	20%
Baked potato	1 whole	0.22	20%	18%
Asparagus	1 cup cooked	0.22	20%	18%
Peanuts	1 oz dry, unsalted	0.19	17%	16%
Black-eyed peas	1 cup cooked	0.17	15%	14%
Watermelon	1 cup fresh	0.13	12%	11%
Sirloin steak	3.5 oz broiled	0.13	12%	11%
Honeydew melon	1 cup fresh	0.13	12%	11%
Orange	1 fresh medium	0.12	11%	10%
Winter squash	1 cup baked	0.12	11%	10%
Tofu	½ cup	0.1	9%	8%
Milk	2%, 8 oz	0.1	9%	8%
Green beans	1 cup cooked	0.1	9%	8%
Broccoli	1 cup cooked	0.1	9%	8%
Bread, whole wheat	1 slice	0.09	8%	8%
Sole/flounder	3 oz cooked	0.08	7%	7%
Cauliflower	1 cup cooked	0.08	7%	7%
Tomato	1 whole raw	0.07	6%	6%

Quick Reference for Patient Teaching
• Include lean pork in menus
• Use green peas, split peas, black peas, black-eyed peas, kidney beans in soups
• Choose enriched pasta and bread products
• Breakfast: Oatmeal or fortified cereal
• Side dish: Boiled or baked squash

L. Vitamin A

Food	Portion size	Vitamin A (RE)	% DRI
Beef liver	3 oz fried	9,123	1,042
Pumpkin	1 cup canned	5,424	620
Sweet potato	1 whole baked	2,486	284
Carrot	1 whole fresh	2,024	231
Spinach	1 cup cooked	1,474	168
Butternut squash	1 cup baked	1,435	164
Mango	1 medium fresh	806	92
Papaya	1 medium fresh	612	70
Cantaloupe	1 cup fresh	516	59
Turnip greens	½ cup chopped	396	45
Collard greens	1 cup chopped	349	40
Apricot halves	10 halves	253	29
Winter squash	½ cup cubes	235	27
Mustard greens	½ cup chopped	212	24
Broccoli	½ cup frozen	174	20
Parsley	½ cup chopped	156	18
Milk	2%, 8 oz	140	16
Egg	1 whole fresh	95	11
Cheddar cheese	1 oz	86	10

Watermelon	1 cup fresh	58	7
Margarine	Tub-type 1 tsp	47	5
Sole/flounder	3 oz cooked	28	3
Orange	1 medium fresh	26	3
Green beans	½ cup canned	24	3
Corn	½ cup canned	13	2
Apple	1 medium fresh	7	1
Chicken breast	½ roasted w/o skin	5	0.5
Sirloin steak	3.5 oz broiled	0	0
Brewer's yeast	1 oz	0	0
Bread, whole wheat	1 slice	0	0

Quick Reference for Patient Teaching

- Use fresh spinach, romaine lettuce, carrots, and tomatoes in salads
- Use canned pumpkin in cookies, pies, and desserts
- Serve baked sweet potatoes in place of baked potatoes
- Breakfast: fruit salad of mango, papaya, and cantaloupe
- Snack: Dried peaches and apricots

M. Vitamin D

Food	Portion Size	Vitamin D (µg)	% DRI
Milk	2%, 8 oz	1.6	33%
Cornflakes	1 cup	0.81	16%
Cod liver oil	1 Tbs	0.55	11%
Egg	1 whole fresh	0.41	8%
Margarine	1 tsp, tub type	0.34	7%
Frankfurter	1 beef frank	0.18	4%
Braunschweiger	1 oz tube type	0.15	3%
Rice, wild	⅔ cup instant	0.07	1%

Rice, white	⅔ cup instant	0.03	<1%
Cheddar cheese	1 oz	0.02	<1%

Quick Reference for Patient Teaching

- Drink three 8-oz glasses of milk per day
- 10 to 15 minutes of sunlight exposure three times per week
- Breakfast: Vitamin-D-fortified cereals with milk
- Snacks: Pudding made with low-fat milk or yogurt
- Use vitamin-D-fortified margarine instead of butter

N. Vitamin E

Food	Portion Size	Vitamin E (mg)	% DRI
Wheat germ oil	1 tablespoon	20.3	102%
Sunflower seeds	1 oz dry roasted	14.2	71%
Mayonnaise	1 Tbs	11	55%
Almonds	1 oz dried	6.7	34%
Dried filberts	1 oz	6.7	34%
Sunflower seed oil	1 Tbs	6.3	32%
Sweet potato	1 medium raw	5.9	30%
Almond oil	1 Tbs	5.3	27%
Cottonseed oil	1 Tbs	4.8	24%
Safflower oil	1 Tbs	4.6	23%
Wheat germ	¼ cup toasted	4.1	20%
Peanut butter	2 Tbs	3	15%
Shrimp	3 oz boiled	3	15%
Canola oil	1 Tbs	2.5	13%
Asparagus	1 cup cooked	2.4	12%
Mango	1 raw medium	2.3	12%
Avocado	½ cup	2.3	12%

Peanuts	1 oz dry roasted	2.2	11%
Brazil nuts	1 oz dried	2.1	11%
Salmon	3 oz baked	2	10%
Corn oil	1 Tbs	1.9	10%
Olive oil	1 Tbs	1.7	8%
Peanut oil	1 Tbs	1.6	8%
Soybean oil	1 Tbs	1.5	8%
Apple	1 fresh medium	1.5	8%
Brussels sprouts	1 cup cooked	1.3	7%
Spinach	1 cup raw	1.1	5%
Macaroni	1 cup cooked	1	5%
Parsley	1 Tbs	1	5%
Pear	1 fresh medium	0.83	4%
Cheddar cheese	1 oz	0.5	3%

Quick Reference for Patient Teaching

- Use wheat germ or sunflower oil in salad dressings or baked goods
- Serve baked sweet potato slices instead of regular chips (slice thin and bake)
- Replace cream cheese with peanut butter on bagels
- Add wheat germ to cereal or yogurt
- Snack: Sunflower seeds, peanuts, or almonds

O. Vitamin K

Food	Portion Size	Vitamin K (µg)	% DRI
Turnip greens	1 cup chopped raw	364	455%
Green tea	1 oz dry	199	249%
Spinach	1 cup raw	148	185%
Broccoli	1 cup cooked	126	158%
Beef liver	3.5 oz raw	104	104%

Cauliflower	1 cup raw	96	120%
Soybean oil	1 Tbs	76	95%
Chickpeas	1 oz dry	74	93%
Asparagus	1 cup cooked	69	86%
Lentils	1 oz dry	62	78%
Soybeans	1 oz	53	66%
Cabbage	1 cup raw shredded	52	65%
Mung beans	1 oz dry	48	60%
Green beans	1 cup boiled	44	55%
Wheat flour	Whole wheat, 1 cup	36	45%
Tomato	1 whole fresh	28	35%
Egg	1 whole fresh	25	31%
Peas	1 oz dry	23	29%
Wheat bran	1 oz	23	29%
Lettuce	1 leaf iceberg	22	28%
Strawberries	1 cup raw	21	26%
Watercress	1 cup chopped	20	25%
Oats	1 oz dry	18	23%
Wheat germ	1 oz	10	13%
Carrot	1 medium raw	9	11%
Corn oil	1 Tbs	8	10%
Orange	1 fresh medium	7	9%
Potato	1 whole baked	6	8%
Cucumber	1 cup raw	6	8%

Quick Reference for Patient Teaching

- Add turnip greens or kale to soup or eat as side dish

- Entree: Stir-fry of broccoli, cauliflower, spinach, carrots, and asparagus

- Add spinach, watercress, and tomatoes to sandwiches

• Use soybean oil to make salad dressing
• Salad: Spinach and lettuce with tomatoes and chickpeas
• Appetizer: Coleslaw with low-fat or fat-free dressing

United States Department of Agriculture, Agricultural Research Service. USDA Food composition databases. Available at: https://ndb.nal.usda.gov/ndb/search/list. Accesses January 3, 2018.

National Institutes of Health, Office of Dietary Supplements. U.S. Department of Health and Human Services. Available at: https://ods.od.nih.gov/Health_Information/Dietary_Reference_Intakes.aspx. Accessed December 17, 2018.

APPENDIX E:
LABORATORY ASSESSMENT

L aboratory and other diagnostic tests are tools used by clinicians to gain valuable, objective information about their patients. When used in conjunction with other patient information, such as anthropometric data, a thorough history, and a physical examination, laboratory tests can provide valuable information about a patient's nutritional status and their response to medical nutrition therapy.

This appendix contains an alphabetical list of common laboratory (lab) measurements that are relevant to nutrition assessment. This list is not meant to be comprehensive; rather, it is a quick reference to the lab tests most commonly used by dietitians in the clinical setting.

Normal values are listed, but it must be noted that normal ranges of lab test results vary significantly, depending on the lab and their methods of testing. It is important to always check the normal values at the facility where the test is performed. This information is almost always given directly adjacent to the patient's specific lab result. In this book, Reference Ranges for blood tests are reported in the conventional US system first, then in the SI system (International System of Units, or Système Internationale d'Unités), if available. Critical values are also listed, if applicable. All values given are for adults. Conditions that may cause test results to be increased or decreased are listed under the heading "Clinical Implications."

TYPICAL LAB CHARTING

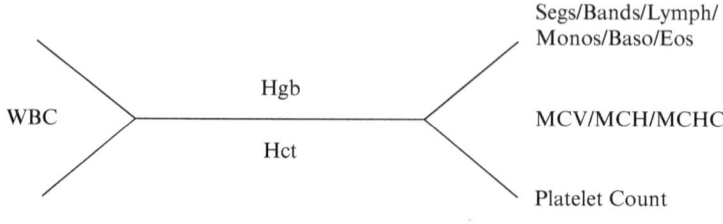

FIGURE A-1. Complete blood count.

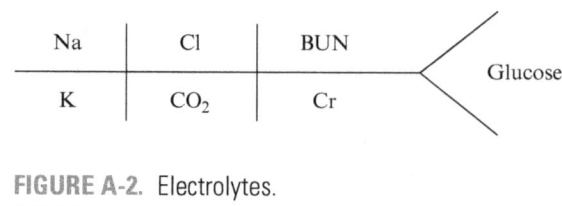

FIGURE A-2. Electrolytes.

LABORATORY VALUES FOR ASSESSING NUTRITIONAL STATUS

ALBUMIN

Reference Range
3.5–5.0 g/dL or 35–50 g/L

Clinical Implications
Increased Levels
Dehydration.

Decreased Levels
Malnutrition; pregnancy; acute and chronic inflammation and infections; cirrhosis, liver disease, alcoholism; nephrotic syndrome, renal disease; burns; third-space losses; protein-losing enteropathies, such as Crohn's disease; overhydration.

ARTERIAL BLOOD GASES (BLOOD GASES, ABG)

Reference Range
pH: 7.35–7.45 (critical values: <7.25 or >7.55)
PCO_2: 35–45 mm Hg (critical values: <20 or >60 mm Hg)
HCO_3: 21–28 mEq/L (critical values: <15 or >40)
PO_2: 80–100 mm Hg (critical values: <40)
O_2 Saturation: 95%–100% (critical values: 75% or lower)

Clinical Implications: pH
Increased Levels (Alkalosis)
Metabolic: Hypokalemia; hypochloremia; chronic vomiting; aldosteronism; chronic and high-volume gastric suctioning; sodium bicarbonate administration.
Respiratory: Hypoxemic states (e.g., congestive heart failure [CHF], cystic fibrosis [CF], carbon monoxide poisoning, pulmonary emboli, shock, acute pulmonary diseases); anxiety, neuroses, psychoses; pain; pregnancy.

Decreased Levels (Acidosis)
Metabolic: Ketoacidosis (diabetes and starvation); lactic acidosis; severe diarrhea; renal failure; strenuous exercise.
Respiratory: Respiratory failure; neuromuscular depression; pulmonary edema.

Clinical Implications: PCO_2
Increased Levels
Chronic obstructive pulmonary disease (COPD; bronchitis, emphysema); oversedation; head trauma; other causes of hypoventilation (e.g., Pickwickian syndrome).

Decreased Levels
Hypoxemia; pulmonary emboli; anxiety; pain; pregnancy; other causes of hyperventilation.

Clinical Implications: HCO$_3$
Increased Levels
Chronic vomiting or high-volume gastric suction; aldosteronism; COPD; use of mercurial diuretics.

Decreased Levels
Chronic or severe diarrhea; chronic use of loop diuretics; starvation; acute renal failure; diabetic ketoacidosis.

Clinical Implications: PO$_2$
Increased Levels
Polycythemia; increased inspired O$_2$; hyperventilation.

Decreased Levels
Anemias; mucous plug; bronchospasm; atelectasis

BLOOD UREA NITROGEN (BUN)

Reference Range
10–20 mg/dL or 3.6–7.1 mmol/L
(Critical values: >100 mg/dL indicates serious impairment of renal function)

Clinical Implications
Increased Levels
Prerenal (hypovolemia, shock, burns, dehydration, congestive heart failure (CHF), myocardial infarction (MI), gastrointestinal bleeding (GI bleed), excessive protein ingestion, and/or catabolism, starvation, sepsis); renal (renal disease or failure, nephrotoxic drugs); postrenal (urethral obstruction from stones/tumors/congenital anomalies, bladder outlet obstruction from prostatic hypertrophy, cancer, or congenital anomalies.

Decreased Levels
Liver failure; acromegaly; malnutrition; overhydration; negative nitrogen balance; syndrome of inappropriate secretion of antidiuretic hormone (SIADH); pregnancy; nephrotic syndrome; anabolic steroid use; impaired absorption (celiac disease)

CALCIUM (CA)—TOTAL AND IONIZED CALCIUM

Reference Range
Total Ca: 9.0–10.5 mg/dL or 2.25–2.75 mmol/L
(Critical values: <6 or >13 mg/dL or <1.5 or >3.25 mmol/L)
Ionized Ca: 4.5–5.6 mg/dl or 1.05–1.30 mmol/L
(Critical values: <2.2 or >7 mg/dL or <0.78 or >1.58 mmol/L)

Clinical Implications
Increased Levels (Hypercalcemia)
Hyperparathyroidism; cancer with parathyroid hormone (PTH)–
producing tumors (metastatic bone cancers, Hodgkin lymphoma,
leukemia, and non-Hodgkin lymphoma); Paget disease of the bone;
prolonged immobilization; milk-alkali syndrome; excessive intake of
vitamin D, milk, antacids; Addison disease; granulomatous infections
(e.g., sarcoidosis, tuberculosis).

Decreased Levels (Hypocalcemia)
Pseudohypocalcemia due to low albumin levels;[1] hypoparathyroidism;
renal failure; hyperphosphatemia secondary to renal failure; rickets;
vitamin D deficiency; osteomalacia; malabsorption; pancreatitis;
malnutrition; alkalosis.

CHLORIDE (CL)

Reference Range
98–106 mEq/L or 98–106 mmol/L
(Critical values: <80 or >115 mEq/L)

Clinical Implications
Increased Levels (Hyperchloremia)
Dehydration; Cushing syndrome; hyperparathyroidism; renal tubular
acidosis; metabolic acidosis; eclampsia; hyperventilation, which causes
respiratory alkalosis

---

1   Because about one-half of blood calcium is bound to albumin, when albumin
levels are low, the serum calcium will also be low. Calcium levels can be adjusted
with the following equation when serum albumin is low: Corrected calcium =
total calcium mg/dL + 0.8 [4 – serum albumin g/dL].

Decreased Levels
Overhydration; prolonged vomiting or gastric suctioning; CHF; chronic diarrhea or high-output GI fistula; metabolic alkalosis; burns; Addison disease; salt-losing nephritis; SIADH; fever; ulcerative colitis.

CHOLESTEROL

Reference Range
Desirable: 140–199 mg/dL or 3.63–5.17 mmol/L
Borderline high: 200–239 mg/dL or 5.18–6.21 mmol/L
High: >240 mg/dL or >6.22 mmol/L

Clinical Implications
Increased Levels (Hypercholesterolemia)
Familial hypercholesterolemia and/or hyperlipidemia; hypothyroidism; poorly controlled diabetes mellitus; nephrotic syndrome; cholestasis; pregnancy (third trimester); obesity; high dietary intake; Werner syndrome; acute myocardial infarction; atherosclerosis; biliary cirrhosis; pancreatectomy

Decreased Levels
Malabsorption; malnutrition; advanced cancer; hyperparathyroidism; chronic anemias; severe burns; sepsis/stress; liver disease.

CREATININE (SERUM CREATININE)

Reference Range
Female: 0.5–1.1 mg/dL or 44–97 μmol/L
Male: 0.6–1.2 mg/dL or 53–106 μmol/L
(Critical values for female and male: >4 mg/dL)[2]

---

2   Note: Reduced muscle mass in elderly and young patients may cause decreased values, which may mask renal disease in these age groups.

Clinical Implications

Increased Levels

Impaired renal function (e.g., glomeruloneprhitis, pyelonephritis, acute tubular necrosis, urinary tract obstruction); muscle disease (gigantism, acromegaly); rhabdomyolysis; shock (prolonged); diabetic nephropathy; CHF

Decreased Levels

Debilitation; decreased muscle mass (e.g., muscular dystrophy, myasthenia gravis); advanced and severe liver disease; with age proportional to decrease in muscle mass.

ERYTHROPOIETIN (EPO)

Reference Range

5–35 IU/L

Clinical Implications

Increased Levels

Anemia (iron deficiency, megaloblastic, hemolytic); myelodysplasia; chemotherapy; AIDS; renal cell carcinoma; adrenal carcinoma; pregnancy.

Decreased Levels

Polycythemia vera; rheumatoid arthritis; multiple myeloma.

Folic Acid (Folate)

Reference Range

5–25 mg/mL or 11–57 mmol/L

Clinical Implications

Increased Levels

Pernicious anemia, vitamin B_{12} deficiency; vegetarianism; recent massive blood transfusion; blind loop syndrome.

Decreased Levels

Inadequate intake (malnutrition, chronic disease, alcoholism, anorexia, diet devoid of fresh vegetables); malabsorption (e.g., small bowel disease); pregnancy; megaloblastic anemia; hemolytic anemia; malignancy; chronic renal disease; drugs that are folic antagonists (phenytoin, aminopterin, methotrexate, antimalarials, alcohol, oral contraceptives).

GLUCOSE (BLOOD SUGAR, FASTING BLOOD SUGAR [FBS])

Reference Range

110 mg/dL or <6.1 mmol/L
(Critical values: <40 and >400 mg/dL)

Clinical Implications

Increased Levels (Hyperglycemia)

Diabetes mellitus (DM); Cushing syndrome; acute stress response (MI, cerebrovascular accident [CVA], burns, infection, surgery); pheochromocytoma, acromegaly, gigantism; chronic renal failure; glucagonoma; acute pancreatitis; pregnancy; corticosteroid therapy.

Decreased Levels (Hypoglycemia)

Pancreatic islet cell carcinoma; Addison disease; hypothyroidism; hypopituitarism; liver disease; starvation; insulin overdose.

GLUCOSE, POSTPRANDIAL (2-HOUR POSTPRANDIAL GLUCOSE [2-HOUR PPG])

Reference Range

0–50 years: 40 mg/dL or <7.8 mmol/L
50–60 years: <150 mg/dL
>60 years: <160 mg/dL

Clinical Implications

Increased Levels

DM; gestational diabetes mellitus (GDM); malnutrition; hyperthyroidism; acute stress response (MI, CVA, burns, infection, surgery);

Cushing syndrome; pheochromocytoma; chronic renal failure; glucagonoma; diuretic therapy; corticosteroid therapy; liver disease.

Decreased Levels
Insulinoma; hypothyroidism; hypopituitarism; insulin overdose; Addison disease.

GLUCOSE TOLERANCE (GT, ORAL GLUCOSE TOLERANCE TEST [OGTT])

Reference Range
Fasting: <110 mg/dL or <6.1 mmol/L
30 minutes: <200 mg/dL or <11.1 mmol/L
1 hour: <200 mg/dL or <11.1 mmol/L
2 hours: <140 mg/dL or <7.8 mmol/L
3 hours: 70–115 mg/dL or <6.4 mmol/L

Clinical Implications
Increased Levels
DM; acute stress response (MI, CVA, burns, infection, surgery); Cushing syndrome; pheochromocytoma; chronic renal failure; glucagonoma; diuretic therapy; corticosteroid therapy; liver disease; acute pancreatitis; myxedema; Somogyi response to hypoglycemia.

GLYCOSYLATED HEMOGLOBIN (GHB; GLYCOHEMOGLOBIN [GHB], HEMOGLOBIN A$_{1c}$ [HBA$_{1c}$] OR [A1C])

Reference Range
Nondiabetic adult: 2.2%–4.8%
Good diabetic control: 2.5%–5.9%
Fair diabetic control: 6%–8%
Poor diabetic control: >8%

Clinical Implications
Increased Levels
Newly diagnosed DM; pregnancy; nondiabetic hyperglycemia (acute stress response, Cushing syndrome, pheochromocytoma, glucagonoma, corticosteroid therapy).

Decreased Levels
Hemolytic anemia or other diseases with shortened red blood cell life span such as sickle-cell disease and glucose-6-dehydrogenase deficiency; chronic blood loss; chronic renal failure.

HEMATOCRIT (HCT; PACKED CELL VOLUME [PCV])

Reference Range[3]
Male: 42%–52% or 0.42–0.52 volume fraction
Female: 37%–47% or 0.37–0.47 volume fraction

Clinical Implications
Increased Levels
Erythrocytosis; congenital heart disease; polycythemia vera; severe dehydration; severe COPD; diabetic acidosis; transient cerebral ischemia (TIA); trauma; burns.

Decreased Levels
Anemia; hemoglobinopathy; cirrhosis; hemolytic anemia; hemorrhage; dietary deficiency ; renal disease; pregnancy; leukemias, lymphomas, Hodgkin lymphoma; peptic ulcer disease; rheumatoid arthritis.

HEMOGLOBIN (HGB, HB)

Reference Range[4]
Male: 14–18 g/dL or 8.7–11.2 mmol/L
Female: 12–16 g/dL or 7.4–9.9 mmol/L
(Critical values: <5 g/dL or >20 g/dL)

Clinical Implications
Increased Levels
Erythrocytosis; congenital heart disease; polycythemia vera; severe dehydration; severe COPD; high altitudes; severe burns.

---

3   Note: Values may be slightly decreased in the elderly.
4   Note: Values may be slightly decreased in the elderly.

Decreased Levels
Anemia; hemoglobinopathy; cirrhosis; hemolytic anemia; hemorrhage; dietary deficiency; bone marrow failure; renal disease; pregnancy; leukemias, lymphomas, Hodgkin lymphoma.

HOMOCYSTEINE (HCY)

Reference Range
4–14 μmol/L

Clinical Implications
Increased Levels
Vascular diseases (cardiac, cerebral, peripheral); cystinuria; vitamin B_6 or B_{12} deficiency; folate deficiency; malnutrition.

IRON LEVEL (FE)

Reference Range
Male: 80–100 μg/dL or 14–32 μmol/L
Female: 60–60 μg /dL or 11–29 μmol/L

Clinical Implications
Increased Levels
Hemosiderosis or hemochromatosis; iron poisoning; hemolytic anemia; multiple or massive blood transfusions; hepatitis; lead poisoning; nephritis.

Decreased Levels
Iron-deficiency anemia; chronic blood loss; insufficient dietary iron intake; third-trimester pregnancy; inadequate intestinal absorption of iron.

MAGNESIUM (MG)

Reference Range
1.3–2.1 mEq/L or 0.65–1.05 mmol/L
(Critical values: <0.5 or >3 mEq/L)

Clinical Implications
Increased Levels
Renal insufficiency; Addison disease; hypothyroidism; dehydration; use of magnesium-containing antacids or salts.

Decreased Levels
Malnutrition; malabsorption; hypoparathyroidism; alcoholism; chronic renal tubular disease; diabetic acidosis; excessive loss of body fluids (sweating, lactation, diuretic abuse, chronic diarrhea); cirrhosis of the liver; hypokalemia.

OSMOLALITY (SERUM OSMOLALITY)

Reference Range
285–295 mOsm/kg H_2O or 285–295 mmol/kg
(Critical values: <265 mOsm/kg or >320 mOsm/kg)

Clinical Implications
Increased Levels
Dehydration; hypernatremia; hypercalcemia; DM, hyperglycemia, diabetic ketoacidosis; azotemia; mannitol therapy; alcohol ingestion (ethanol, methanol, ethylene glycol); uremia; diabetes insipidus.

Decreased Levels
Overhydration; SIADH; hyponatremia; acute kidney injury; continuous IV D5W

PHOSPHATE (PO_4), PHOSPHORUS (P)

Reference Range
3.0–4.5 mg/dL or 0.97–1.45 mmol/L
(Critical values: <1 mg/dL)

Clinical Implications

Increased Levels

Renal failure; hypoparathyroidism; acromegaly; bone metastasis; sarcoidosis; hypocalcemia; Addison disease; rhabdomyolysis; healing fractures, hypervitaminosis D.

Decreased Levels

Hyperparathyroidism; hypercalcemia; rickets; malnutrition; gram-negative sepsis; hyperinsulinism; alkalosis; IV glucose administration (phosphorus follows glucose into cells); starvation; malabsorption syndrome; hypomagnesemia; chronic alcoholism; vitamin D deficiency; nasogastric suctioning; vomiting.

POTASSIUM (K)

Reference Range

3.5–5.0 mEq/L or 3.5–5.0 mmol/L
(Critical values: <2.5 or >6.5 mEq/L)

Clinical Implications

Increased Levels (Hyperkalemia)

Excessive dietary or IV intake; acute or chronic renal failure; Addison disease; hypoaldosteronism; aldosterone-inhibiting diuretics (spironolactone, triamterene); crush- or cell-damaging injuries (accidents, burns, surgery, chemotherapy); hemolysis; acidosis; dehydration.

Decreased Levels (Hypokalemia)

Deficient dietary or IV intake; burns/trauma/surgery; diarrhea/vomiting/sweating; diuretics; hyperaldosteronism; Cushing syndrome; licorice ingestion; alkalosis; glucose administration; cystic fibrosis.

PREALBUMIN (PAB; THYROXINE-BINDING PREALBUMIN [TBPA], THYRETIN, TRANSTHYRETIN)

Reference Range

15–36 mg/dL or 150–360 mg/L
(Critical values: <10.7 mg/dL indicates severe nutritional deficiency)

Clinical Implications
Increased Levels
Hodgkin lymphoma; pregnancy

Decreased Levels
Malnutrition; liver damage; burns; inflammation.

PROTHROMBIN TIME (PT; PRO-TIME, INTERNATIONAL NORMALIZED RATIO [INR])

Reference Range
11.0–13.0 seconds; 85%–100% of control
Full anticoagulant therapy: <1.5–2 times control value; 20%–30% of control
(Critical values: >20 seconds; full anticoagulant therapy: 3 times control values)

Clinical Implications
Increased Levels (Prolonged PT)
Liver disease (hepatitis, cirrhosis); hereditary factor deficiency (factors II, V, VII, X); vitamin K deficiency; bile duct obstruction; coumarin ingestion; massive blood transfusion; salicylate intoxication.

Decreased levels
Thrombophlebitis, myocardial infarction, pulmonary embolism

RED BLOOD CELL COUNT (RBC COUNT; ERYTHROCYTE COUNT)

Reference Range
RBC × 10^6/μL or RBC × 10^{12}/L
Male: 4.7–6.1; Female: 4.2–5.4

Clinical Implications
Increased Levels
Erythrocytosis; congenital heart disease; severe COPD; polycythemia vera; severe dehydration; hemoglobinopathies; high altitude.

Decreased Levels
Anemia; cirrhosis; hemorrhage; Addison disease; renal disease; bone marrow failure; pregnancy; rheumatoid/collagen-vascular diseases (rheumatoid arthritis [RA], systemic lupus erythematosus [SLE], sarcoidosis); lymphoma/leukemia/Hodgkin lymphoma; chronic infections, excessive IV fluids.

SODIUM (NA)

Reference Range
136–145 mEq/L or 136–145 mmol/L
(Critical values: <120 or >160 mEq/L)

Clinical Implications
Increased Levels (Hypernatremia)
Increased sodium intake (dietary or IV); decreased sodium loss (Cushing syndrome, hyperaldosteronism); excessive free body water loss (GI, excessive sweating, extensive burns, diabetes insipidus, osmotic diuresis).

Decreased Levels (Hyponatremia)
Decreased sodium intake (deficient dietary or IV sodium); increased sodium loss (Addison disease, diarrhea/vomiting, intraluminal bowel loss, diuretic administration, chronic renal insufficiency, gastric suctioning); increased free body water (excessive oral or IV water intake, hyperglycemia, CHF, peripheral edema, pleural effusion, SIADH).

TOTAL IRON-BINDING CAPACITY (TIBC)

Reference Range
250–460 µg/dL or 45–82 µmol/L

Clinical Implications
Increased Levels
Estrogen therapy; polycythemia vera; pregnancy (late); iron-deficiency anemia; acute and chronic blood loss; acute hepatitis.

Decreased Levels
Hypoproteinemia (malnutrition or burns); inflammatory diseases; cirrhosis; hemolytic, pernicious, and sickle-cell anemias; thalassemia.

TRANSFERRIN

Reference Range
Male: 215–365 mg/L or 2.15–3.65 g/L
Female: 250–380 mg/dL or 2.50–3.80 g/L

Clinical Implications
Increased Levels
Estrogen therapy; polycythemia vera; pregnancy (late); iron-deficiency anemia.

Decreased Levels
Hypoproteinemia (malnutrition or burns); inflammatory diseases; cirrhosis; hemolytic, pernicious, and sickle-cell anemias; renal disease; acute liver disease.

TRANSFERRIN SATURATION

Reference Range
Male: 20%–50%
Female: 15%–50%

Clinical Implications
Increased Levels
Hemochromatosis; increased iron intake; hemolytic anemia; thalassemia; acute liver disease.

Decreased Levels
Iron-deficiency anemia; anemia of infection and chronic diseases; malignancy.

VITAMIN B$_{12}$ (CYANOCOBALAMIN)

Reference Range
160–950 pg/mL or 118–701 mmol/L

Clinical Implications
Increased Levels
Leukemia, polycythemia vera; severe liver dysfunction; diabetes; myeloproliferative disease.

Decreased Levels
Pernicious anemia; malabsorption syndromes and inflammatory bowel disease (IBD); intestinal worm infestation; Zollinger-Ellison syndrome; folic acid deficiency; vitamin C deficiency; achlorydria; large proximal gastrectomy.

WHITE BLOOD COUNT AND DIFFERENTIAL COUNT (WBC WITH DIFFERENTIAL)

Reference Range
Total WBCs: 5,000–10,000/mm^3 or 5–10 (10^9/L
(Critical values: <2,500 or >30,000/mm^3)
Lymphocytes: 1,000–4,000/mm^3 (comprise 20%–40% of the total WBC; in malnutrition, lymphocyte count is reduced).

Clinical Implications
Increased WBC Count (Leukocytosis)
Infection; leukemic neoplasia or other myeloproliferative disorders; trauma/stress/hemorrhage; tissue necrosis; inflammation; thyroid storm; steroid use.

Decreased WBC Count (Leukopenia)
Drug toxicity; bone marrow failure; dietary deficiency of vitamin B$_{12}$ or iron; autoimmune disease; hypersplenism.

LABORATORY TEST PANELS

Laboratory tests are often ordered as panels that are disease or organ specific. Next are some common test panels that have significance to the registered dietitian (RD). Note that panels may be modified or expanded at different clinical facilities.

Anemia Panel

CBC; RBC indices; reticulocyte count:
Microcytic: erythrocyte sedimentation rate (ESR); iron panel
Normocytic: ESR; hemolysis profile
Macrocytic: vitamin B_{12}; folate; thyroid-stimulating hormone (TSH)

Basic Metabolic Panel (7 Channel/Chem 7/SMA-7)

Carbon dioxide content; chloride, blood; creatinine, blood; glucose, blood; potassium, blood; sodium, blood; urea nitrogen, blood (BUN).

Complete Blood Cell Count (CBC) with Differential (Diff)

RBC; Hgb; Ht; red blood cell indices (mean corpuscular volume [MCV], mean corpuscular hemoglobin [MCH], mean corpuscular hemoglobin concentration [MCHC], red blood cell distribution width [RDW]); WBC and Diff count (neutrophils; lymphocytes; monocytes; eosinophils; basophils); blood smear; platelet count; mean platelet volume (MPV).

Comprehensive Metabolic Panel (12 Channel/Chem 12)

Albumin; alkaline phosphatase; AST (SGOT); bilirubin-total; BUN; calcium; chloride; creatinine; glucose; potassium; protein-total; sodium.

The old Comprehensive Metabolic Panel or "Chem 20" includes all the above labs plus:

ALT (SGPT); bilirubin-direct; carbon dioxide; cholesterol; GGT; LDH; phosphorus; uric acid.)

Diabetes Mellitus Management

Anion gap; basic metabolic panel; hemoglobin A_{1C}; lipid profile.

Hepatic Function
ALT; albumin; alkaline phosphatase; AST; bilirubin-direct; bilirubin-total; GGT; protein, total; prothrombin time (PT).

Lipid Panel
Cholesterol-total; high-density lipoprotein (HDL); triglyceride; low-density lipoprotein (LDL); very-low-density lipoprotein (VLDL).

Pancreatic Panel
Amylase; calcium; glucose; lipase; triglyceride.

Renal Panel
Albumin; basic metabolic panel; calcium; CBC; creatinine clearance; magnesium; phosphorus; protein-total; protein-urine; protein-24-hour urine.

References
U.S. National Library of Medicine, Medline Plus. Laboratory Tests. Available at:
https://www.nlm.nih.gov/medlineplus/laboratorytests.html. Accessed February 1, 2018.

Mayo Clinic. Tests and Procedures. Available at:
http://www.mayoclinic.org/tests-procedures. Accessed February 1, 2018.

APPENDIX F:
COMMON MEDICAL ABBREVIATIONS

~	Approximately
ABG	Arterial blood gas
ABW	Actual body weight
ac; a.c.	Before a meal
ad lib.	ad libitum, freely, as desired
ADLs	Activities of daily living
AFib	Atrial fibrillation
AKA	Above knee amputation
AKI	Acute kidney injury
ALP	Alkaline phosphatase
ALT	Alanine aminotransferase
AMA; a.m.a.	Against medical advice
AMI	Acute myocardial infarction
AMS	Altered mental status
A&O	Alert and oriented
ARDS	Acute respiratory distress syndrome
ARF	Acute renal failure; acute respiratory failure
ASA	Aspirin
ASCVD	Atherosclerotic cardiovascular disease
ASHD	Arteriosclerotic heart disease
AST	Aspartate aminotransferase
A-V; AV	Arteriovenous; atrioventricular

BG	Blood glucose
bid; b.i.d.	Twice a day
BiPAP	Bi-level positive airway pressure
BKA	Below knee amputation
BM	Bowel movement
BMI	Body mass index
BMR	Basal metabolic rate
BP	Blood pressure
BPA	Best practice alert
bpm	Beats per minute
BS	Blood sugar
BSA	Body surface area
BUN	Blood urea nitrogen
Bx	Biopsy
C	Celsius; kilocalorie
c̄	With
CA	Cancer; cardiac arrest
CABG	Coronary artery bypass graft
CAD	Coronary artery disease
Cal	kilocalorie
CAP	Community-acquired pneumonia
cath	Catheter
CBC	Complete blood count
CC; C.C.	Chief complaint
cc	Cubic centimeter
CCU	Coronary care unit; critical care unit

C. diff	*Clostridium difficile*
CHD	Coronary heart disease
CHF	Congestive heart failure
CHI	Closed head injury
CHO	Carbohydrate
CKD	Chronic kidney disease
CNS	Central nervous system
CO	Cardiac output
c/o	Complains of
COPD	Chronic obstructive pulmonary disease
CPAP	Continuous positive airway pressure
Cr	Creatinine
CPR	Cardiopulmonary resuscitation
CRP	C-reactive protein
CRRT	Continuous renal replacement therapy
CT	Computerized tomography
CV	Cardiovascular
CVA	Cerebrovascular accident
D5	5% dextrose
D5W	5% dextrose in water
/d	Per day
DBP	Diastolic blood pressure
dc	Discontinue
DEXA	Dual-energy X-ray absorptiometry
DKA	Diabetic ketoacidosis
dL	Deciliter

DM	Diabetes mellitus
DNR	Do not resuscitate
DO	Doctor of osteopathy
DOB	Date of birth
DOE	Dyspnea on exertion
DRI	Dietary reference intake
DTs	Delirium tremens
DVT	Deep vein thrombosis
Dx	Diagnosis
ECF	Extended care facility
ECG	Electrocardiogram
ECHO	Echocardiography
ECMO	Extracorporeal membrane oxygenation
ED	Emergency department; eating disorder
EEG	Electroencephalogram
EENT	Eye, ear, nose, and throat
EF	Ejection fraction
EGD	Esophagogastroduodenoscopy
EHR	Electronic health record
EKG	Electrocardiogram
EMR	Electronic medical record
EMS	Emergency medical service
EMT	Emergency medical technician
EN	Enteral nutrition
Endo	Endocrine; endoscopy
ENT	Ear, nose, and throat

ER	Emergency room
ERCP	Endoscopic retrograde cholangio-pancreatography
ESRD	End-stage renal disease
ETOH; EtOH	Ethyl alcohol
EPO	Erythropoietin
F	Fahrenheit
FBG	Fasting blood glucose
FBS	Fasting blood sugar
Fe	Iron
FFP	Fresh frozen plasma
Fld	Fluid
FTT	Failure to thrive
F/U	Follow-up
FUO	Fever of unknown origin
Fx	Fracture
G; Glu	Glucose
g; gm	Gram
GB	Gallbladder; Guillain-Barré
GCS	Glasgow coma scale
GDM	Gestational diabetes mellitus
GERD	Gastroesophageal reflux disease
GFR	Glomerular filtration rate
GI	Gastrointestinal
GP	General practitioner
GSW	Gunshot wound
GTT	Glucose tolerance test

GU	Genitourinary
H&H	Hematocrit and hemoglobin
H&P	History and physical
Hb; hgb	Hemoglobin
HCAP	Health-care associated pneumonia
HCT; Hct	Hematocrit
HD	Hemodialysis
HDL	High-density lipoprotein
HEENT	Head, eye, ear, nose, and throat
HF	Heart failure
HIPAA	Health Insurance Portability and Accountability Act
h/o	History of
HOB	Head of bed
h.s.	Bedtime
HPI	History of present illness
HR	Heart rate
HTN	Hypertension
Hx	History
I&O	Intake and output
IBD	Inflammatory bowel disease
IBS	Irritable bowel syndrome
IBW	Ideal body weight
ICD	Implantable cardioverter defibrillator
ICU	Intensive care unit
ID	Infectious disease
IDDM	Insulin-dependent diabetes mellitus

IF	Intrinsic factor
IM	Internal medicine
inj.	Injection
INR	International normalized ratio
IV	Intravenous
K	Potassium
kcal	Kilocalorie
kg	Kilogram
KVO	Keep vein open
L; l	Liter
L&D	Labor and delivery
lab	Laboratory
lb	Pound
LBW	Low birth weight
LDL	Low-density lipoprotein
LE	Lower extremity
LES	Lower esophageal sphincter
LFT	Liver function test
LGA	Large for gestational age
LLE	Left lower extremity
LLQ	Left lower quadrant
LOS	Length of stay
LUE	Left upper extremity
LUQ	Left upper quadrant
MAP	Mean arterial pressure
MBSS	Modified barium swallow study

mcg	Microgram
MCH	Mean corpuscular hemoglobin
MCHC	Mean corpuscular hemoglobin concentration
MCV	Mean corpuscular volume
MD	Doctor of medicine; muscular dystrophy
mEq	Milliequivalent
mg	Milligram
Mg	Magnesium
MI	Myocardial infarction
ml	Milliliter
MM	Mucous membrane; multiple myeloma
mm	Millimeter
mm Hg	Millimeters of mercury
MRA	Magnetic resonance angiography
MRI	Magnetic resonance imaging
MRN	Medical record number
MRSA	Methicillin-resistant *Staphylococcus aureus*
MVA	Motor vehicle accident
N/A	Not applicable
Na	Sodium
NaCl	Sodium chloride
NAD	No acute distress
NC	Nasal cannula
NG; ng	Nasogastric
NGT	Nasogastric tube
NICU	Neonatal intensive care unit

NIDDM	Noninsulin-dependent diabetes mellitus
NKA	No known allergies
NP	Nurse practitioner
NPO; n.p.o.	Nothing by mouth
NS	Normal saline
NSAID	Nonsteroidal anti-inflammatory drug
NSTEMI	Non-ST-elevation myocardial infarction
N&V; N/V	Nausea and vomiting
OB/GYN	Obstetrics and gynecology
OP	Outpatient
OR	Operating room
ORIF	Open reduction with/and internal fixation
OSHA	Occupational Safety and Health Administration
OT	Occupational therapy
OTC	Over the counter
oz	Ounce
P	Phosphorus
PA	Physician assistant
PACU	Post-anesthesia care unit
PAD	Peripheral arterial disease
PCA	Patient-controlled analgesia
PCP	Primary care physician
PD	Parkinson's disease; peritoneal dialysis
PE	Physical examination; pulmonary embolism
PEG	Percutaneous endoscopic gastrostomy
per	Through; by

PERRLA	Pupils equal, regular, react to light and accommodation
PET	Positron emission tomography
Pharm; Phar.	Pharmacy
PICC	Peripherally inserted central catheter
PMH	Past medical history
PN	Parenteral nutrition
PNS	Peripheral nervous system
PO; p.o.	Orally
PRBCs	Packed red blood cells
PRN	As needed
PT	Physical therapy
Pt	Patient
q	Every
RA	Room air; rheumatoid arthritis
RBC	Red blood cell; red blood count
RDA	Recommended dietary allowance
RDS	Respiratory distress syndrome
RFT	Renal function test
RLE	Right lower extremity
RLQ	Right lower quadrant
RN	Registered nurse
R/O	Rule out
ROM	Range of motion
ROS	Review of systems
RQ	Respiratory quotient
RR	Respiratory rate

R/T	Related to
RUE	Right upper extremity
RUQ	Right upper quadrant
Rx	Prescription
S-A; SA	Sinoatrial
SARS	Severe acute respiratory syndrome
SB	Small bowel
SBO	Small bowel obstruction
SBP	Systolic blood pressure
SCI	Spinal cord injury
SCD	Sequential compression device
SGA	Small for gestational age
SLP	Speech-language pathology
SOB	Shortness of breath
S/P; s/p	Status post
s/s	Signs and symptoms
Staph	*Staphylococcus*
STAT; stat	Immediately
STEMI	ST-elevation myocardial infarction
Strep	*Streptococcus*
Sx	Symptoms; surgery
T	Temperature
TB	Tuberculosis
TBI	Traumatic brain injury
TEE	Transesophageal echocardiogram
TF	Tube feeding

TIA	Transient ischemic attack
TIBC	Total iron-binding capacity
tid; t.i.d.	Three times a day
TPN	Total parenteral nutrition
TSH	Thyroid-stimulating hormone
Tx	Treatment
UA	Urinalysis
UBW	Usual body weight
UC	Ulcerative colitis
UE	Upper extremity
UGIS	Upper gastrointestinal series
URI	Upper respiratory infection
U/S; US	Ultrasound
UTI	Urinary tract infection
VDRF	Ventilator-dependent respiratory failure
VF	Ventricular fibrillation
VLBW	Very low birth weight
VLDL	Very low density lipoprotein
VT	Ventricular tachycardia
WBC	White blood cell; white blood count
WDWN	Well-developed, well-nourished
WNL	Within normal limits
wt.	Weight
XR; X-ray	Radiograph
yo	Years old

APPENDIX G:
NUTRITIONALLY RELEVANT MEDICATIONS

The following table of medications is not meant to be comprehensive, but instead lists common medications that have significant nutritional implications. The list is alphabetical by generic name (in *italics*) and cross-referenced by brand or trade name.

Medication	Class & Action	Side Effects	Nutritional Implications
Adalat	See *nifedipine*		
Aldactone	See *spironolactone*		
Apresoline	See *hydralazine*		
Atenolol Tenormin	Beta-blocker, antiadrenergic, antiarrhythmic	Diarrhea, constipation, nausea, and vomiting. Possible hypoglycemia. Signs of sympathetic response to hypoglycemia may be masked. May have a decreased insulin release in response to hyperglycemia. Concurrent use of beta-adrenergic blockers and St John's wort or yohimbine may result in a decrease in beta-adrenergic blocker effectiveness. Concurrent use of beta-adrenergic blockers and ma huang may result in reduced hypotensive effect of beta-adrenergic blockers.	Adherence necessary for those following diabetic diet. Monitor blood glucose levels. Be cautious of nonsympathetic signs of hypoglycemia. Consider fluid and electrolyte replacement for diarrhea and vomiting.

Medication	Class & Action	Side Effects	Nutritional Implications
Atorvastatin Lipitor	Inhibitor of HMG-CoA reductase	Constipation, diarrhea, gas, upset stomach, and upper right stomach pain. Coenzyme Q10 may be significantly reduced. Concurrent use of atorvastatin and niacin may result in an increased risk of myopathy or rhabdomyolysis. St John's wort may result in reduced effectiveness of atorvastatin. Black cohosh may result in elevated liver enzymes. Grapefruit juice or grapefruit-containing foods may result in increased bioavailability of atorvastatin resulting in an increased risk of myopathy or rhabdomyolysis.	Avoid intake large quantities of grapefruit juice or grapefruit-containing foods for it increases the absorption of statins (>1 qt/day). Eat a low-cholesterol, low-fat diet for best results. Gastrointestinal problems generally transient.
Azithromycin Zithromax	Antibiotic Bacteriostatic or bactericidal	Occasional nausea, vomiting, diarrhea, abdominal pain, anorexia, stomatitis, bad taste in mouth.	Take with food to avoid GI disturbances. Azithromycin oral suspension should be taken 1 hr before or 2 hrs after meals. Eat small, frequent meals to avoid anorexia. Consider fluid and electrolyte replacement for diarrhea. Avoid alcohol.
Bactrim, Bactrim DS	See *sulfamethoxazole*		

(Continued)

Medication	Class & Action	Side Effects	Nutritional Implications
Benazepril Lotensin	Antihypertensive ACE Inhibitor	May increase serum potassium. May decrease serum sodium. Nausea, salty or metallic taste, mouth sores. Concurrent use of angiotensin-converting enzyme inhibitors and yohimbine or ma huang may result in reduced effectiveness of angiotensin-converting enzyme inhibitors.	Caution with foods high in potassium or potassium supplements. Avoid salt substitutes. Maintain adequate hydration.
Betaloc	See *metoprolol*		
Biaxin	See *clarithromycin*		
Bumetanide Bumex	Diuretic Loop diuretic	Ginkgo biloba may cause increased blood pressure. Licorice can increase the risk of hypokalemia. May increase blood glucose, uric acid, cholesterol, LDL, calcium, and triglycerides. May decrease urinary excretion of calcium and increase excretion of magnesium, sodium, and potassium levels.	Consume foods high in potassium and magnesium. Avoid consumption of natural licorice. Monitor electrolyte levels and consider supplementation. Caution with calcium supplements.
Bupropion Wellbutrin, Zyban	Antidepressant Serotonin & norepinephrine reuptake inhibitor	Dry mouth, upset stomach, vomiting, weight loss, and constipation. Alcohol may increase side effects.	Monitor weight. Use ice chips or chew gum for dry mouth. Avoid alcohol.
Bumex	See *bumetanide*		

Medication	Class & Action	Side Effects	Nutritional Implications
Calan	See *verapamil*		
Calcijex	See *calcitriol*		
Calcium salts PhosLo, Caltrate, Dicarbosil, OsCal, Titralac, Tums, Citracal, Calcitrate	Calcium-based phosphorus binder	Hypercalcemia, stomach pains, nausea, vomiting, constipation, dry mouth, thirst, and frequent urination. Concurrent use of calcium and oxalic acid foods (spinach, rhubarb, beet greens, asparagus etc.) may result in decreased calcium exposure. Concurrent use of calcium and phytic acid foods (beans, seeds, nuts, whole grains etc.) may result in decreased calcium effectiveness.	Maintain adequate hydration, serum magnesium, phosphate, potassium levels, and urine calcium levels.
Calcitrate	See *calcium salts*		
Calcitriol Calcijex, Rocaltrol	Vitamin D	May increase aluminum concentration, hypercalcemia, serum cholesterol, serum phosphorous, and magnesium concentration. Upset stomach, vomiting, dry mouth, constipation, metallic taste in mouth, increased thirst, decreased appetite, weight loss, and fatty stools.	Avoid use of antacids. Only works in conjunction with appropriate intake of calcium. Consider low-phosphate diet if on dialysis.
Caltrate	See *calcium salts*		
Capoten	See *captopril*		

(Continued)

Medication	Class & Action	Side Effects	Nutritional Implications
Capozide	See *captopril*		
Captopril	Antihypertensive ACE Inhibitor	May increase serum potassium. May decrease serum sodium. Nausea, salty or metallic taste, mouth sores. Concurrent use of angiotensin-converting inhibitors and yohimbine or ma huang may result in reduced effectiveness of angiotensin converting enzyme inhibitors.	Caution with foods high in potassium or potassium supplements. Avoid salt substitutes. Maintain adequate hydration.
Catapres	See *clonidine*		
Celexa	See *citalopram*		
Cholestyramine Questran, Prevalite	Bile acid sequestrant	May decrease serum potassium and calcium. Binds fat-soluble vitamin A, D, E, and K, folic acid, and beta-carotene. Constipation, nausea, vomiting, abdominal pain, indigestion. Occasional diarrhea.	Mix with 3 to 6 oz of liquid, such as juice, milk, or water for powdered form. Irritating to GI tract. Take before meals. Take fat-soluble vitamins in a water miscible form or take a supplement prior to initial daily dose of drug. Monitor nutrient levels if long-term use of drug is indicated. Consider high-fiber diet for constipation.

Medication	Class & Action	Side Effects	Nutritional Implications
Cinacalcet Sensipar	Calcimimetic	High-fat intake may increase cinacalcet concentration of plasma. Nausea, vomiting, and diarrhea. Concurrent use of cinacalcet and food may result in increased bioavailability of cinacalcet. Concurrent use of cinacalcet and grapefruit juice or grapefruit-containing foods may increase the effects of cinacalcet.	Avoid taking with grapefruit juice or grapefruit-containing foods.
Ciprofloxacin	Antibacterial	Upset stomach, vomiting, stomach pain, indigestion. Inflammation of the stomach leading to possible diarrhea. Aluminum, magnesium, calcium, ferrous sulfate, and zinc are thought to form chelation complexes preventing the drugs from being absorbed. Concurrent use of fluoroquinolones and dandelion may result in decreased fluoroquinolone effectiveness. Concurrent use of ciprofloxacin and iron may result in decreased ciprofloxacin effectiveness. Fennel may result in decreased bioavailability of ciprofloxacin and possible antibiotic treatment failure. Zinc may result in decreased ciprofloxacin effectiveness. Caffeine may result in increased caffeine concentrations and enhanced CNS stimulation.	Take with 8 oz of water. Ensure adequate fluid intake. Consider fluid and electrolyte replacement for vomiting and diarrhea. Should not be taken with dairy products or calcium-containing fluids. Do not need to avoid foods containing these products.

(Continued)

Medication	Class & Action	Side Effects	Nutritional Implications
Cisplatin Platinol, Platinol-AQ	Alkylating agent	Loss of appetite, weight loss, diarrhea, nausea, vomiting, and altered taste.	Drink plenty of fluids for drug; irritates the kidney. Vomiting is severe. May consider anti-emetic therapy. Monitor weight. Encourage food intake when patient feels best; e.g., morning.
Citalopram Celexa	Antidepressant Selective serotonin reuptake inhibitor (SSRI)	Nausea, diarrhea, vomiting, anorexia, dry mouth, and dyspepsia. May decrease serum sodium. Concurrent use of SSRIs and St John's wort or ginkgo biloba may result in an increased risk of serotonin syndrome (hypertension, hyperthermia, myoclonus, mental status changes).	Consider fluid and electrolyte replacement for diarrhea and vomiting. Use ice chips or chew gum for dry mouth. Avoid alcohol.
Citracal	See *calcium salts*		
Clarithromycin Biaxin	Antibiotic Bacteriostatic or bactericidal	Occasional nausea, vomiting, diarrhea, abdominal pain, anorexia, stomatitis, bad taste in mouth.	Take with food to avoid GI disturbances. Eat small, frequent meals to avoid anorexia. Consider fluid and electrolyte replacement for diarrhea. Avoid alcohol.

Medication	Class & Action	Side Effects	Nutritional Implications
Clonidine Catapres, Duraclon	Alpha-antiadrenergic	Constipation, nausea, vomiting, dry mouth, and drowsiness. Concurrent use of clonidine and yohimbine may result in reduced clonidine effectiveness. Concurrent use of clonidine and ma huang may result in increased blood pressure.	Avoid alcohol intake for it can exacerbate drowsiness. Use ice chips or chew gum for dry mouth.
Clopidogrel Plavix	Anti-platelet	Upset stomach, stomach pain, diarrhea, and constipation. Ginger may increase the possibility of bleeding. Concurrent use of clopidogrel and ginkgo biloba, chaparral (also known as creosote bush), bladder wrack (type of seaweed), vitamin A, kava, licorice, clove oil, garlic, anise, boldo, motherwort, cat's claw, bilberry, bogbean, curcumin, celery, evening primrose, black currant, borage, feverfew, dandelion, angelica, meadowsweet, astragalus, tan-shen (red sage), skullcap, guggul, hawthorn, arnica, and ginger may result in an increased risk of bleeding. Concurrent use of clopidogrel and grapefruit juice or grapefruit-containing foods may result in reduced exposure of the active clopidogrel metabolite.	Consider small, frequent meals for anorexia. Consider fluid and electrolyte replacement for diarrhea. Consistency in dietary and supplemental intake must be consistent to achieve steady level of anticoagulation. Those on long-term use should be monitored for bone density. Avoid taking with grapefruit juice or grapefruit-containing foods.

(Continued)

Medication	Class & Action	Side Effects	Nutritional Implications
Co-trimoxazole/ trimethoprim/ Sulfamethoxazole Bactrim, Bactrim DS	Bactericidal	May cause anorexia, nausea, vomiting, diarrhea, abdominal pain, or stomatitis. May hinder folate metabolism.	Take with 8 oz of water on an empty stomach. Eat small, frequent meals to avoid anorexia. Take a folate supplement. Consider fluid and electrolyte replacement for diarrhea.
Coumadin	See *warfarin*		
Covera-HS	See *verapamil*		
Cyclophosphamide Cytoxan	Alkylating agent, nitrogen mustard	Nausea, vomiting, loss of appetite, and weight loss. Concurrent use of cyclophosphamide and St. John's wort may result in reduced cyclophosphamide effectiveness.	Drink plenty of fluids for drug; irritates bladder and kidneys. Encourage food intake when patient feels best; e.g., morning.
Cytoxan	See *cyclophosphamide*		
Dialyvite Diatx, Nephrocaps, Nephrovite	B-complex with vitamin C and Biotin	Abdominal pain, cramps, dyspepsia, and nausea.	Taken when vitamins inadequate, usually after dialysis when fluid is removed. Used to replace water-soluble vitamin losses.
Diatx Dicarbosil	See *dialyvite* See *calcium salts*		

Medication	Class & Action	Side Effects	Nutritional Implications
Digoxin Lanoxin	Antiarrhythmic, cardiac glycoside	Occasional diarrhea, loss of appetite, lower stomach pain, nausea, and/or vomiting. May reduce potassium levels and increase urinary excretion of magnesium. Concurrent use of digoxin and St. John's wort, khella, charcoal, and kaolin may result in reduced digoxin efficacy. Concurrent use of digoxin and calcium may result in a serious risk of arrhythmia and cardiovascular collapse. Concurrent use of digoxin and oleander, sea cucumber, carob, licorice, lily of the valley, pheasant's eye, Chan-Su, cascara sagrada (buckthorn), aloe, or senna may result in increased risk of digoxin toxicity. The use of Siberian ginseng, tan-shen, or ashwagandha may result in falsely elevated digoxin levels.	Hypomagnesemia, hypokalemia, and hypercalcemia elevate drug toxicity. Ensure consumption adequate potassium and magnesium. Care should be taken with calcium supplements and antacids.
Doxercalciferol	See *calcitriol*		
Hectorol			
Duraclon	See *clonidine*		
Dyrenium	See *triamterene*		
Effexor, Effexor XR	See *venlafaxine*		

(Continued)

Medication	Class & Action	Side Effects	Nutritional Implications
Enalapril Vasotec	Antihypertensive ACE Inhibitor	May increase serum potassium. May decrease serum sodium. Nausea, salty or metallic taste, mouth sores. Concurrent use of angiotensin-converting enzyme inhibitors and yohimbine or ma huang may result in reduced effectiveness of angiotensin-converting enzyme inhibitors.	Caution with foods high in potassium or potassium supplements. Avoid salt substitutes. Maintain adequate hydration.
Ery-Tab	See *erythromycin*		
Erythromycin Ery-Tab	Antibiotic Bacteriostatic or bactericidal	Occasional nausea, vomiting, diarrhea, abdominal pain, anorexia, stomatitis, bad taste in mouth Concurrent use of erythromycin and autumn crocus (colchicine) may result in increased plasma levels of colchicine and increased risk of toxicity. Concurrent use of erythromycin and grapefruit juice or grapefruit-containing foods may result in increased erythromycin bioavailability.	Take with food to avoid GI disturbances. Eat small, frequent meals to avoid anorexia. Consider fluid and electrolyte replacement for diarrhea. Avoid alcohol. Avoid taking with grapefruit or grapefruit-containing foods.
Effexor	See *venlafaxine*		
Eskalith, Eskalith CR	See *lithium*		
Extentabs	See *quinidine*		
Femiron	See *ferrous fumarate*		

Medication	Class & Action	Side Effects	Nutritional Implications
Fenofibrate	See *gemfibrozil*		
Tricor			
Feosol	See *ferrous sulfate*		
Feostat	See *ferrous fumarate*		
Feratab	See *ferrous sulfate*		
Fergon	See *ferrous sulfate*		
Ferrex	See *ferrous sulfate*		
Ferrlecit	See *sodium ferric gluconate*		
Ferrous fumarate Femiron, Feostat	Iron supplement	Constipation, diarrhea, and abdominal discomfort, dark stools.	Emphasize iron-rich food in a well-balanced diet.
Ferrous sulfate Feosol, Feratab, Fergon, Ferrex, Hemocyte, Nephro-Fer, Niferex	Iron supplement	Constipation and stomach upset. Concurrent use of iron and zinc may result in decreased gastrointestinal absorption of iron and/or zinc. Concurrent use of iron and dairy foods may result in decreased iron bioavailability. Concurrent use of iron and phytic acid foods (beans, seeds, nuts, some whole grains) may result in reduced iron absorption.	Emphasize iron-rich food in a well-balanced diet.

(*Continued*)

Medication	Class & Action	Side Effects	Nutritional Implications
Ferrous gluconate	See *ferrous sulfate*		
Flagyl	See *metronidazole*		
Fluoxetine Prozac	Antidepressant Selective serotonin reuptake inhibitor (SSRI)	Alcohol may increase depression. Nausea, diarrhea, decreased appetite, dry mouth, vomiting, constipation, and abdominal pain. Concurrent use of SSRIs and St John's wort or ginkgo biloba may result in increased risk of serotonin syndrome (hypertension, hyperthermia, myoclonus, mental status changes).	Avoid alcohol. Consider fluid and electrolyte replacement for diarrhea and vomiting. Use ice chips or chew gum for dry mouth. Consider small, frequent meals for decreased appetite.
Fluvastatin	See *atorvastatin*		
Lescol *Furosemide* Lasix	Diuretic Loop diuretic	Ginkgo biloba may cause increased blood pressure. Licorice can increase the risk of hypokalemia. May increase blood glucose, uric acid, cholesterol, LDL, calcium, and triglycerides. May decrease urinary excretion of calcium and increase excretion of magnesium, sodium, and potassium levels. Loss of appetite. Concurrent use of loop diuretics and ginseng or geranium may result in increased risk of diuretic resistance. Concurrent use of loop diuretics and yohimbine may result in reduced diuretic effectiveness.	Consume foods high in potassium and magnesium. Avoid consumption of natural licorice. Monitor electrolyte levels and consider supplementation. Caution with calcium supplements.

Medication	Class & Action	Side Effects	Nutritional Implications
Gemfibrozil Lopid	Fibric acid derivative	Stomach pain, diarrhea, constipation, vomiting, and gas.	Eat a low-cholesterol, low-fat, low-sucrose diet for best results. Avoid alcohol. Consider fluid and electrolyte replacement for diarrhea and vomiting.
Hectorol	See *doxercalciferol*		
Hydralazine Apresoline	Antiarrhythmic, Antiprotozoal	Nausea, vomiting, diarrhea, fluid retention, and edema. Impedes metabolism of pyridoxine (vitamin B_6). Concurrent use of hydralazine and yohimbine or ma huang may result in reduced hydralazine effectiveness.	Doctor may prescribe a low-salt or low-sodium diet. Take with food. Monitor for pyridoxine deficiency. Consume diet high in pyridoxine. Consider supplementation.
Hemocyte	See *ferrous sulfate*		
Imfed	See *iron dextran*		
Iron *dextran* Imfed	IV iron, Hematinic	Nausea, vomiting, and metallic taste. Concurrent use of iron and zinc may result in decreased gastrointestinal absorption of iron and/or zinc. Concurrent use of iron and phytic acid foods (beans, seeds, nuts, some whole grains) may result in reduced iron absorption.	Avoid taking oral iron. Emphasize iron-rich food in a well-balanced diet.
Iron sucrose Venofer	IV iron, Hematinic	Diarrhea.	Avoid taking oral iron. Emphasize iron-rich food in a well-balanced diet.

(Continued)

Medication	Class & Action	Side Effects	Nutritional Implications
Isocarboxazid Marplan	Antidepressant monoamine oxidase inhibitor (MAOI)	Sudden high blood pressure may occur with ingestion of certain foods. Alcohol may increase depressant effect. Caffeine may increase blood pressure and cardiac arrhythmias. Concurrent use of MAOIs and yerba mate, guarana, or bitter orange may result in acute headache and increase in blood pressure. Kava, ma huang, licorice, ginkgo biloba or nutmeg may result in increased risk of adverse effects from excessive monoamine oxidase inhibition. St John's wort may result in an increased risk of serotonin syndrome (hypertension, hyperthermia, myoclonus, mental status changes) and/or an increased risk of hypertensive crisis. Ginseng may result in insomnia, tremor, headache, agitation, and worsening of depression.	Avoid foods high in tyramine: cheeses, fava, or broad-bean pods; yeast or meat extracts, smoked or pickled meat, poultry, or fish; fermented sausage such as bologna, pepperoni, salami, or other fermented meat; avocados; bananas; beer; wine; and raisins. Avoid excess amounts of caffeine, tea, or chocolate. Avoid alcohol.
Isoptin, Isoptin SR	See *verapamil*		
Keflex	See *cephalexin*		
Kinidine	See *quinidine*		
Lanoxin	See *digoxin*		

Medication	Class & Action	Side Effects	Nutritional Implications
Lasix	See *furosemide*		
Lescol	See *fluvastatin*		
Lipitor	See *atorvastatin*		
Lisinopril Prinivil, Zestril	Antihypertensive ACE inhibitor	May increase serum potassium. May decrease serum sodium. Nausea, salty or metallic taste, mouth sores.	Caution with foods high in potassium or potassium supplements. Avoid salt substitutes. Maintain adequate hydration.
Lithane	See *lithium*		
Lithium Eskalith, Eskalith CR, Lithobid, Lithane, Lithonate, Lithotabs	Antimanic agent	Drug interferes with the regulation of sodium and water levels in the body and may lead to dehydration. Toxicity may result from sodium depletion. Caffeine appears to reduce serum lithium concentrations and increase side effects. Loss of appetite, stomach pain or bloating, gas, indigestion, weight gain or loss, dry mouth, excessive saliva in the mouth, tongue pain, change in the ability to taste food, swollen lips, and constipation. Concurrent use of lithium and yohimbine may result in increased risk of manic episodes. Psyllium may result in decreased plasma levels and effectiveness of lithium. Guarana or yerba mate may result in alterations in serum lithium levels.	Maintain steady salt and fluid intake. Avoid salt-free diet or sodium depletion. Avoid caffeine.

(Continued)

Medication	Class & Action	Side Effects	Nutritional Implications
Lithobid	See *lithium*		
Lithonate	See *lithium*		
Lithotabs	See *lithium*		
Lopid	See *gemfibrozil*		
Lopressor	See *metoprolol*		
Marplan	See *isocarboxazid*		
Methotrexate	Antimetabolite, folate antagonist	Nausea, vomiting, diarrhea, stomach pain, mouth sores, and loss of appetite. Inhibitor of dihydrofolate reductase, thus decreasing availability of active folate. Concurrent use of methotrexate and cola may result in increased methotrexate serum levels and increased risk of toxicity.	Consume high Vitamin B_{12} diet. Consider fluid and electrolyte replacement for diarrhea and vomiting. Encourage food intake when patient feels best; e.g., morning. Drink extra fluids to pass more drug through the urine. Leucovorin should be considered to reverse toxic effect of folic acid antagonists.

Medication	Class & Action	Side Effects	Nutritional Implications
Metoprolol Betaloc, Lopressor, Toprol XL	Beta-blocker, antiadrenergic, antiarrhythmic	Diarrhea, constipation, nausea, and vomiting. Possible hypoglycemia. Signs of sympathetic response to hypoglycemia may be masked. May have a decreased insulin release in response to hyperglycemia. Concurrent use of beta-adrenergic blockers and St John's wort or yohimbine may result in decreased effectiveness of beta-adrenergic blockers. Dong quai may result in low blood pressure. Ma huang may result in* reduced hypotensive effect of beta-adrenergic blockers.	Adherence necessary for those following diabetic diet. Monitor blood glucose levels. Be cautious of nonsymphathetic signs of hypoglycemia. Consider fluid and electrolyte replacement for diarrhea and vomiting.
Metronidazole Flagyl	Antibacterial, antiprotozoal	Anorexia, nausea, dry mouth, stomatitis, diarrhea or constipation, vomiting, and metallic taste. Concurrent use of metronidazole and milk thistle may result in reduced metronidazole and active metabolite exposure.	Avoid alcohol and alcohol-containing products during and at least 5 days after treatment. Avoid hot and spicy foods. Consider fluid and electrolyte replacement for diarrhea. Take with food to prevent GI distress. Consider small, frequent meals for anorexia. Use ice chips or chew gum for dry mouth.
Nardil	See *phenelzine*		
Nephrocaps	See *dialyvite*		
Nephro-Fer	See *ferrous sulfate*		
Nephrovite	See *dialyvite*		

(Continued)

Medication	Class & Action	Side Effects	Nutritional Implications
Niacin Niacor, Niaspan, Nicotinex, Slo-Niacin	Nicotinic acid derivative	Alcohol may increase side effects of niacin. Occasional gas, nausea, vomiting, and diarrhea. May increase blood uric acid and glucose levels.	Caution with diabetes. Ensure adherence to diabetic diet if necessary. May consider low-purine diet if necessary. Consider fluid and electrolyte replacement for diarrhea and vomiting.
Niacor	See *niacin*		
Niaspan	See *niacin*		
Nicotinex	See *niacin*		
Nifedical	See *nifedipine*		
Nifedipine Adalat, Nifedical, Procardia	Calcium channel blocker	Upset stomach, heartburn, nausea, and constipation. Concurrent use of nifedipine and ginseng or ginkgo biloba may result in an increased risk of nifedipine side effects. Dong quai may result in low blood pressure. Ma huang may result in reduced hypotensive effect of calcium channel blockers. Yohimbine may result in reduced calcium channel blocker effectiveness. Grapefruit juice or grapefruit-containing foods may result in severe hypotension, myocardial ischemia, increased vasodilator side effects.	Avoid drinking grapefruit juice or eating grapefruit 1 hr before or for 2 hrs after taking nifedipine.

Medication	Class & Action	Side Effects	Nutritional Implications
Niferex	See *ferrous sulfate*		
Oncovin	See *vincristine*		
Orlistat Xenical	Lipase inhibitor	Flatulence, fatty stools, nausea, diarrhea. Decreased absorption vitamins A and E.	Side effects are transient. Monitor nutrient levels.
OsCal	See *calcium salts*		
Parnate	See *tranylcypromine*		
Paroxetine Paxeva, Paxil, Paxil CR	Antidepressant Selective serotonin reuptake inhibitor (SSRI)	Nausea, dry mouth, constipation, diarrhea, and decreased appetite. Concurrent use of SSRIs and St John's wort or ginkgo biloba may result in an increased risk of serotonin syndrome (hypertension, hyperthermia, myoclonus, mental status changes).	Consider fluid and electrolyte replacement for diarrhea. Use ice chips or chew gum for dry mouth. Consider small, frequent meals for decreased appetite.
Paxeva	See *paroxetine*		
Paxil, Paxil CR	See *paroxetine*		
Penicillin	Antibiotic Kill or prevent growth of bacteria	GI disturbances including mild diarrhea, nausea, or vomiting (stomatitis, black or hairy tongue has been reported). Some may contain high amounts of sodium or potassium.	Should be taken 1 hr before or 2 hrs after food to facilitate absorption. Consider fluid and electrolyte replacement for diarrhea. Caution if on low-sodium diet. Some strengths of amoxicillin may contain phenylalanine.

(Continued)

Medication	Class & Action	Side Effects	Nutritional Implications
Paricalcitol/Zemplar	See *calcitriol*		
Phenelzine Nardil	Antidepressant Monoamine oxidase inhibitor (MAOI)	Sudden high blood pressure may occur with ingestion of certain foods. Alcohol may increase depressant effect. Caffeine may increase blood pressure and cardiac arrhythmias. Concurrent use of MAOIs and yerba mate, guarana, or bitter orange may result in acute headache and increase in blood pressure. Kava, ma huang, licorice, ginkgo biloba, or nutmeg may result in increased risk of adverse effects from excessive monoamine oxidase inhibition. St John's wort may result in an increased risk of serotonin syndrome (hypertension, hyperthermia, myoclonus, mental status changes) and/or an increased risk of hypertensive crisis. Ginseng may result in insomnia, tremor, headache, agitation, and worsening of depression. Avocado may result in hypertensive crisis (headache, palpitation, neck stiffness).	Avoid foods high in tyramine: cheeses, fava, or broad-bean pods; yeast or meat extracts, smoked or pickled meat, poultry, or fish; fermented sausage such as bologna, pepperoni, salami, or other fermented meat; avocados; bananas; beer; wine; and raisins. Avoid excess amounts of caffeine, tea, or chocolate. Avoid alcohol.
PhosLo	See *calcium salts*		
Platinol, Platinol-AQ	See *cisplatin*		

Medication	Class & Action	Side Effects	Nutritional Implications
Plavix	See *clopidogrel*		
Pravachol	See *pravastatin*		
Pravastatin	Inhibitor of HMG-CoA reductase	Constipation, diarrhea, gas, upset stomach, and upper-right stomach pain. Coenzyme Q10 may be significantly reduced. Concurrent use of HMG-CoA reductase inhibitors and oat bran may result in reduced effectiveness of HMG CoA reductase inhibitors. Concurrent use of Pravastatin and St John's wort may result in reduced effectiveness of Pravastatin.	Avoid intake large quantities of grapefruit juice or grapefruit-containing foods for it increases the absorption of statins (>1 quart/day). Eat a low-cholesterol, low-fat diet for best results. Gastrointestinal problems generally transient.
Prevalite	See *cholestyramine*		
Prinivil	See *lisinopril*		
Procardia	See *nifedipine*		
Propanolol Inderal	See *atenolol*		
Prozac	See *fluoxetine*		
Questran	See *cholestyramine*		
Quinidex	See *quinidine*		

(Continued)

Medication	Class & Action	Side Effects	Nutritional Implications
Quinidine Kinidine, Quinidex, Extentabs	Antiarrhythmic, antiprotozoal	Abdominal pain and cramps, diarrhea, nausea, and vomiting. May cause hypokalemia, hypomagnesemia, and/or hypocalcemia. Concurrent use of quinidine and grapefruit juice may result in decreased metabolic conversion of quinidine to 3-hydroxyquinidine.	Consider fluid and electrolyte replacement for diarrhea and vomiting. Consume diet adequate in potassium, magnesium, and calcium. Supplementation maybe necessary.
Renagel	See *sevelamer*		
Rocaltrol	See *calcitriol*		
Sensipar	See *cinacalcet*		
Sertraline	Antidepressant		
Zoloft	Selective serotonin reuptake inhibitor (SSRI)	May increase serum triglyceride and total cholesterol. May decrease uric acid levels. St John's Wort may increase adverse side effects. Nausea, diarrhea, dry mouth, constipation, altered taste, and dyspepsia. Concurrent use of SSRIs and St John's wort or ginkgo biloba may result in an increased risk of serotonin syndrome (hypertension, hyperthermia, myoclonus, mental status changes). Concurrent use of sertraline and grapefruit juice or grapefruit-containing foods may result in elevated sertraline serum concentrations and an increased risk of adverse side effects.	Monitor blood lipid levels. Consider fluid and electrolyte replacement for diarrhea and vomiting. Use ice chips or chew gum for dry mouth. Avoid alcohol. Avoid grapefruit or grapefruit-containing foods.

Medication	Class & Action	Side Effects	Nutritional Implications
Sevelamer Renagel	Non-calcium-based phosphorus binder	Diarrhea, dyspepsia, gas, constipation, nausea, and vomiting.	Take with food. Use of aluminum should be limited to <14 days. Monitor bicarbonate, chloride, calcium, and phosphorous levels.
Simvastatin Zocor	Inhibitor of HMG-CoA reductase	Constipation, diarrhea, gas, upset stomach, and upper right stomach pain. Coenzyme Q10 may be significantly reduced. Concurrent use of HMG-CoA reductase inhibitors and oat bran may result in reduced effectiveness of HMG CoA reductase inhibitors. Concurrent use of simvastatin and cranberry juice may result in increased risk of hepatitis and myopathy/ rhabdomyolysis. Concurrent use of HMG-CoA reductase inhibitors and pectin may result in reduced effectiveness of HMG CoA reductase inhibitors.	Avoid intake large quantities of grapefruit juice for it increases the absorption of statins (>1 quart/day). Eat a low-cholesterol, low-fat diet for best results. Gastrointestinal problems generally transient.
Slo-Niacin	See *niacin*		
Sodium ferric	See *iron sucrose*		
Gluconate complex			
Ferrlecit			

(Continued)

Medication	Class & Action	Side Effects	Nutritional Implications
Spironolactone Aldactone	Diuretic Potassium-sparing diuretic	Hyperkalemia, dehydration, hyponatremia, nausea, vomiting, anorexia, abdominal cramps, and diarrhea. Concurrent use of diuretics and licorice may result in increased risk of hypokalemia and/or reduced effectiveness of the diuretic. Concurrent use of potassium-sparing diuretics and ma huang may result in reduced hypotensive effect of potassium-sparing diuretics. Concurrent use of diuretics and yohimbine may result in reduced diuretic effectiveness.	Avoid foods high in potassium, potassium supplements, and salt substitutes.
Tenormin	See *atenolol*		
Titralac	See *calcium salts*		
Toprol XL	See *metoprolol*		
Tranylcypromine Parnate	Antidepressant Monoamine oxidase inhibitor (MAOI)	Sudden high blood pressure or increased MAOI activity may occur with ingestion of certain foods and herbals (avocado, yerba mate, guarana, kava, liquorice, ma huang, St John's wort, bitter orange, ginseng, ginkgo biloba, nutmeg, caffeine). Alcohol may increase depressant effect. Caffeine may increase blood pressure and cardiac arrhythmias. GI upset.	Avoid foods high in tyramine: cheeses, fava or broad-bean pods, yeast or meat extracts, smoked or pickled meat, poultry, or fish, fermented sausage such as bologna, pepperoni, salami, or other fermented meat, avocados, bananas, beer, wine, and raisins. Avoid excess amounts of caffeine, tea, or chocolate. Avoid alcohol.

Medication	Class & Action	Side Effects	Nutritional Implications
Triamterene Dyrenium	Diuretic Potassium-sparing diuretic	Hyperkalemia, dehydration, hyponatremia, nausea, vomiting, anorexia, abdominal cramps, and diarrhea. Concurrent use of diuretics and yohimbine may result in reduced diuretic effectiveness. Concurrent use of potassium-sparing diuretics and ma huang may result in reduced hypotensive effect of potassium-sparing diuretics. Concurrent use of triamterene and potassium foods may result in hyperkalemia.	Avoid foods high in potassium, potassium supplements, and salt substitutes.
Tricor	See *fenofibrate*		
Trovafloxacin Trovan	Quinolone	Iron preparations may increase drug absorption. Dandelion may increase drug effect. Fennel seed may decrease drug effect resulting in treatment failure. Diarrhea.	Consider fluid and electrolyte replacement for diarrhea.
Trovan	See *trovafloxacin*		
Tums	See *calcium salts*		
Vasotec	See *enalapril*		
Velban	See *vinblastine*		
Velsar	See *vinblastine*		

(Continued)

Medication	Class & Action	Side Effects	Nutritional Implications
Venlafaxine Effexor, Effexor XR	Antidepressant	Nausea, dry mouth, anorexia, and constipation. St John's Wort may increase sedative effect. Concurrent use of venlafaxine and St John's wort may result in an increased risk of serotonin syndrome (hypertension, hyperthermia, myoclonus, mental status changes).	Use ice chips or chew gum for dry mouth. Monitor weight.
Venofer	See *iron sucrose*		
Verapamil Calan, Verelan, Verelan PM, Isoptin, Isoptin SR, Covera-HS	Calcium channel blocker	Constipation, upset stomach, heartburn. Concurrent use of verapamil and caffeine may result in increased caffeine serum concentrations and enhanced CNS stimulation.	Avoid drinking grapefruit juice or eating grapefruit 1 hr before or for 2 hrs after taking nifedipine.
Verelan, Verelan PM	See *verapamil*		
Vinblastine Velban, Velsar, vinblastine sulfate, VBL	Plant alkaloid	Nausea, vomiting, stomach pain, constipation, and diarrhea.	Drink plenty of fluids to decrease constipation.
Vincristine Oncovin	Plant alkaloid	Nausea, vomiting, stomach pain, stomach cramps, constipation, and diarrhea. Concurrent use of vincristine and grapefruit juice or grapefruit-containing foods may result in increased plasma concentrations of vincristine.	Consider fluid and electrolyte replacement for diarrhea and vomiting. May consider laxatives for constipation. Mild vomiting remedied with antiemetic. Avoid grapefruit or grapefruit-containing foods.

Medication	Class & Action	Side Effects	Nutritional Implications
Warfarin Coumadin	Anticoagulant	Anorexia, nausea, abdominal cramping and diarrhea. Prevents the conversion of vitamin K to its active form. Garlic may increase the risk of bleeding. Mineralization of newly formed bone may be deterred.	Consider small, frequent meals for anorexia. Consider fluid and electrolyte replacement for diarrhea. Dietary and supplemental intake, particularly vitamin K, must be consistent to achieve steady level of anticoagulation. Those on long-term use should be monitored for bone density.
Wellbutrin	See *bupropion*		
Xenical	See *orlistat*		
Zemplar	See *paricalcitol*		
Zestril	See *lisinopril*		
Zithromax	See *azithromycin*		
Zocor	See *simvastatin*		
Zoloft	See *sertraline*		
Zyban	See *bupropion*		

(Continued)

References

Micromedex® (electronic version). Truven Health Analytics, Greenwood Village, Colorado, USA. Available at: https://www.micromedexsolutions.com/ (cited: April 1, 2018).

APPENDIX H: BODY MASS INDEX TABLE

Body Mass Index Table

	Underweight		Normal						Overweight					Obesity Class 1					Class 2				Extreme Obesity Class III
BMI	18	18.5	19	20	21	22	23	24	25	26	27	28	29	30	31	32	33	34	35	36	37	38	39	40
Height (Inches)	Weight (Pounds)																							
58	86	89	91	96	100	105	110	115	119	124	129	134	138	143	148	153	158	162	167	172	177	181	186	191
59	89	92	94	99	104	109	114	119	124	128	133	138	143	148	153	158	163	168	173	178	183	188	193	198
60	92	95	97	102	107	112	118	123	128	133	138	143	148	153	158	163	168	174	179	184	189	194	199	204
61	95	98	100	106	111	116	122	127	132	137	143	148	153	158	164	169	174	180	185	190	195	201	206	211
62	98	101	104	109	115	120	126	131	136	142	147	153	158	164	169	175	180	186	191	196	202	207	213	218
63	101	104	107	113	118	124	130	135	141	146	152	158	163	169	175	180	186	191	197	203	208	214	220	225
64	105	108	110	116	122	128	134	140	145	151	157	163	169	174	180	186	192	197	204	209	215	221	227	232
65	108	111	114	120	126	132	138	144	150	156	162	168	174	180	186	192	198	204	210	216	222	228	234	240
66	111	115	118	124	130	136	142	148	155	161	167	173	179	186	192	198	204	210	216	223	229	235	241	247
67	115	118	121	127	134	140	146	153	159	166	172	178	185	191	198	204	211	217	223	230	236	242	249	255
68	118	122	125	131	138	144	151	158	164	171	177	184	190	197	203	210	216	223	230	236	243	249	256	262
69	122	125	128	135	142	149	155	162	169	176	182	189	196	203	209	216	223	230	236	243	250	257	263	270
70	125	129	132	139	146	153	160	167	174	181	188	195	202	209	216	222	229	236	243	250	257	264	271	278
71	129	133	136	143	150	157	165	172	179	186	193	200	208	215	222	229	236	243	250	257	265	272	279	286
72	133	136	140	147	154	162	169	177	184	191	199	206	213	221	228	235	242	250	258	265	272	279	287	294
73	136	140	144	151	159	166	174	182	189	197	204	212	219	227	235	242	250	257	265	272	280	288	295	302
74	140	144	148	155	163	171	179	186	194	202	210	218	225	233	241	249	256	264	272	280	287	295	303	311
75	144	148	152	160	168	176	184	192	200	208	216	224	232	240	248	256	264	272	279	287	295	303	311	319
76	148	152	156	164	172	180	189	197	205	213	221	230	238	246	254	263	271	279	287	295	304	312	320	328

Data from (i) National Institutes of Health and National Heart, Lung, and Blood Institute. Evidence report of clinical guidelines on the identification, evaluation, and treatment of overweight and obesity in adults. (September 1998). Bethesda, MD: NIH publication number 98-4083.

(ii) Centers for Disease Control and Prevention, Division of Nutrition, Physical Activity, and Obesity. Available at: https://www.cdc.gov/healthyweight/assessing/bmi/adult_bmi/. Accessed April 10, 2018.